AF845231

OCCUPATIONAL STRESS AND WELL-BEING IN MILITARY CONTEXTS

RESEARCH IN OCCUPATIONAL STRESS AND WELL-BEING

Series Editors: Pamela L. Perrewé, Jonathon R. B. Halbesleben and Christopher C. Rosen

Recent Volumes:

Volume 1:	Exploring Theoretical Mechanisms and Perspectives
Volume 2:	Historical and Current Perspectives on Stress and Health
Volume 3:	Emotional and Physiological Processes and Positive Intervention Strategies
Volume 4:	Exploring Interpersonal Dynamics
Volume 5:	Employee Health. Coping and Methodologies
Volume 6:	Exploring the Work and Non-Work Interface
Volume 7:	Current Perspectives on Job-Stress Recovery
Volume 8:	New Developments in Theoretical and Conceptual Approaches to Job Stress
Volume 9:	The Role of Individual Differences in Occupational Stress and Well-Being
Volume 10:	The Role of the Economic Crisis on Occupational Stress and Well-Being
Volume 11:	The Role of Emotion and Emotion Regulation in Job Stress and Well-Being
Volume 12:	The Role of Demographics in Occupational Stress and Well-Being
Volume 13:	Mistreatment in Organizations
Volume 14:	The Role of Leadership in Occupational Stress
Volume 15:	The Role of Power, Politics, and Influence in Occupational Stress and Well-Being

RESEARCH IN OCCUPATIONAL STRESS AND WELL-BEING VOLUME 16

OCCUPATIONAL STRESS AND WELL-BEING IN MILITARY CONTEXTS

EDITED BY

PETER D. HARMS
The University of Alabama, USA

PAMELA L. PERREWÉ
Florida State University, USA

emerald PUBLISHING

United Kingdom – North America – Japan
India – Malaysia – China

Emerald Publishing Limited
Howard House, Wagon Lane, Bingley BD16 1WA, UK

First edition 2018

Copyright © 2018 Emerald Publishing Limited

Reprints and permissions service
Contact: permissions@emeraldinsight.com

No part of this book may be reproduced, stored in a retrieval system, transmitted in any form or by any means electronic, mechanical, photocopying, recording or otherwise without either the prior written permission of the publisher or a licence permitting restricted copying issued in the UK by The Copyright Licensing Agency and in the USA by The Copyright Clearance Center. Any opinions expressed in the chapters are those of the authors. Whilst Emerald makes every effort to ensure the quality and accuracy of its content, Emerald makes no representation implied or otherwise, as to the chapters' suitability and application and disclaims any warranties, express or implied, to their use.

British Library Cataloguing in Publication Data
A catalogue record for this book is available from the British Library

ISBN: 978-1-78756-184-7 (Print)
ISBN: 978-1-78756-183-0 (Online)
ISBN: 978-1-78756-185-4 (Epub)

ISSN: 1479-3555 (Series)

Printed and bound by CPI Group (UK) Ltd, Croydon, CR0 4YY

ISOQAR REGISTERED

ISOQAR certified Management System, awarded to Emerald for adherence to Environmental standard ISO 14001:2004.

Certificate Number 1985
ISO 14001

INVESTOR IN PEOPLE

CONTENTS

About the Authors *vii*

Preface *xi*

Processing War: Similarities and Differences in PTSD Antecedents and Outcomes between Military and Civilian War Survivors
Matthew R. Leon, Holly K. Osburn and Thomas Bellairs *1*

Cold-blooded Killers? Rethinking Psychopathy in the Military
Karen Landay and Rachel E. Frieder *23*

Measuring Job Performance in the Army: Insights from Evidence on Civilian Stress and Health
Stacy Ann Hawkins, Loryana L. Vie, Pedro S. A. Wolf, Paul B. Lester, Kerry S. Whittaker, Jacob N. Hawkins and Alycia L. Perez *49*

Work, Stress, and Health of Military Couples across Transitions
Wylie H. Wan, Sarah N. Haverly and Leslie B. Hammer *69*

Fighting for Family: Considerations of Work–Family Conflict in Military Service Member Parents
Maura J. Mills and Leanne M. Tortez *91*

Examining Veteran Transition to the Workplace through Military Transition Theory
Sara Kintzle and Carl A. Castro *117*

Psychosocial Health Prevention Programs in Military Organizations: A Quantitative Review of the Evaluative Rigor Evidence
Adam J. Vanhove, Tiffany Brutus and Kristin A. Sowden 129

Pain in the Civilian and Military Workplace
Ethan W. Gossett and P. D. Harms 157

Index 187

ABOUT THE AUTHORS

Thomas Bellairs is an active Duty Officer in the US Air Force. He earned his PhD in Management from the University of Alabama. His research interests include job crafting, employee well-being, stress management, and how employees view their future at work.

Tiffany Brutus is a Graduate Student of the Organizational Science and Leadership Concentration in the School of Strategic Leadership Studies at James Madison University. She is interested in exploring the roles of leadership and administration as it relates to the implementation of health education strategies, interventions, and programs.

Carl A. Castro is an Associate Professor and the Director of the Center for Innovation and Research on Veterans & Military Families at USC. His research focuses on assessing factors associated with soldier, family, and unit readiness, and evaluating the process of service members' transitions from military to civilian life.

Rachel E. Frieder is an Assistant Professor of Management in University of North Florida's Coggin College of Business. Her research interests involve how individuals get ahead at work with an emphasis on topics such as adaptive (e.g., political skill) and maladaptive individual differences (e.g., psychopathy), leadership, and work relationship quality.

Ethan W. Gossett received his Bachelor of Science in Psychology from the University of Alabama at Birmingham where he was a member of the Biobehavioral Pain Research Laboratory. His primary research interests include work hazards, emotional well-being, and pain as well as organizational outcomes associated with acute and chronic pain conditions.

Leslie B. Hammer is a Professor in the Department of Psychology at Portland State University and a Professor in the Oregon Institute of Occupational Health Sciences at Oregon Health & Science University. Her work focuses on workplace programs that reduce work–life stress and evaluating the effectiveness of supervisor support training.

P. D. Harms is an Assistant Professor of Management at the University of Alabama. He received his PhD from the University of Illinois, Urbana-Champaign. His current research interests include the assessment and development of personality, psychological well-being, and leadership.

Sarah N. Haverly is a doctoral student of Applied Psychology at the Portland State University. Her research interests include occupational health psychology, self-conscious emotional processes, the unique experience of military service members, and interpersonal relationships as they impact, and are impacted by, workplace factors.

Jacob N. Hawkins is a Research Assistant for the Research Facilitation Laboratory. Jake graduated from the University of California, Santa Barbara, where he worked in research laboratories in evolutionary and developmental psychology. His research interests include mental health, positive psychology strategies, and resilience among children and adolescents.

Stacy Ann Hawkins received her PhD from Claremont Graduate University. She is currently a Behavioral Research Scientist and Family Resilience Division Chief at the Research Facilitation Laboratory. Her work has explored relationships and well-being among a wide variety of populations, including parents of infants, same-sex couples, and military families.

Sara Kintzle is an Associate Research Professor in the USC Suzanne Dworak-Peck School of Social Work Center for Innovation and Research on Veterans & Military Families. Kintzle's research involves the experience of service members and veterans, including risk and protective factors related to successful military transition.

Karen Landay is a Doctoral Student in the Culverhouse College of Commerce at the University of Alabama. Her primary research interests include leadership and dark personality, the interaction of gender differences with dark personality, and the effects of music on outcomes such as training and development.

Matthew R. Leon is an Assistant Professor of Management at the University of Central Oklahoma. Leon has also worked as a Civilian Research Scientist across three different universities and as an Applications Analyst for the US Navy's Naval Aerospace Medical Research Laboratory and Naval Medicine Operational Training Center.

Paul B. Lester is an Officer in the US Army and serves as the Director of the Research Facilitation Laboratory in Monterey, CA. His research interests include resilience, psychological health, positive psychology, leadership, courage, and Big Data. He has served in the Army since 1991.

Maura J. Mills is an Assistant Professor of Management at the Culverhouse College of Commerce, University of Alabama. Her research focuses on the work–non-work interface, related gender considerations, and positive organizational behavior, including employee attitudes, well-being, and work engagement.

Holly K. Osburn is an Assistant Professor of Management at the University of Central Oklahoma. She received her PhD in Industrial and Organizational Psychology from the University of Oklahoma. Her primary areas of interest include leadership, planning, creativity, and business ethics.

Alycia L. Perez received her PhD in Industrial and Organizational Psychology from the University of Akron. Her research largely focuses on leadership, organizational well-being, employee positive functioning, and gender issues. Dr. Perez has been working in support of US Army Initiatives with the Research Facilitation Laboratory since 2012.

Kristin A. Sowden holds a Bachelor of Arts in English and Secondary Education from the College of New Jersey and a Master's degree in Education in Counseling Psychology from the James Madison University. She is currently pursuing her PhD in Strategic Leadership at James Madison University.

Leanne M. Tortez is an adjunct Faculty Member in the Organizational and Leadership Psychology Department at William James College, and recently worked as a Research Analyst for Northwell Health in Manhasset, New York. Her research interests include the work–family interface, leadership, community-based participatory research, and qualitative methods.

Adam J. Vanhove is an Assistant Professor in the School of Strategic Leadership Studies at the James Madison University. He received PhD in Industrial–Organizational Psychology from the Colorado State University. His research focuses on occupational health, resilience, and well-being.

Loryana L. Vie serves as the Senior Project Director of the Positive Soldier Health Project, a military-civilian collaboration between the University of Pennsylvania and the U.S. Army, funded by the Robert Wood Johnson Foundation (Principal Investigator: Dr. Martin E. P. Seligman). She received her PhD in Social and Personality Psychology from the University of California, Riverside. Her research interests include military health, individual differences in health and health behavior engagement, and quantitative methods for studying changes in health. Dr. Vie has worked with the Research Facilitation Laboratory since 2012.

Wylie H. Wan completed her PhD in Developmental Psychology at the University of Michigan and conducted postdoctoral work at the Oregon Institute of Occupational Health Sciences at Oregon Health & Science University. Her research focuses on close relationships, living and working environments, and health and well-being across the life course.

Kerry S. Whittaker is a member of the Research Facilitation Laboratory. She received her Doctorate in Medical Psychology from the Uniformed Services University of Health Sciences. Her research has focused on exploring the relationship between stress and other psychosocial factors in the etiology and progression of cardiovascular disease.

Pedro S. A. Wolf is a Behavioral Scientist at the Research Facilitation Laboratory. He earned a Doctorate Degree in Psychology from the University of Arizona. Before attending college, he served in the US Army as an Airborne Infantryman with the 75th Ranger Regiment.

PREFACE

In the 16th volume of *Research in Occupational Stress and Well-Being*, we have eight chapters that cover topics related to the causes, consequences, and experiences associated with stress and well-being of soldiers, veterans, and their family members. Our first three chapters cover topics related to the antecedents and processes related to the experiences of stress and post-traumatic stress disorder in military personnel and how research in this area can inform both the future military research and stress-related research in civilian settings. In the lead chapter, Matthew R. Leon, Holly K. Osburn, and Thomas Bellairs review research on the link between combat experiences and the development of post-traumatic stress, the factors that increase or decrease the likelihood of developing stress-related disorders, and how these processes compare to those of civilian war survivors. In the second chapter, Karen Landay and Rachel E. Frieder investigate how trait psychopathy may explain why certain individuals are attracted to professions wherein the likelihood of experiencing violence is more likely and how such characteristics may influence the manner in which such individuals cope with combat-related experiences. In the third chapter, a team from the US Army's Research Facilitation Laboratory discusses current practices in terms of how the US Army measures and monitors mental health in soldiers and its link with performance metrics.

The theme of the second section concerns issues surrounding how the stress-related experiences of soldiers can influence those around them and how veterans cope with stress when their service ends. In the fourth chapter of this volume, Wylie H. Wan, Sarah N. Haverly, and Leslie B. Hammer use the life course perspective to examine the experiences of military couples across stress-inducing events such as relocations and deployments. In the fifth chapter, Maura J. Mills and Leanne M. Tortez review the literature surrounding military families with a focus on parenting issues and how the military family lifestyle can impact child's well-being. The sixth chapter by Sara Kintzle and Carl A. Castro follows the theme of examining stressors outside and after life as a soldier by introducing the military transition theory and reviewing the literature surrounding how soldiers transition to life after active service.

The final section of this volume deals more specifically with the processes surrounding how military personnel cope with stress on their jobs. In the seventh chapter, Adam J. Vanhove, Tiffany Brutus, and Kristin A. Sowden review the state of the literature on interventions designed to improve soldier well-being in terms of its scientific rigor. In the final chapter, Ethan W. Gossett and P. D. Harms make the argument that there is a need to move beyond stress and well-being in both military and civilian literature and to address more directly the role of pain in terms of understanding the acute and chronic disorders often experienced by military personnel both during and after their service.

We are thrilled to bring these chapters together to address such a significant issue and are particularly proud that our authors were able to reflect successfully how stress and well-being shape the experiences of military personnel both in and out of the combat zone. We hope that these chapters will help shape the future research in both military and civilian research literatures. Finally, we would like to thank the authors for contributing to this volume, the reviewers who helped develop the chapters, and especially to the former and current service members who shared their insights concerning the topics that were needed to accurately reflect issues of importance to them as well as those who contributed as authors.

Peter D. Harms and
Pamela L. Perrewé

PROCESSING WAR: SIMILARITIES AND DIFFERENCES IN PTSD ANTECEDENTS AND OUTCOMES BETWEEN MILITARY AND CIVILIAN WAR SURVIVORS

Matthew R. Leon, Holly K. Osburn and Thomas Bellairs

ABSTRACT

Post-traumatic stress disorder (PTSD) affects both civilian and military populations following wartime experiences. However, despite an abundance of research investigating civilian and military populations separately, much less focus has been given to synthesizing and integrating findings to describe how civilian and military war survivors are comparatively affected by PTSD. This review is broken down into three sections covering (1) risk factors associated with PTSD, (2) relationships between PTSD and mental health outcomes, and (3) protective factors that can attenuate PTSD and its effects. Each section covers findings for civilians and military personnel and highlights similarities and differences between groups.

Keywords: Post-traumatic stress disorder; military war survivors; civilian war survivors

Occupational Stress and Well-being in Military Contexts
Research in Occupational Stress and Well-being, Volume 16, 1–22
Copyright © 2018 by Emerald Publishing Limited
All rights of reproduction in any form reserved
ISSN: 1479-3555/doi:10.1108/S1479-355520180000016001

INTRODUCTION

The mental health consequences of wartime experiences are heavily documented and widely recognize the impact of post-traumatic stress disorder (PTSD) on both military and civilian war survivors. However, the PTSD process impacts these groups differently, including variation in risk factors (Brewin, Andrews, & Valentine, 2000), severity of mental health outcomes such as depression (O'Campo et al., 2006), and presence of protective factors (e.g., social camaraderie; Allden et al., 1996). Despite a glut of research investigating civilian and military populations separately, much less focus has been given to synthesizing and integrating findings to describe how civilian and military war survivors are comparatively affected by PTSD. The purpose of this manuscript is to draw attention to similarities and differences in PTSD antecedents and outcomes associated with wartime in both civilian and military populations. Understanding the unique impact of PTSD in the context of civilian and military status will (1) increase our ability to provide insight and intervention to families with mixed military/civilian status dealing with PTSD, (2) bolster the effectiveness of existing PTSD treatment by providing more targeted information for differing demographics, and (3) identify differences in the power of various antecedents and outcomes of PTSD across military and civilian populations.

When discussing PTSD throughout this manuscript, we reference its description by the American Psychiatric Association in the Diagnostic and Statistical Manual of Mental Disorders, Fifth Edition (DSM-5; American Psychiatric Association, 2013), where PTSD is categorized as a trauma- and stressor-related disorder. Criteria include all of the following: (a) exposure to death, threatened death, actual or threatened serious injury, or actual or threatened sexual violence, (b) persistently re-experiencing the traumatic event, (c) avoidance of trauma-related stimuli, (d) negative thoughts or feelings that begin or worsen after the trauma, and (e) trauma-related arousal and reactivity that began or worsened after the trauma; additionally, symptoms must, (f) last for more than one month, (g) create distress or functional impairment, and (h) not be due to medication, substance use, or other illness. Note that before the formalization of the PTSD diagnosis in 1980, psychologists categorized the diagnosis under names such as combat exhaustion, shell shock, and traumatic war neurosis (Friedman, Schnurr, & McDonagh-Coyle, 1994).

Based on the DSM-5 criteria, research suggests that PTSD affects up to 8.3% of US adults over their lifetime (Kilpatrick et al., 2013), but this number almost doubles for military war survivors (14–16%; Gates et al., 2012). While PTSD statistics on US civilian war survivors is sparse due to lack of data, research on various international populations suggests extraordinarily high prevalence of PTSD. Moisander and Edston (2003) found rates of 69–92% among refugees from six different nations. Similarly, Wenzel, Griengl, Stompe, Mirzaei, and Keiffer (2000) reported PTSD rates of 91% over a three-year study of exiled survivors. More conservative estimates suggest rates between 20% (Eisenman, Gelberg, Liu, & Shapiro, 2003) and 31% (Ramsay, Gorst-Unsworth, & Turner, 1993). A recent review by Johnson and Thompson (2008) suggests that prevalence rates vary based on study methodology, which may explain the wide range of findings. Well-documented outcomes of PTSD include suicide (Krysinska & Lester, 2010; Tarrier & Gregg, 2004), drug and alcohol abuse (McFarlane, 1998; Shipherd, Staffer, & Tanner, 2005), and behavioral problems at work (Smith, Schnurr, & Rosenheck, 2005) and home (Riggs, Byrne, Weathers, & Litz, 1998). Moreover, PTSD is often comorbid with other mental health disorders such as depression and anxiety (Silove, Sinnerbrink, Field, Manicavasagar, & Steel, 1997).

This manuscript contains three sections. First, we will review risk factors associated with PTSD and their impact on civilian and military war survivors. Demographic factors such as education, gender, race, and age at trauma will be explored in conjunction with individual variables such as psychiatric history, previous trauma, and coping strategies. Second, we will discuss relationships between PTSD and mental health outcomes, including comorbidity with states such as depression and anxiety and likelihood of long-term psychological issues. Finally, in conjunction with the discussion on mental health outcomes, we will explore the power of protective factors in attenuating PTSD and its effects. Specifically, we will focus on differences in post-trauma responses due to previous training and individual traits. For example, Meichenbaum (1994) urged researchers to consider how the expectation of violence can impact the likelihood of PTSD. Regarding military war survivors, the expectation of combat is high and satisfies professional duties whereas that same expectation can shatter feelings of normalcy and safety among civilians. Further, military war survivors may be more likely to find high levels of social support from their peers who share similar experiences. Conversely, expectation of violence among civilians may violate norms of safety, pose threats to their homes and families, and be a catalyst for displacement as refugees (Silove et al., 1997).

We hope this research provides a more nuanced approach to help prevent a wide variety of negative outcomes such as divorce, suicide, and ongoing mental health issues based on more deeply detailed data about the target populations. Further, we hope this manuscript serves as the first step for researchers as they conceive and design studies in this area and the practitioners that apply research findings. We believe that developing a deeper understanding of the PTSD process in varying contexts will benefit scholars and practitioners seeking to predict a broad range of PTSD antecedents and outcomes and, potentially, explain otherwise unaccounted for variance across military and civilian war survivors.

RELATIONSHIPS BETWEEN PTSD AND MENTAL HEALTH OUTCOMES

Research findings of over 20 years suggest that individuals experiencing interpersonal violence or military combat have the highest conditional probability of experiencing PTSD (Breslau, Chilcoat, Kessler, & Davis, 1999; Kessler et al., 2005; Kilpatrick et al., 2013; Resnick, Kilpatrick, Dansky, Saunders, & Best, 1993). According to the United Nations High Commissioner for Refugees (UNHCR,

2008), this group includes an estimated 50 million civilians each year in addition to countless military personnel. While there is no universal response to PTSD, common outcomes include anxiety and depression, behavioral issues, and cognitive and emotional consequences. In the following section, we review the literature on PTSD and mental health outcomes in military and civilian populations. Given the similarities in mental health outcomes, civilian and military groups are reviewed together.

Comorbidity with Anxiety and Depression

One of the largest challenges facing researchers and clinicians is untangling comorbid symptoms such as anxiety and depression from PTSD. Most commonly, PTSD victims suffer from comorbid anxiety, depression, or a triple comorbidity of PTSD, anxiety, and depression simultaneously (Ginzburg, Ein-Dor, & Solomon, 2010). A meta-analysis of 161 studies and roughly 82,000 research participants identified rates of depression ranging from 3% to 85.5% in various PTSD samples (Steel et al., 2009). An additional review by Ginzburg et al. (2010) reported estimates between 21% and 94% for depression and PTSD (e.g., Frayne et al., 2005; Ginzburg, 2007), 39–97% for anxiety and PTSD (e.g., Hashemian et al., 2006; Sundquist, Johansson, DeMarinis, & Johansson-Sundquist, 2005), and 11–67% for triple comorbidity (Brady & Clary, 2004; Hashemian et al., 2006). That is, military veterans suffering from PTSD have, at a minimum, a one in five likelihood of also suffering from depression or anxiety.

Comorbidity of symptoms increases the likelihood of long-term psychological complications in military and civilian war survivors (Blair, 2000). The DSM-5 lists intrusion, avoidance, and alterations or arousal in mood or cognition as behavioral criteria associated with PTSD. Intrusion is the involuntary manifestation of thoughts, images, feelings, or nightmares into one's consciousness. Intrusions are associated with previous trauma and can re-create combat stress reactions (Solomon & Mikulincer, 2007), resulting in intensive feelings of fear, anxiety, or aggression. These feelings may result in negative behavioral reactions such as increased likelihood of suicidal ideations, depression, or anxiety.

In most cases, intrusion is followed by avoidance (Horowitz, 1982). While intrusion is exclusively a psychological phenomenon (although it can lead to behavioral reactions), avoidance manifests itself both cognitively and behaviorally. Cognitive symptoms include the tendency to deny meaning and consequences of trauma and negatively evaluate unwanted feelings (Hayes, Wilson, Gifford, Follette, & Strosahl, 1996). Behavioral avoidance strategies include inhibition and engagement in counter-phobic activities (e.g., shunning large crowds, identifying all exits before entering public spaces; Solomon & Mikulincer, 2007). Kashdan, Morina, and Priebe (2009) found that partial avoidance mediates the relationship between PTSD and quality of life. Specifically, avoidance habits developed by PTSD victims exacerbate anticipatory anxiety and interfere with potential disconfirming evidence that may alleviate feelings of avoidance (e.g., walking through a crowd may not be as anxiety-inducing as an individual initially believes; Barlow, 2000; Salters-Pedneault, Tull, & Roemer, 2004). As such, habitually engaging in avoidance behaviors inhibits quality of life by constraining day-to-day functions of individuals with PTSD.

Relationships between PTSD and mental health outcomes are further complicated by the reciprocal nature of PTSD and disorders such as depression (Breslau et al., 1998). Prior psychiatric history (especially depression) can obfuscate the relationship between PTSD and psychological or behavioral outcomes. Studies examining the causal relationship between PTSD and major depression have suggested that the association may have multiple explanations. First, depression increases the individual probability that one will be vulnerable to stressors that may cause PTSD (Breslau, Davis, Andreski, Peterson, & Schultz 1997; Bromet, Sonnega, & Kessler, 1998; Connor & Davidson 1997). Conversely, PTSD increases the chance of first-time depression (Breslau et al., 1997; Kessler, Sonnega, Bromet, Hughes, & Nelson, 1995). These findings suggest that the presence of either PTSD or depression makes one vulnerable to the other (Breslau et al., 1997). Scholars continue to struggle with delineating the causal relationship between PTSD and depression (Breslau & Davis, 1987; Breslau, Davis, Andreski, & Peterson, 1991; Kendler et al., 1995; Kessler, 1997; Yehuda & McFarlane, 1995).

Anxiety is often comorbid with depression and/or PTSD (Ginzburg et al., 2010) and manifests itself as nervousness, worry, or unease about an event. For PTSD victims, anxiety can be triggered by any stimuli that remind them of PTSD-related experiences or trauma. Behavioral reactions are often similar to fear cues in individuals without anxiety (Grillon, 2002). Further, anxiety triggers similar biological responses to those of PTSD patients (Etkin & Wager, 2007). Due to these types of confounding factors, it remains difficult to distinguish causality between PTSD and anxiety (similar to the relationship between PTSD and depression). However, research of samples of war survivors often shows differences in the antecedents of anxiety and depression. For example, Silove et al. (1997) found moderate positive correlations between PTSD and anxiety, but different predictors. Antecedents of anxiety included being female and experiencing recent conflict, while PTSD was related to pre-trauma and loneliness. A meta-analysis of adult refugees reported PTSD rate of 10%, depression rate of 5%, and generalized anxiety rate of 4%, with high probability of overlapping symptoms (Fazel, Wheeler, & Danesh, 2005). Similar to depression, comorbidity complicates diagnoses and the ability to make causal claims.

RISK FACTORS ASSOCIATED WITH THE DEVELOPMENT OF PTSD

The US government has indicated a strong interest in managing PTSD and its outcomes among veterans. However, challenges abound due to the varied demographics, socioeconomic status, and needs of the 21.8 million veterans of the US Armed Forces. In the following section, we review veteran susceptibility to PTSD based on demographic data, individual and situational factors contributing to PTSD, and briefly discuss coping strategies.

Military War Survivors

Demographic Predictors of PTSD

Several demographic factors play a major role in the likelihood of PTSD development. In this section, we will discuss pre-military (i.e., factors present before enlistment) and military (i.e., factors present after enlistment) variables contributing to or attenuating the likelihood of PTSD. Pre-enlistment issues can often cause negative outcomes both during and after military service; as such, it is important to identify these obstacles and target these individuals for preventative interventions (Nock et al., 2014). Specifically, we will discuss commonly studied variables, including age, gender, race, and pre-trauma risk factors.

Previous research suggests that age of enlistment is linked with PTSD development (where younger enlistees are more likely to develop PTSD; Breslau et al., 1999). A meta-analysis of 13 studies reported younger age at trauma was – despite a small effect size – a significant predictor of PTSD among military samples (Brewin et al., 2000). Similarly, Smith et al. (2008) found higher self-reports of new-onset PTSD in younger members of US soldiers deployed to Iraq and Afghanistan. Providing appropriate training to young military personnel on identification of symptoms, coping, and the value of social support may reduce risks for these individuals. This could include an emphasis on problem-focused coping, providing information on support options (e.g., counseling), and relationship-building among squad-mates.

Gender effects are an intensely studied correlate of PTSD. Direct comparisons suggest that women are more likely than men to develop PTSD following combat exposure (Brewin et al., 2008; Smith et al., 2008; Wolfe & Kimmerling, 1997). Data from the Veteran's Affairs office suggest about 10 of every 100 women (or 10%) develop PTSD sometimes in their lives compared with about four of every 100 men (or 4%; Department of Veterans Affairs, 2016). In general, women experience higher levels of stress in deployment despite similar exposure to deployment stressors (Vogt, Pless, King, & King, 2005). However, not all stressors are created equal. The same study reported that sexual harassment had a more negative impact on men's mental health, while concerns about family and relationship disruptions were harder on women.

Minorities have a slightly higher rate of PTSD than non-minority veterans, with 5.8% of minority veterans and 5.0% of non-minority veterans reporting PTSD as a service-connected disability (Department of Veterans Affairs, 2017). This makes PTSD the second most prevalent reported disability for minority veterans, following tinnitus (roughly 7%). According to the Department of Veterans Affairs National Center for PTSD, some demographics, including African-Americans and Hispanics, may be more likely than Whites to develop PTSD because these groups are more likely to go through a trauma. For example, Vietnam veterans self-reporting a minority status were in combat more than Whites (Department of Veterans Affairs, 2017).

In addition to Veterans Affairs data, academic evidence also suggests that race may predict risk of PTSD onset (Sutker, Davis, Uddo, & Ditta, 1995; Vasterling et al., 2002). Effect sizes are reportedly small, although meta-analytic data suggest that race may have a larger impact on PTSD development in civilian rather than military populations (Brewin et al., 2000). In some cases, race may act as a moderator rather than a main effect (e.g., Breslau et al., 2014; Brewin et al., 2000). More research is needed into the moderating and main effects of race before making conclusive statements. With that in mind, the general consensus is that demographic factors such as race and gender are weak predictors of PTSD development (Ozer, Best, Lipsey, & Weiss, 2003). Scholars also caution against confounding issues with demographic variables such as race and socioeconomic status (King, King, Foy, Keane, & Fairbank, 1999). In a meta-analytic review, Brewin et al. (2000) found a stronger effect size for low socioeconomic status than gender, race, and education level. However, they noted that all these variables produced low effect sizes (between 0.05 and 0.14).

Individual Factors Predicting PTSD

Individual characteristics can act as pre-dispositional risk factors in the role of PTSD development. Surveys have shown that a majority of research participants who experience any trauma have experienced multiple traumas, and individuals with PTSD are likely to report multiple childhood traumas (Berntsen et al., 2012; Breslau et al., 1999; Galea et al., 2002; Resnick, Yehuda, Pitman, & Foy, 1995) compared with adult trauma victims who do not display symptoms of PTSD. Pre-dispositional factors fall into one of the three categories: intra-individual psychopathological factors, normal pre-existing traits, and exposure to external stressors/situations (Emery, Emery, Shama, Quiana, & Jassani, 1991). Psychopathological factors include emotional problems or other mental disorders (e.g., anxiety and depression), normal pre-existing traits include personality and intelligence, and exposure to external stressors/situations includes episodes such as car accidents or parental alcoholism. Pre-dispositional factors often remain undisclosed by applicants or unidentified by recruiters. As such, it is difficult to measure frequency of pre-trauma risk in military populations. In addition, external stressors such as childhood trauma or family instability are related to gender, race, or socioeconomic status – further muddying the relationship between pre-dispositional factors and PTSD development (King et al., 1999). Regardless of type of trauma, the current consensus is that early stressors produce greater responsiveness to stressors later in life (Breslau et al., 2014). This idea of sensitization guides research on early indicators of PTSD, particularly when studying early life stressors surrounding family issues.

Trauma in family of origin is a consistent predictor of PTSD among veterans (Emery et al., 1991; King et al., 1999). Broadly, research suggests that household instability, lack of control, and familial disorganization have the strongest impacts on PTSD development (Berntsen et al., 2012; Breslau, Troost, Bohnert, & Luo, 2013; Koenen et al., 2002). Specifically, childhood adversity predicts likelihood of PTSD following deployment as well as the likelihood of becoming less resilient to deployment stressors over time (Berntsen et al., 2012). These findings are particularly concerning for two reasons: (1) deployment stressors such as war trauma and resettlement are already highly consistent with PTSD development (Blair, 2000) and (2) these findings suggest the nullification of existing levels of resilience that individuals may rely on to combat PTSD and combat stressors in general. For example, Maguen et al. (2008) – in a study of pre-deployment stressors and their relationship to the future resilience – suggested that a history of trauma outweighs the otherwise positive benefits of a resilient personality or resilient training. That is, the findings indicated that pre-deployment stressors and lifetime trauma had a stronger relationship with the development of PTSD than resilience did with attenuating PTSD. Finally, the relationship between prior trauma and PTSD is similar across demographics and does not differ in time elapsed since trauma or in method of PTSD assessment (Ozer et al., 2003). This is an unusual finding because it shows that prior trauma consistently predicts PTSD almost regardless of other contextual variables.

How individuals interpret early trauma also plays a large factor in the future likelihood of manifesting PTSD (Emery et al., 1991). For example, Koenen et al. (2002) suggested that pre-existing psychopathology mediates the relationship between early age at trauma and development of PTSD, which affects interpretation of and response to trauma. Similarly, family history of psychopathology acts as a small to moderate predictor of PTSD development in adults (Ozer et al., 2003). This relationship varied by type of traumatic experience (with non-combat violence having the strongest relationship) suggesting that interpretation and variance in events is a probable factor in development of PTSD. To combat PTSD susceptibility, data suggest that perceptions of structure (e.g., a regular schedule imposed by parents and regular school attendance) and feelings of responsibility at a young age can mitigate the potential for negatively interpreting traumatic events (Emery et al., 1991).

Coping with PTSD

It is almost impossible that a military war survivor will not have encountered at least one of the many PTSD antecedents discussed in this manuscript. Therefore, it is important to discuss potential coping mechanics for these populations. Coping is a broad concept and refers to a trait that denotes a person's general emotional and physiological stability or a state focused on handling reactions to environmental stimuli (Lazarus & Folkman, 1984). PTSD research focuses primarily on the second definition of coping with an emphasis on individual and social factors that help manage the resource demands of PTSD (Besser, Weinberg, Zeigler-Hill, & Neria, 2014; Priebe et al., 2010). Toward this end, coping actions require (1) effort from the individual, (2) behaviors or cognitive action, and (3) an appraisal of the stressor (Schwarzer & Schwarzer, 1996). Considerable evidence associates coping responses with psychological well-being and functionality in military samples. Historically, PTSD research in a military context draws heavily from clinical and military psychology and identifies three primary coping mechanisms that reduce impact of PTSD and risk of PTSD development: social support, utilizing psychological counseling services, and problem-focused coping strategies (Summerfield, 2000; Zeidner, 1994).

Scholars operationalize perceived social support as one's perceptions of helpful and unhelpful social interactions (Pietrzak, Johnson, Goldstein, Malley, & Southwick, 2009). Multiple meta-analyses suggest that perceptions of social support are negatively associated with PTSD in military personnel regardless of generation (Brewin et al., 2000; Ozer, et al., 2003). The importance of social support in combating negative mental health outcomes such as PTSD cannot be understated. For example, a study of Iraqi asylum seekers found that poor social support was a stronger prediction of depression than history of torture (Gorst-Unsworth & Goldenberg, 1998). Further, Brewin et al. (2000), in their meta-analysis of PTSD predictors, found lack of social support to have the strongest effect size of all correlates with a weighted effect size of 0.40 (race was the weakest with a weighted effect size of 0.05). A more recent meta-analysis yielded an effect size of –0.28 between perceived social support and PTSD (Ozer et al., 2003). This meta-analysis found that the perceived social support–PTSD relationship became stronger over time. Specifically, studies with more than three years of time lapse between the traumatic event and PTSD assessment exhibited the strongest effect size ($r = -0.42$), while studies in the six month to three-year period were lower ($r = -0.16$) and those with one to six months between assessment were lower still ($r = 0.01$). Finally, this relationship had a larger effect size in studies of combat trauma ($r = -0.26$) than noncombat violence ($r = -0.11$). Together, these data suggest that the effect of social support may be cumulative over time and be especially important for war survivors.

Social support helps shape the post-trauma environment by acting as a secondary level of prevention by protecting against the development and consequences of trauma-related psychopathology such as PTSD (Ozbay et al., 2007; Ozer, 2003). Studies exploring the impact of social support on health outcomes suggest that social support promotes the use of available medical programs, increases early detection of illness, and decreases morbidity (Ozbay et al., 2007). The absence of social support can be particularly detrimental to those veterans needing treatment for PTSD; for example, in a study of veterans returning from Vietnam, Johnson et al. (1997) found that lack of social support (as an indicator of homecoming stress) increased feelings of isolation as well as frequency and intensity of PTSD symptoms.

Fortunately, military members have a clear support group in their peers, officer structure, and through the efforts of programs based out of Veterans Affairs, among other government-sanctioned and non-profit organizations. Research suggests that veteran peers (e.g., members of one's unit) are viewed as providing high levels of social support (Laffaye, Cavella, Drescher, & Rosen, 2008; Pietrzak et al., 2010). In fact, Laffaye et al.'s (2008) suggested that veterans view their peers as providing more social support and less interpersonal stress than any other group, including spouses, relatives, and nonveteran friends. While sources of social support remain understudied, it appears to be a fruitful area of future inquiry. In addition to informal and formal support groups, research shows that participating in professional psychological treatments (e.g., counseling and cognitive therapy) provides benefits to military war survivors (Resick, 2001).

Organizations such as the American Psychological Association, US Department of Veterans Affairs, and the US Department of Defense have created clinical guidelines for psychological treatments of PTSD. Most commonly, counselors and clinicians utilize exposure therapy, cognitive therapy, and cognitive behavioral therapy in patients with severe PTSD. These trauma-focused therapies are broadly available to veterans, commonly taught to clinicians, and have exhibited high levels of success as empirically based PTSD treatments. In this manuscript, we will provide general overviews of these three types of treatments. However, many variants exist.

Exposure therapy includes directly addressing thoughts, feelings, and memories of a traumatic event through guided reflection in order to reduce symptom severity. Exposure treatment is considered a first-line treatment (i.e., a standard, first approach solution) for PTSD and is considered a highly efficacious method for treating a large majority of PTSD victims (Committee on Treatment of Posttraumatic Stress Disorder, & Institute of Medicine, 2008; Cusack et al., 2016). Given the intensity of exposure therapy, it is often utilized in short periods and in conjunction with other types of therapies. The necessary brevity of exposure therapy is a considerable advantage for victims who are unwilling to devote large amounts of time to other types of counseling programs (e.g., behavioral modification). In fact, even a single session of exposure therapy has been shown to reduce fear and PTSD in earthquake survivors (Basoglu, Salcioglu, & Livanuo, 2007).

Cognitive therapy is another first-line treatment that helps clients change unhelpful thinking patterns to improve functioning (e.g., using mindfulness techniques to be aware of one's own stress, identifying and coping with obsessive thoughts). The goal of cognitive therapy is to help individuals regulate emotional responses to their interpretation of different situations. Often, this includes exercises designed to identify distorted or negative thinking patterns and modify existing beliefs to cope more effectively with the surrounding environment. This therapy is brief, goal-oriented, and time-limited (Cusack et al., 2016). Evidence supports the idea that cognitive therapy can attenuate PTSD symptoms, completely remove PTSD diagnosis, and improve severity of depression and anxiety among adults with PTSD (Cusack et al., 2016).

Cognitive-behavioral therapy combines facets of exposure and cognitive therapy with behavioral therapy techniques (Harvey, Bryant, & Terrier, 2003). It is based on behavioral conditioning and is a fairly resource-intensive therapy – it requires eight to 12 weekly sessions of up to 90 minutes (Cusack et al., 2016). However, given the more mixed and general nature of this therapy, it can be employed in a wide variety of settings, including in a group format, with a focus on correcting specific behaviors, and to target a wide variety of PTSD outcomes (Committee on Treatment of Posttraumatic Stress Disorder, & Institute of Medicine, 2008; Foa, Keane, Friedman, & Cohen, 2008). Research shows low rates of remission for military veterans utilizing cognitive behavioral therapy and show that it is just as effective as other types of intensive counseling programs (Levi, Bar-Haim, Kreiss, & Fruchter, 2016).

While all three of these types of therapies are effective, PTSD victims and their counselors must consider other issues before committing to a program. Factors include clinical judgment about the intervention's appropriateness for the client, patient preferences, and ease of access to treatment. For example, exposure therapy is still a specialized program that is not available at many community-based mental health facilities (Cusack et al., 2016). At this time, studies show promise for integrative multiple types of therapies, but more research is needed (Mills et al., 2012; Sannibale et al., 2013).

Civilian War Survivors

This section mirrors the previous portions of this manuscript – we will discuss commonly studied variables, including age, gender, race, and pre-trauma risk factors. However, this section focuses exclusively on civilian war survivors, who are different in several key ways. First, there are many more studies dedicated to responding to tragedy and trauma as a community. This is obviously something unique to civilians since they often remain with their community where the war and trauma occurred. On the other hand, soldiers are removed from the communities with which they shared the trauma upon returning home (Norris, Stevens, Pfefferbaum, Wyche, & Pfefferbaum, 2008; Pfefferbaum et al., 2008). Second, civilians are often unprepared for combat experiences and wartime trauma. Unlike military war survivors, civilians lack resilience training, are not pre-selected or screened for protective traits, and often do not have government entities such as Veterans Affairs who specialize in helping victims to recover. Moreover, military war survivors prepare for wartime trauma due to its nature as a regular work duty. Finally, civilian research naturally covers a broader age range. Children and elderly are just as likely to experience wartime trauma as middle-aged adults, where military samples naturally do not include youth and rarely include elderly outside of retrospective inter-generational studies (e.g., comparisons of Vietnam veterans vs operation enduring freedom (OEF) veterans). Given these differences, research suggests that external factors such as trauma severity and injury play a more powerful role in PTSD for civilians than military (Abenhai, Dab, & Salmi, 1992). On the other hand, demographic variables such as race, age, and gender yield similar results (e.g., Ai, Peterson, & Ubelhor, 2002; Cheung, 1994; Reppesgaard, 1997; Scholte et al., 2004).

Demographic Predictors of PTSD

Civilians aged over 65 years are at an increased risk of developing PTSD following wartime experiences (Cardozo, Vergara, Agani, & Gotway, 2000; Eytan, Gex-Fabry, Toscani, Deroo, & Bovier, 2004). This research has been consistent across research participants in European, Middle Eastern, and Asian populations, but almost no data currently exist for war survivors in North America. One notable exception are the data covering the 9/11 terrorist attacks which showed consistent results with other research (e.g., DiGrande, Neria, Brackbill, Pulliam, & Galea, 2011). Johnson and Thompson (2008) conducted a meta-analysis of civilian PTSD development among war survivors and noted that older adults were at higher risk of PTSD development, but cautioned that the age differences may have been attributable to differences in type of trauma, lack of social support, or refugee status. As such, more research targeting elderly populations needs to occur before making strong conclusions.

On the opposite end of the spectrum, children also struggle with wartime experiences. About 11% of child refugees report PTSD, and are 10 times more likely to have PTSD than a child not exposed to wartime trauma (Fazel, Wheeler, & Danesh, 2005). Here, data are similar to military populations where childhood trauma is a predictor of PTSD development in adulthood. This is an incredibly vulnerable population requiring special care due to the difficulty of identifying PTSD through traditional self-report techniques.

Gender studies are also similar to military samples showing that women are more likely to develop PTSD (e.g., Ekblad, Prochazka, & Roth, 2002; Morina et al., 2016). However, civilian research suggests that this may be due to an increased likelihood of rape and the increased risk of becoming a single parent or widow from losing a spouse who was in the military (Johnson & Thompson, 2008). However, similar results exist regardless of presence of rape or death of spouses (e.g., DiGrande et al., 2011). Other scholars propose that women may be more likely to engage in emotion-focused coping (instead of more effective problem-focused coping) or that women are merely more likely to report PTSD symptoms than men (McNally, 2003).

Individual Factors Predicting PTSD

Given the harmful outcomes of war on civilians, a large amount of time and energy has been spent identifying variables that put civilians at risk of developing PTSD. Broadly, research suggests that war experiences themselves are incredibly strong predictors (Michultka, Blanchard, & Kalous 1998). Specifically, exposure to situational factors seem to be the most predictive of civilian PTSD development with findings showing that severe injury (Abenhaim et al., 1992), number of war experiences (Michultka, et al., 1998), and severity of trauma (Carlson & Rosser-Hogan, 1993) all strongly predicting PTSD development. A recent review of the mental health of wartime survivors confirms these findings and shows that mental health issues remain prevalent for many years following wartime trauma (Bogic, Njoku, & Priebe, 2015). It is possible that trauma exposure is more impactful for civilians because these experiences destroy assumptions of safety. As such, civilians may be more likely to experience intrusive thoughts about the experiences and less emotional numbing. Conversely, military veterans are less likely to experience intrusive thoughts and receive training to deal with them (Meichenbaum, 1994).

Another unique factor for civilians is refugee status. By definition, refugees are displaced during wartime, which results in particular vulnerability to PTSD due to lack of coping resources, social support, and the stress associated with forced removal from one's home and possibly from country (Steel et al., 2009). Compared to non-refugee war survivors, refugees experience moderately worse mental health outcomes (Porter & Haslam, 2005). These outcomes are due to post-displacement accommodation, lack of economic opportunity, and loss of social support (Eisenbruch, 1991). Refugees are one of the most difficult populations to study due to practical obstacles. Populations are often inaccessible to researchers physically due to injury, and linguistic and cultural differences; aid receives justified priority over scientific investigation (Porter & Haslam, 2005). Unfortunately, this results in a dearth of empirically rigorous studies in this area and more exploratory or methodologically compromised work. Finally, it is difficult to draw generalizable conclusions due to the extremely localized circumstances that refugees face – there is no standardized refugee or refugee experience. Regardless, data show that refugee war survivors are at a distinct disadvantage even compared to other civilian war survivors.

Coping with PTSD

Clinicians use many of the same coping techniques employed with military war survivors to aid civilian survivors. However, given the additional issues civilians often have with recurring and intrusive thoughts about their war trauma, some researchers also suggest reducing experiential avoidance as a coping strategy to mitigate PTSD symptoms (Kashdan et al., 2015). Experiential avoidance is the tendency to evaluate negatively intrusive or unwanted feelings and thoughts, being unable to tolerate these thoughts, and desire to control or remove them (Hayes et al., 1996). Individuals exhibiting high levels of experiential avoidance have a difficult time managing unpleasant emotions and thoughts. Helping civilians through this process is paramount in reducing PTSD and its symptoms over time.

Avoidance-based strategies sit on the opposite end of the spectrum of recommended therapies such as the previously discussed exposure therapy and cognitive therapy, which recommend individuals confront and accept their emotions and thoughts in order to work through them. Individuals unable to accept and manage their thoughts are often constricted in their behaviors. For example, they may be unable to maintain social relationships, leave home, or hold a job due to the constant anxiety they experience from fear of intrusive thoughts (Hayes et al., 1996). This anxiety acts as a constant resource drain due to the substantial efforts expended by victims who structure their life around avoiding potentially triggering experiences. As such, a clinician's top priority with civilians is making them comfortable addressing their negative thoughts and emotions in order to move forward to more advanced programs (e.g., cognitive-behavioral therapy) that can reduce the impact of their PTSD.

Both civilians and military personnel are at risk of PTSD development following wartime experiences. However, the primary antecedents differ between each group. When studying and treating military war survivors, clinicians and scholars must be particularly wary of childhood trauma, family history of psychopathology, and focus on guiding victims in interpreting war trauma in a constructive fashion (e.g., minimizing survivor guilt). Treatment targeted for civilian war survivors should be based on amount and severity of witnessed trauma and focus on providing clear structures of social support that may not exist for these groups.

INDIVIDUAL PROTECTIVE FACTORS IN POST-TRAUMA RESPONSE

Each person processes trauma in a unique way. In this manuscript, we have discussed individual characteristics that can increase the likelihood of PTSD (e.g., childhood trauma), but many streams of research focus on individual characteristics that protect against PTSD. Clinicians and scholars have shown particular interest in individual ability to overcome stress (e.g., resilience), personality traits such as altruism and extroversion, and self-regulation. Given that these traits act similarly in both military and civilian populations (Bonanno, Galea, Bucciarelli, & Vlahov, 2006; Campbell-Sills, Cohan, & Stein, 2006), we will discuss both groups simultaneously in this section. In addition, we will provide an overview of the literature and findings related to individual characteristics that attenuate the effects of PTSD following trauma exposure.

Research on resilience suggests that it can act as a protective factor against stressors and PTSD development in military populations (e.g., King, King, Fairbank, Keane, & Adams, 1998; Meredith et al., 2011; Tsai, Harpez-Rotem, Pietrzak, & Southwick, 2012). While no universal definition of resilience exists, it encompasses the ability to recover from stress or trauma. Resilient individuals are more likely to perceive traumatic events as challenges or growth opportunities instead of threats, exhibit lower amounts of emotional fluctuation when under stress, and maintain a more positive mindset (Bartone, 2006).

Additional traits, including altruism and extraversion, correlate with reduced likelihood of PTSD (Meredith et al., 2011). Scholars posit that altruistic and extroverted individuals are more likely to develop strong social support networks, which – as discussed previously – play a large role in reducing PTSD (Foa et al., 2008). For example, results from a study of Vietnam War veterans suggested that altruism significantly decreased PTSD symptomatology over time (Kishon-Barash, Midlarsky, & Johnson, 1999). Vollhardt (2009) also provides a detailed account of the benefits of altruism and prosocial behaviors following trauma, emphasizing the importance of trauma victims pro-actively helping others. Extraversion has been tied to resilience (Campbell-Sills, 2006) and social support (Cohen & Wills, 1985), which buffer effects of PTSD. For example, extraverted individuals tend to easily form attachments with others, seek interaction, and utilize support networks (Costa & McCrae, 1992).

Finally, emotional regulation is often emphasized in therapy (Ford & Russo, 2006). Individuals with high levels of emotional regulation are less likely to experience emotional numbing, social detachment, and intrusive thoughts (American Psychiatric Association, 2013). This is particularly important in aiding with recovery from trauma. Currently, emotional regulation is integrated into several types of cognitive therapy, given its strong empirical associations with recovery in a wide range of trauma victims.

DISCUSSION

As expected, antecedents of PTSD differ in strength between civilians and military war survivors (see Table 1 for overview). High risk of exposure to multiple traumas and a lack of reporting trauma are particularly impactful for military. Given the general duties of many military personnel, it is likely that cumulative exposure to trauma occurs. Potential trauma events (e.g., combat exposure) should be documented for military war survivors as a potential early indicator of PTSD development. Civilians are especially susceptible to war experiences, including witnessing injury or being injured. Moreover, civilians are much more likely to develop PTSD if they lack social support or have their communities disrupted (e.g., refugees). As such, the most important strategy for PTSD civilians is to build and maintain a strong support network. Across military and civilian groups, age of trauma is strongly related to PTSD development, and extra care should be given to monitor young enlistees and civilian children and elderly. Finally, demographics are small but significant predictors of PTSD, with both military and civilian women displaying a larger propensity to develop PTSD than men do.

Although PTSD outcomes are similar between groups, coping and therapeutic strategies should emphasize different areas based on the unique needs

Table 1. Overview of PTSD Antecedents and Coping Effectiveness.

	Military	Civilian
Age	Younger age at trauma more likely to develop PTSD; younger age at trauma has larger effect size for men than women	Civilians over 65 years old have higher risk than children or younger adults of developing PTSD after wartime experience; children exposed to wartime experience 10× more likely to develop PTSD than other children
Gender	Women more likely to report PTSD following combat than men; however, meta-analytic data suggest there may be no significant gender effect in military samples	Women more likely to develop PTSD following wartime experience than men; may be due to exposure to additional trauma such as rape; meta-analytic data suggest substantial gender effect
Race	Minorities report slightly higher rates of PTSD (0.8% higher report rate)	Weak to nonexistent relationship between race and PTSD development following combat exposure
Pre-trauma	Childhood trauma increases likelihood of PTSD development	Childhood trauma increases likelihood of PTSD development
Exposure to wartime trauma	High risks associated with exposure to multiple traumas	High risks associated with severity of trauma and witnessing trauma
Coping techniques	Experiential avoidance often impossible – exposure therapy can be effective instead; problem-focused coping effective; social support effective; encourage reporting of trauma and PTSD symptoms	Experiential avoidance effective in severe cases – exposure therapy often difficult for civilians; problem-focused coping effective; social support effective (especially with refugees)

of military and civilian war survivors. Broadly, coping strategies should directly address emotional and cognitive triggers and emphasize the importance of support networks. However, civilians may be more sensitive to direct confrontation of their feelings and memories (e.g., exposure therapy); whereas it may be particularly effective in terms of time and cost resources for many military war survivors. Civilian-coping strategies should lean more on providing a stable and normal external environment – this may be particularly effective for displaced civilians such as refugees.

Limitations and Future Directions

This manuscript is limited in that it shows only a broad overview of the decades of PTSD research. However, it is valuable to gain and compare "big picture" knowledge of the mechanisms of PTSD development in one of the most vulnerable populations in the world – war survivors. In this manuscript, we have identified high-level similarities and differences in antecedents and provided a starting point for the future research. In addition, we did not explore pharmacotherapy components of PTSD in this manuscript (e.g., changes in brain chemistry, pharmaceutical treatments for PTSD). However, existing books, reviews, and meta-analytic studies cover this topic (e.g., Foa et al., 2008; Mohamed & Rosenheck, 2008; Watts et al., 2013). Finally, it is difficult to generalize existing results, given the large variation in geography, demographics, and the unique characteristics of each war's survivors. While broad statements can be made (e.g., social support is important, PTSD will likely affect children differently than adults, symptoms change over time), it is difficult and empirically unsound to believe that effect sizes or causal relationships will remain the same as the nature of war and worldwide demographics continue to change. At best, previous research in this area acts as guideposts for practical solutions and the future research.

The future research can delve more deeply into the nuances of effective coping strategies and further measures the efficacy of different types of therapy and support. Moreover, counselors and researchers in this area should not shy away from replicating previous studies to clarify the generalizability of existing data. Additional research is also needed to provide more nuanced data in areas such as social support (e.g., exploring different sources of social support), therapeutic options (behavioral vs pharmaceutical), and how PTSD manifests itself in different cohorts (e.g., OEF vs Operation Iraqi Freedom veterans). Finally, the review of the literature yielded no studies directly studying agency as a protective factor against PTSD. Scholars allude to research participants' sense of agency when discussing displacement of refugees or as a facet of other clinical issues (e.g., external locus of control), but – to our knowledge – there are no articles directly addressing the role of agency in attenuating PTSD following combat experiences. This may prove to be a fruitful area of the future research as locus of control is often tied to clinical recovery.

CONCLUSION

We hope this research can provide a more nuanced approach to help prevent a wide variety of negative outcomes such as divorce, suicide, and ongoing mental health issues based on more deeply detailed data about the target populations. With this in mind, we hope this manuscript has served as a first step for researchers as they conceive and design studies in this area and the practitioners that apply research findings. We believe that developing a deeper understanding of this phenomenon in varying contexts will benefit scholars and practitioners seeking to predict a broad range of PTSD antecedents and outcomes and, potentially, explain otherwise unaccounted for variance in PTSD outcomes across military and civilian war survivors.

REFERENCES

Abenhaim, L., Dab, W., & Salmi, L. R. (1992). Study of civilian victims of terrorist attacks (France 1982–1987). *Journal of Clinical Epidemiology*, *45*, 103–109.

Ai, A. L., Peterson, C., & Ubelhor, D. (2002). War-related trauma and symptoms of posttraumatic stress disorder among adult Kosovar refugees. *Journal of Traumatic Stress*, *15*, 157–160.

Allden, K., Poole, C., Chantavanich, S., Ohmar, K., Aung, N. N., & Mollica, R. F. (1996). Burmese political dissidents in Thailand: Trauma and survival among young adults in exile. *American Journal of Public Health*, *86*, 1561–1569.

American Psychiatric Association. (2013). *Diagnostic and statistical manual of mental disorders: DSM-5*. Washington, DC: American Psychiatric Association.

Barlow D. H. (2000). Unraveling the mysteries of anxiety and its disorders from the perspective of emotion theory. *American Psychologist*, *55*,1247–1263.

Bartone, P. T. (2006). Resilience under military operational stress: Can leaders influence hardiness?. *Military Psychology*, *18*(S), S131.

Basoglu, M., Şalcioglu, E., & Livanou, M. (2007). A randomized controlled study of single-session behavioural treatment of earthquake-related post-traumatic stress disorder using an earthquake simulator. *Psychological Medicine*, *37*(2), 203–213. doi:10.1017/S0033291706009123

Berntsen, D., Johannessen, K. B., Thomson, Y. D., Bertelsen, M., Hoyle, R. H., & Rubin, D. C. (2012). Peace and war: Trajectories of posttraumatic stress disorder symptoms before, during, and after military deployment in Afghanistan. *Psychological Science*, *23*(12), 1557–1565.

Besser, A., Weinberg, M., Zeigler-Hill, V., & Neria, Y. (2014). Acute symptoms of posttraumatic stress and dissociative experiences among female Israeli civilians exposed to war: The roles of intrapersonal and interpersonal sources of resilience. *Journal of Clinical Psychology*, *70*(12), 1227–1239.

Blair, R. G. (2000). Risk factors associated with PTSD and major depression among Cambodian refugees in Utah. *Health & Social Work*, *25*(1), 23–30.

Bogic, M., Njoku, A., & Priebe, S. (2015). Long-term mental health of war-refugees: A systematic literature review. *BMC International Health and Human Rights*, *15*(1), 29.

Bonanno, G. A., Galea, S., Bucciarelli, A., & Vlahov, D. (2006). Psychological resilience after disaster: New York City in the aftermath of the September 11th terrorist attack. *Psychological Science*, *17*(3), 181–186.

Brady, K. T., & Clary, C. M., (2004). Affective and anxiety comorbidity in posttraumatic stress disorder treatment trials of sertraline. *Community Psychiatry*, *44*, 360–369.

Breslau, N., Chilcoat, H. D., Kessler, R. C., & Davis, G. C. (1999). Previous exposure to trauma and PTSD effects of subsequent trauma: Results from the Detroit area survey of trauma. *American Journal of Psychiatry*, *156*(6), 902–907.

Breslau, N., & Davis, G. C. (1987). Posttraumatic stress disorder: The stressor criterion. *The Journal of Nervous and Mental Disease*, *175*(5), 255–264.

Breslau, N., Davis, G. C., Andreski, P., & Peterson, E. (1991). Traumatic events and posttraumatic stress disorder in an urban population of young adults. *Archives of General Psychiatry*, *48*(3), 216–222.

Breslau, N., Davis, G. C., Andreski, P., Peterson, E. L., & Schultz, L. R. (1997). Sex differences in posttraumatic stress disorder. *Archives of General Psychiatry*, *54*(11), 1044–1048.

Breslau, N., Kessler, R. C., Chilcoat, H. D., Schultz, L. R., Davis, G. C., & Andreski, P. (1998). Trauma and posttraumatic stress disorder in the community: The 1996 Detroit area survey of trauma. *Archives of General Psychiatry*, *55*(7), 626–632.

Breslau, N., Koenen, K. C., Luo, Z., Agnew-Blais, J., Swanson, S., Houts, R. M., … Moffitt, T. E. (2014). Childhood maltreatment, juvenile disorders and adult post-traumatic stress disorder: A prospective investigation. *Psychological Medicine*, *44*(9), 1937–1945.

Breslau, N., Troost, J. P., Bohnert, K., & Luo, Z. (2013). Influence of predispositions on post-traumatic stress disorder: Does it vary by trauma severity?. *Psychological Medicine*, *43*(2), 381–390.

Brewin, C. R., Andrews, B., & Valentine, J. D. (2000). Meta-analysis of risk factors for posttraumatic stress disorder in trauma-exposed adults. *Journal of Consulting and Clinical Psychology*, *68*(5), 748–766.

Brewin, C. R., Scragg, P., Robertson, M., Thompson, M., d'Ardenne, P., & Ehlers, A. (2008). Promoting mental health following the London bombings: A screen and treat approach. *Journal of Traumatic Stress*, *21*(1), 3–8.

Bromet, E., Sonnega, A., & Kessler, R. C. (1998). Risk factors for DSM-III-R posttraumatic stress disorder: Findings from the National Comorbidity Survey. *American Journal of Epidemiology*, *147*(4), 353–361.

Campbell-Sills, L., Cohan, S. L., & Stein, M. B. (2006). Relationship of resilience to personality, coping, and psychiatric symptoms in young adults. *Behaviour Research and Therapy*, *44*(4), 585–599.

Cardozo, B. L., Vergara, A., Agani, F., & Gotway, C. A. (2000). Mental health, social functioning, and attitudes of Kosovar Albanians following the war in Kosovo. *The Journal of the American Medical Association*, *284*, 569–577.

Carlson, E. B., & Rosser-Hogan, R. (1993). Mental health status of Cambodian refugees ten years after leaving their homes. *American Journal of Orthopsychiatry*, *63*(2), 223.

Cheung, P. (1994). Posttraumatic stress disorder among Cambodian refugees in New Zealand. *The International Journal of Social Psychiatry*, *40*, 17–26.

Cohen, S., & Wills, T. A. (1985). Stress, social support, and the buffering hypothesis. *Psychological Bulletin*, *98*(2), 310.

Committee on Treatment of Posttraumatic Stress Disorder, & Institute of Medicine. (2008). *Treatment of posttraumatic stress disorder: An assessment of the evidence*. Washington, DC: National Academies Press.

Connor, K. M., & Davidson, J. R. (1997). Familial risk factors in posttraumatic stress disorder. *Annals of the New York Academy of Sciences*, *821*(1), 35–51.

Costa, P. T., & McCrae, R. R. (1992). Four ways five factors are basic. *Personality and Individual Differences*, *13*(6), 653–665.

Cusack, K., Jonas, D. E., Forneris, C. A., Wines, C., Sonis, J., Middleton, J. C., … Weil, A. (2016). Psychological treatments for adults with posttraumatic stress disorder: A systematic review and meta-analysis. *Clinical Psychology Review*, *43*, 128–141.

Department of Veterans Affairs. (2016). Retrieved from http://www.ptsd.va.gov. Accessed June 17, 2017.

Department of Veterans Affairs. (2017). *Minority veterans report: Military Service History and VA benefit utilization statistics*. Washington, DC: Data Governance and Analytics.

DiGrande, L., Neria, Y., Brackbill, R. M., Pulliam, P., & Galea, S. (2011). Long-term posttraumatic stress symptoms among 3,271 civilian survivors of the September 11, 2001, terrorist attacks on the World Trade Center. *American Journal of Epidemiology*, *173*(3), 271–281.

Eisenbruch, M. (1991). From post-traumatic stress disorder to cultural bereavement: Diagnosis of Southeast Asian refugees. *Social Science & Medicine*, *33*(6), 673–680.

Eisenman, D. P., Gelberg, L., Liu, H., & Shapiro, M. F. (2003). Mental health and health-related quality of life among adult Latino primary care patients living in the United States with previous exposure to political violence. *The Journal of the American Medical Association*, *290*, 627–634.

Ekblad, S., Prochazka, H., & Roth, G. (2002). Psychological impact of torture: A 3-month follow-up of mass-evacuated Kosovan adults in Sweden. Lessons learnt for prevention. *Acta Psychiatrica Scandinavica, 106*, 30–37.

Emery, V. O., Emery, P. E., Shama, D. K., Quiana, N. A., & Jassani, A. K. (1991). Predisposing variables in PTSD patients. *Journal of Traumatic Stress, 4*(3), 325–343.

Etkin, A., & Wager, T. D. (2007). Functional neuroimaging of anxiety: A meta-analysis of emotional processing in PTSD, social anxiety disorder, and specific phobia. *American Journal of Psychiatry, 164*(10), 1476–1488.

Eytan, A., Gex-Fabry, M., Toscani, L., Deroo, L., & Bovier, P. A. (2004). Determinants of postconflict symptoms in Albanian Kosovars. *Journal of Nervous and Mental Disease, 192*, 664–671.

Fazel, M., Wheeler, J., & Danesh, J. (2005). Prevalence of serious mental disorder in 7000 refugees resettled in western countries: A systematic review. *The Lancet, 365*(9467), 1309–1314.

Foa, E. B., Keane, T. M., Friedman, M. J., & Cohen, J. A. (Eds.). (2008). *Effective treatments for PTSD: Practice guidelines from the International Society for Traumatic Stress Studies*. New York, NY: Guilford Press.

Ford, J. D., & Russo, E. (2006). Trauma-focused, present-centered, emotional self-regulation approach to integrated treatment for posttraumatic stress and addiction: Trauma adaptive recovery group education and therapy (TARGET). *American Journal of Psychotherapy, 60*(4), 335–355.

Frayne, S. M., Seaver, M. R., Loveland, S., Christansen, C., Spiro, A., Parker, V. A., Skinner, K. M. (2005). Burden of medical illness in women with depression and posttraumatic stress disorder. *Archives of International Medicine, 164*, 1306–1312.

Friedman, M. J., Schnurr, P. P., & McDonagh-Coyle, A. (1994). Post-traumatic stress disorder in the military veteran. *Psychiatric Clinics of North America, 17*(2), 265–278.

Galea, S., Ahern, J., Resnick, H., Kilpatrick, D., Bucuvalas, M., Gold, J., & Vlahov, D. (2002). Psychological sequelae of the September 11 terrorist attacks in New York City. *New England Journal of Medicine, 346*(13), 982–987.

Gates, M. A., Holowka, D. W., Vasterling, J. J., Keane, T. M., Marx, B. P., & Rosen, R. C. (2012). Posttraumatic stress disorder in veterans and military personnel: Epidemiology, screening, and case recognition. *Psychological Services, 9*(4), 361–382.

Ginzburg, K. (2007). Comorbidity of PTSD and depression following myocardial infarction. *Journal of Affective Disorders, 94*, 135–143.

Ginzburg, K., Ein-Dor, T., & Solomon, Z. (2010). Comorbidity of posttraumatic stress disorder, anxiety and depression: A 20-year longitudinal study of war veterans. *Journal of Affective Disorders, 123*(1), 249–257.

Grillon, C. (2002). Startle reactivity and anxiety disorders: Aversive conditioning, context, and neurobiology. *Biological Psychiatry, 52*(10), 958–975.

Gorst-Unsworth, C., & Goldenberg, E. (1998). Psychological sequelae of torture and organised violence suffered by refugees from Iraq. Trauma-related factors compared with social factors in exile. *The British Journal of Psychiatry, 172*(1), 90–94.

Harvey, A. G., Bryant, R. A., & Tarrier, N. (2003). Cognitive behaviour therapy for posttraumatic stress disorder. *Clinical Psychology Review, 23*(3), 501–522.

Hashemian, F., Khoshnood, K., Desai, M. M., Falahati, F., Kasl, S., Southwick, S. (2006). Anxiety, depression, and posttraumatic stress in Iranian survivors of chemical warfare. *JAMA, 296*, 560–566.

Hayes S. C., Wilson K. G., Gifford E. V., Follette V. M., Strosahl K. (1996). Experiential avoidance and behavioral disorders: A functional dimensional approach to diagnosis and treatment. *Journal of Consulting and Clinical Psychology, 64*, 1152–1168.

Horowitz, M. J. (1982). Psychological processes induced by illness, injury, and loss. In T. Milon, C. Green, & R. Meagher (Eds.), *Handbook of clinical health psychology* (pp. 53–68). New York, NY: Plenum Press.

Johnson, D. R., Lubin, H., Rosenheck, R., Fontana, A., Sonthwick, S., & Charney, D. (1997). The impact of the homecoming reception on the development of posttraumatic stress disorder: The West Haven Homecoming Stress Scale (WHHSS). *Journal of Traumatic Stress, 10*(2), 259–277.

Johnson, H., & Thompson, A. (2008). The development and maintenance of post-traumatic stress disorder (PTSD) in civilian adult survivors of war trauma and torture: A review. *Clinical Psychology Review, 28*(1), 36–47.

Kashdan, T. B., Morina, N., & Priebe, S. (2009). Post-traumatic stress disorder, social anxiety disorder, and depression in survivors of the Kosovo War: Experiential avoidance as a contributor to distress and quality of life. *Journal of Anxiety Disorders*, *23*(2), 185–196.

Kendler, K. S., Walters, E. E., Neale, M. C., Kessler, R. C., Heath, A. C., & Eaves, L. J. (1995). The structure of the genetic and environmental risk factors for six major psychiatric disorders in women. Phobia, generalized anxiety disorder, panic disorder, bulimia, major depression, and alcoholism. *Archives of General Psychiatry*, *52*(5), 374–383.

Kessler, R. C. (1997). The effects of stressful life events on depression. *Annual Review of Psychology*, *48*(1), 191–214.

Kessler, R. C., Berglund, P., Demler, O., Jin, R., Merikangas, K. R., & Walters, E. E. (2005). Lifetime prevalence and age-of-onset distributions of DSM-IV disorders in the National Comorbidity Survey Replication. *Archives of General Psychiatry*, *62*(6), 593–602.

Kessler, R. C., Sonnega, A., Bromet, E., Hughes, M., & Nelson, C. B. (1995). Posttraumatic stress disorder in the National Comorbidity Survey. *Archives of General Psychiatry*, *52*(12), 1048–1060.

Kilpatrick, D. G., Resnick, H. S., Milanak, M. E., Miller, M. W., Keyes, K. M., & Friedman, M. J. (2013). National estimates of exposure to traumatic events and PTSD prevalence using DSM-IV and DSM-5 criteria. *Journal of Traumatic Stress*, *26*(5), 537–547.

King, L. A., King, D. W., Fairbank, J. A., Keane, T. M., & Adams, G. A. (1998). Resilience–recovery factors in post-traumatic stress disorder among female and male Vietnam veterans: Hardiness, postwar social support, and additional stressful life events. *Journal of Personality and Social Psychology*, *74*(2), 420.

Kishon-Barash, R., Midlarsky, E., & Johnson, D. R. (1999). Altruism and the Vietnam War veteran: The relationship of helping to symptomatology. *Journal of Traumatic Stress*, *12*(4), 655–662.

Koenen, K. C., Harley, R., Lyons, M. J., Wolfe, J., Simpson, J. C., Goldberg, J., … Tsuang, M. (2002). A twin registry study of familial and individual risk factors for trauma exposure and posttraumatic stress disorder. *The Journal of Nervous and Mental Disease*, *190*(4), 209–218.

Krysinska, K., & Lester, D. (2010). Post-traumatic stress disorder and suicide risk: A systematic review. *Archives of Suicide Research*, *14*(1), 1–23.

Laffaye, C., Cavella, S., Drescher, K., & Rosen, C. (2008). Relationships among PTSD symptoms, social support, and support source in veterans with chronic PTSD. *Journal of Traumatic Stress*, *21*(4), 394–401.

Lazarus, R. S., & Folkman, S. (1984). Coping and adaptation. In *The handbook of behavioral medicine* (pp. 282–325).

Levi, O., Bar-Haim, Y., Kreiss, Y., & Fruchter, E. (2016). Cognitive–behavioural therapy and psychodynamic psychotherapy in the treatment of combat-related post-traumatic stress disorder: A comparative effectiveness study. *Clinical Psychology & Psychotherapy*, *23*(4), 298–307.

Maguen, S., Turcotte, D. M., Peterson, A. L., Dremsa, T. L., Garb, H. N., McNally, R. J., & Litz, B. T. (2008). Description of risk and resilience factors among military medical personnel before deployment to Iraq. *Military Medicine*, *173*(1), 1–9.

McFarlane, A. C. (1998). Epidemiological evidence about the relationship between PTSD and alcohol abuse: The nature of the association. *Addictive Behaviors*, *23*(6), 813–825.

McNally, R. J. (2003). Progress and controversy in the study of posttraumatic stress disorder. *Annual Review of Psychology*, *54*, 229–252.

Meichenbaum, D. (1994). *A clinical handbook/practical therapist manual for assessing and treating adults with post-traumatic stress disorder (PTSD)*. Canada: Institute Press.

Meredith, L. S., Sherbourne, C. D., Gaillot, S. J., Hansell, L., Ritschard, H. V., Parker, A. M., & Wrenn, G. (2011). Promoting psychological resilience in the US military. *Rand Health Quarterly*, *1*(2), 2.

Michultka, D., Blanchard, E. B., & Kalous, T. (1998). Responses to civilian war experiences: Predictors of psychological functioning and coping. *Journal of Traumatic Stress*, *11*(3), 571–577.

Mills, K. L., Teesson, M., Back, S. E., Brady, K. T., Baker, A. L., Hopwood, S., … Ewer, P. L. (2012). Integrated exposure-based therapy for co-occurring posttraumatic stress disorder and substance dependence: A randomized controlled trial. *JAMA*, *308*(7), 690–699.

Moisander, P. A., & Edston, E. (2003). Torture and its sequel – A comparison between victims from six countries. *Forensic Science International*, *137*, 133–140.

Mohamed, S., & Rosenheck, R. A. (2008). Pharmacotherapy of PTSD in the US department of veterans affairs: Diagnostic-and symptom-guided drug selection. *Journal of Clinical Psychiatry*, *69*(6), 959–965.

Morina, N., Sulaj, V., Schnyder, U., Klaghofer, R., Müller, J., Martin-Sölch, C., & Rufer, M. (2016). Obsessive-compulsive and posttraumatic stress symptoms among civilian survivors of war. *BMC Psychiatry*, *16*(1), 115.

Nock, M. K., Stein, M. B., Heeringa, S. G., Ursano, R. J., Colpe, L. J., Fullerton, C. S., ... Zaslavsky, A. M. (2014). Prevalence and correlates of suicidal behavior among soldiers: Results from the army study to assess risk and resilience in service members (Army STARRS). *JAMA Psychiatry*, *71*(5), 514–522.

Norris, F. H., Stevens, S. P., Pfefferbaum, B., Wyche, K. F., & Pfefferbaum, R. L. (2008). Community resilience as a metaphor, theory, set of capacities, and strategy for disaster readiness. *American Journal of Community Psychology*, *41*(1–2), 127–150.

O'campo, P., Kub, J., Woods, A., Garza, M., Jones, A. S., Gielen, A. C., ... Campbell, J. (2006). Depression, PTSD, and comorbidity related to intimate partner violence in civilian and military women. *Brief Treatment and Crisis Intervention*, *6*(2), 99.

Ozbay, F., Johnson, D. C., Dimoulas, E., Morgan III, C. A., Charney, D., & Southwick, S. (2007). Social support and resilience to stress: From neurobiology to clinical practice. *Psychiatry (Edgmont)*, *4*(5), 35.

Ozer, E. J., Best, S. R., Lipsey, T. L., & Weiss, D. S. (2003). Predictors of posttraumatic stress disorder and symptoms in adults: A meta-analysis. *Psychological Bulletin*, *129*(1), 52.

Pfefferbaum, R. L., Reissman, D. B., Pfefferbaum, B., Wyche, K. F., Norris, F. H., & Klomp, R. W. (2008). Factors in the development of community resilience to disasters. In *Intervention and Resilience after Mass Trauma* (49–68).

Pietrzak, R. H., Johnson, D. C., Goldstein, M. B., Malley, J. C., Rivers, A. J., Morgan, C. A., & Southwick, S. M. (2010). Psychosocial buffers of traumatic stress, depressive symptoms, and psychosocial difficulties in veterans of Operations Enduring Freedom and Iraqi Freedom: The role of resilience, unit support, and postdeployment social support. *Journal of Affective Disorders*, *120*(1), 188–192.

Porter, M., & Haslam, N. (2005). Predisplacement and postdisplacement factors associated with mental health of refugees and internally displaced persons: A meta-analysis. *JAMA*, *294*(5), 602–612.

Priebe, S., Bogic, M., Ajdukovic, D., Franciskovic, T., Galeazzi, G. M., Kucukalic, A., ... Schützwohl, M. (2010). Mental disorders following war in the Balkans: A study in 5 countries. *Archives of General Psychiatry*, *67*(5), 518–528.

Ramsay, R., Gorst-Unsworth, C., & Turner, S. (1993). Psychiatric morbidity in survivors of organised state violence including torture. *British Journal of Psychiatry*, *162*, 55–59.

Reppesgaard, H. O. (1997). Studies on psychosocial problems among displaced people in Sri Lanka. *European Journal of Psychiatry*, *11*, 223–234.

Resick, P. A. (2001). *Stress and trauma*. London: Psychology Press.

Resnick, H. S., Kilpatrick, D. G., Dansky, B. S., Saunders, B. E., & Best, C. L. (1993). Prevalence of civilian trauma and posttraumatic stress disorder in a representative national sample of women. *Journal of Consulting and Clinical Psychology*, *61*(6), 984.

Resnick, H. S., Yehuda, R., Pitman, R. K., & Foy, D. W. (1995). Effect of previous trauma on acute plasma cortisol level following rape. *The American Journal of Psychiatry*, *152*(11), 1675.

Riggs, D. S., Byrne, C. A., Weathers, F. W., & Litz, B. T. (1998). The quality of the intimate relationships of male Vietnam veterans: Problems associated with posttraumatic stress disorder. *Journal of Traumatic Stress*, *11*(1), 87–101.

Salters-Pedneault, K., Tull, M. T., & Roemer, L. (2004). The role of avoidance of emotional material in the anxiety disorders. *Applied and Preventive Psychology*, *11*, 95–114.

Sannibale, C., Teesson, M., Creamer, M. C., Sitharthan, T., Bryant, R. A., Sutherland, K., ... Peek-O'Leary, M. (2013). Randomized controlled trial of cognitive behaviour therapy for comorbid post-traumatic stress disorder and alcohol use disorders. *Addiction*, *108*(8), 1397–1410.

Scholte, W. F., Olff, M., Ventevogel, P., De Vries, G., Jansveld, E., Cardozo, B. L., & Crawford, C. A. (2004). Mental health symptoms following war and repression in Eastern Afghanistan. The *Journal of the American Medical Association*, *292*, 585–593.

Schwarzer, R., & Schwarzer, C. (1996). A critical survey of coping instruments. In M. Zeidner, & N. S. Endler (Eds.), *Handbook of coping: Theory, research, applications*. Oxford: Wiley.

Shipherd, J. C., Stafford, J., & Tanner, L. R. (2005). Predicting alcohol and drug abuse in Persian Gulf War veterans: What role do PTSD symptoms play?. *Addictive Behaviors*, *30*(3), 595–599.

Silove, D., Sinnerbrink, I., Field, A., Manicavasagar, V., & Steel, Z. (1997). Anxiety, depression and PTSD in asylum-seekers: Assocations with pre-migration trauma and post-migration stressors. *The British Journal of Psychiatry*, *170*(4), 351–357.

Smith, T. C., Ryan, M. A., Wingard, D. L., Slymen, D. J., Sallis, J. F., & Kritz-Silverstein, D. (2008). New onset and persistent symptoms of post-traumatic stress disorder self-reported after deployment and combat exposures: Prospective population-based US military cohort study. *British Medical Journal* (*BMJ*), *336*(7640), 366–371.

Smith, M. W., Schnurr, P. P., & Rosenheck, R. A. (2005). Employment outcomes and PTSD symptom severity. *Mental Health Services Research*, *7*(2), 89–101.

Solomon, Z., & Mikulincer, M. (2007). Posttraumatic intrusion, avoidance, and social functioning: A 20-year longitudinal study. *Journal of Consulting and Clinical Psychology*, *75*(2), 316.

Steel, Z., Chey, T., Silove, D., Marnane, C., Bryant, R. A., & Van Ommeren, M. (2009). Association of torture and other potentially traumatic events with mental health outcomes among populations exposed to mass conflict and displacement: A systematic review and meta-analysis. *JAMA*, *302*(5), 537–549.

Summerfield, D. (2000). Conflict and health: War and mental health: A brief overview. *British Medical Journal* (*BMJ*), *321*(7255), 232.

Sundquist, K., Johansson, L., DeMarinis, V., Johansson-Sundquist, J. (2005). Posttraumatic stress disorder and psychiatric co-morbidity: symptoms in a random sample of female Bosnian refugees. *European Psychiatry*, *20*, 158–164.

Sutker, P. B., Davis, J. M., Uddo, M., & Ditta, S. R. (1995). War zone stress, personal resources, and PTSD in Persian Gulf War returnees. *Journal of Abnormal Psychology*, *104*(3), 444.

Taft, C. T., King, L. A., King, D. W., Leskin, G. A., & Riggs, D. S. (1999). Partners' ratings of combat veterans' PTSD symptomatology. *Journal of Traumatic Stress*, *12*(2), 327–334.

Tarrier, N., & Gregg, L. (2004). Suicide risk in civilian PTSD patients. *Social Psychiatry and Psychiatric Epidemiology*, *39*(8), 655–661.

Tsai, J., Harpaz-Rotem, I., Pietrzak, R. H., & Southwick, S. M. (2012). The role of coping, resilience, and social support in mediating the relation between PTSD and social functioning in veterans returning from Iraq and Afghanistan. *Psychiatry: Interpersonal & Biological Processes*, *75*(2), 135–149.

United Nations High Commissioner for Refugees (UNHCR). (2008). *Statistical yearbook 2007: Trends in displacement, protection and solutions*. Geneva, Switzerland: United Nations High Commissioner for Refugees.

Vasterling, J. J., Duke, L. M., Brailey, K., Constans, J. I., Allain, A. N., Jr, & Sutker, P. B. (2002). Attention, learning, and memory performances and intellectual resources in Vietnam veterans: PTSD and no disorder comparisons. *Neuropsychology*, *16*(1), 5.

Vogt, D. S., Pless, A. P., King, L. A., & King, D. W. (2005). Deployment stressors, gender, and mental health outcomes among Gulf War I veterans. *Journal of Traumatic Stress*, *18*(2), 115–127.

Vollhardt, J. R. (2009). Altruism born of suffering and prosocial behavior following adverse life events: A review and conceptualization. *Social Justice Research*, *22*(1), 53–97.

Watts, B. V., Schnurr, P. P., Mayo, L., Young-Xu, Y., Weeks, W. B., & Friedman, M. J. (2013). Meta-analysis of the efficacy of treatments for posttraumatic stress disorder. *The Journal of Clinical Psychiatry*, *74*(6), e541–e550.

Wenzel, T., Griengl, H., Stompe, T., Mirzaei, S., & Kieffer, W. (2000). Psychological disorders in survivors of torture: Exhaustion, impairment and depression. *Psychopathology*, *33*, 292–296.

Wolfe, J., & Kimerling, R. (1997). Gender issues in the assessment of posttraumatic stress disorder.

Yehuda, R., & McFarlane, A. C. (1995). Conflict between current knowledge about posttraumatic stress disorder and its original conceptual basis. *American Journal of Psychiatry*, *152*(12), 1705–1713.

Zeidner, M. (1994). Personal and contextual determinants of coping and anxiety in an evaluative situation: A prospective study. *Personality and Individual Differences*, *16*(6), 899–918.

COLD-BLOODED KILLERS? RETHINKING PSYCHOPATHY IN THE MILITARY

Karen Landay and Rachel E. Frieder

ABSTRACT

Stress and the military go hand-in-hand, particularly in combat environments. While some personality traits or types weaken relationships between stress and performance, others, such as psychopathy, may strengthen them. In the present chapter, we consider the ramifications of individuals with high levels of psychopathy or psychopathic tendencies in the military with regard to both their own stress and performance and that of those around them. We discuss different reactions to psychological and physical stress, as well as the implications of psychopathic tendencies as they relate to current military issues, including gender, leadership, teamwork, turnover, post-traumatic stress disorder, and suicide. By juxtaposing relevant research findings on stress and psychopathy, we conclude that psychopathic tendencies should have neither uniformly negative nor positive effects on stress and performance in the military. Rather, effects on such individuals and the peripheral others with whom they interact will likely vary greatly depending on numerous factors.

Keywords: Military; psychopathy; stress; strain; teamwork; turnover; post-traumatic stress disorder

The military presents a unique working environment with correspondingly unique stressors, ranging from work and information overload to extreme temperatures or sleep deprivation (Brusher, 2007). Such stressors can impair physical, cognitive,

Occupational Stress and Well-being in Military Contexts
Research in Occupational Stress and Well-being, Volume 16, 23–47
Copyright © 2018 by Emerald Publishing Limited
All rights of reproduction in any form reserved
ISSN: 1479-3555/doi:10.1108/S1479-355520180000016002

and psychological performance (Orasanu & Backer, 1996), and negatively impact general well-being. For instance, Brusher (2007, p. 112) noted that, "within US military operations, COSR [Combat and Operational Stress Reactions] have accounted for up to one-half of all battlefield casualties, depending upon the difficulty of the conditions." In addition, 20–30% of personnel returning from deployment report suffering from psychological strain (Brusher, 2007). Stress can also have long-term negative ramifications for service members. Since the Vietnam War, an estimated 80,000 US veterans have received "other than honorable" discharges due to post-traumatic stress disorder (PTSD), leaving them ineligible for valuable benefits such as college education, health care, and home loans (Philpott, 2014).

Nonetheless, organizational research suggests that individual differences moderate stress-performance and stressor–strain relationships (e.g., Harms, Krasikova, Vanhove, Herian, & Lester, 2013; Liu, Liu, Mills, & Fan, 2013; Sinclair & Tucker, 2006). For example, desirable characteristics such as conscientiousness (Bowling & Eschleman, 2010), hardiness (Westman, 1990), self-efficacy (Jex & Bliese, 1999), and emotional intelligence (Wu, 2011) have been shown to attenuate the negative relationship between stress and performance. Perhaps of greater concern to stakeholders, however, is the possibility that certain *maladaptive* individual differences may also attenuate these associations.

Along these lines, one notable individual difference that has gained recent attention in the management literature is psychopathy, which along with narcissism and Machiavellianism forms the Dark Triad (Paulhus & Williams, 2002). Psychopathy has bewildered the military community for some time, with concerns including how this aberrant combination of attitudinal and behavioral tendencies affects critical military functions (e.g., fitness for duty; Walker & Bourgeois, 2007). Psychopathy may also affect military-specific job performance both positively and negatively, and its impact warrants further consideration.

For instance, Hare (1999) noted that World War II (WWII) fighter pilots with elevated levels of psychopathic tendencies earned reputations for fearlessly and single-mindedly pursuing their targets. Nonetheless, these same pilots frequently died, taking their crewmates along with them, from avoidable causes such as running out of fuel or interfering with others' flight paths. Accordingly, the impulsivity and remorselessness characteristics of psychopathy are unlikely to be universally beneficial in the demanding and teamwork-focused environment of the military. In support, research has found that bomb disposal experts high in psychopathy "lacked the perfectionism and attention to detail needed to stay alive on the job" (Hare, 1999, p. 62). Nonetheless, psychopathic individuals are thought to remain characteristically calm under pressure (Cleckley, 1950/2015), a trait that seems highly suited to unpredictable, high-stress combat environments.

Moreover, the benefits of psychopathy may be more pronounced in instances of close-quarters personal combat. Prior to the use of psychological conditioning post-WWII, only an estimated 2% of soldiers – supposedly those predisposed to psychopathic tendencies – felt no resistance to, or after-effects of, face-to-face killing (Grossman, 2014). Nonetheless, psychopathy is strongly associated with instrumental, or proactive, violence, which is performed not as a response to provocation but instead quite deliberately in the service of achieving a goal (e.g., murder for an insurance payoff; Reidy, Shelley-Tremblay, & Lilienfeld, 2011). Accordingly, individuals with psychopathic tendencies may be distinctly advantaged in that they may be more willing to wound or even kill their enemy as the opportunity for close-quarters combat brings them face-to-face with the sight, smell, and feel of a human adversary. Thus, as the foregoing examples illustrate, psychopathic personality represents quite the double-edged sword within the military context and should give pause to the military community.

Despite these long-standing concerns, we still know very little about psychopathy as it pertains to today's military settings. Given the continued recurrence of rogue soldiers killing civilians (e.g., McGreal, 2011), it seems possible that a substantial number of individuals with high levels of psychopathy are employed within the military (e.g., Anestis, Green, Arnau, & Anestis, in press; Skeem, Polaschek, Patrick, & Lilienfeld, 2011). This may be explained at least in part by the argument that individuals tend to seek out organizational contexts that align with their own interests and personalities (Schneider, 1987). Thus, individuals with high levels of psychopathy may perceive the military as one such context.

Nonetheless, there is extreme difficulty in assessing the prevalence of psychopathy in the military due to inadequate screening measures. Current US military policy mandates that service members are screened (via self-reported mental health history) for existing mental health disorders at the time of enlistment; however, functional impairment, not simply diagnosis, is required for disqualification from service (Walker & Bourgeois, 2007). For instance, while the symptoms of most personality disorders (e.g., paranoia) would make it difficult for such individuals to complete even basic training, the hallmarks of psychopathy (e.g., fearlessness and composure under pressure) may instead cast such recruits as ideal soldiers (Walker & Bourgeois, 2007). This perception likely further complicates the ability to estimate the prevalence of psychopathy within the military.

While organizational scientists have found that the presence of a psychopathic supervisor results in increased bullying, stress, and burnout (e.g., Boddy, 2011a; Volmer, Koch, & Göritz, 2016) as well as decreased job satisfaction and well-being (e.g., Boddy, 2014; Mathieu & Babiak, 2016a), research has yet to determine whether similar effects exist in the military context. Considering the high-stress and high-stakes nature of these conditions, consequences of psychopathy could be substantially more severe for both individuals themselves and peripheral others. Therefore, we will consider the existing literature on stress and well-being in relation to military settings to offer insights into how psychopathic tendencies might affect the well-being and performance of both individuals in possession of these traits and those with whom such individuals interact.

PSYCHOPATHY

Psychopathy Defined

Psychopathy has been the focus of numerous popular press books, including *Snakes in Suits* (Babiak & Hare, 2006), *Working with Monsters* (Clarke, 2005), and *The Wisdom of Psychopaths* (Dutton, 2012). Psychopathy has also been glorified in movies such as *American Psycho*, *The Silence of the Lambs*, and *A Clockwork Orange*. Psychopathy was originally recognized as a clinical disorder characterized by attributes such as superficial charm, lack of remorse, pathological lying, callousness, and impulsivity (Cleckley, 1950/2015; Hare et al., 1990). More recently, psychopathy was identified as an aberrant personality characteristic whose hallmarks include poor or limited effect (e.g., low anxiety), grandiose interpersonal style (e.g., superficial charm), and impulsivity (e.g., irresponsible behavior).

Psychopathy comprises one-third of the Dark Triad, along with Machiavellianism and narcissism (Paulhus & Williams, 2002). Although all three Dark Triad traits are characterized by extremely low levels of agreeableness, psychopathy exhibits several distinctions (Paulhus & Williams, 2002). Both psychopathy and Machiavellianism are characterized by low levels of conscientiousness, while both psychopathy and narcissism are characterized by high levels of extraversion and openness to experience (Paulhus & Williams, 2002). In contrast, individuals with psychopathic personality traits exhibit low levels of neuroticism, especially as compared to Machiavellians and narcissists (Paulhus & Williams, 2002).

Since its inception, research on psychopathy has suffered from substantial divisiveness within the literature. This dissent is in large part due to the disparate characterizations of psychopathy as both clinical disorder and constellation of aberrant personality traits. More specifically, Hervey Cleckley (1941), considered the father of the scientific study of psychopathy, first identified a clinical profile of psychopathy based on case studies of his hospital patients. The 21 features that Cleckley (1941) identified included superficial charm, disregard for the truth, egocentricity, and inability to accept blame, as well as a total lack of anxiety, feelings of responsibility, impulse control, and empathy. Clinical practice has historically utilized this conceptualization, which maintains that psychopathy is a group of characteristic behavioral, interpersonal, and affective traits (Hare, 1998a; Lilienfeld & Widows, 2005).

However, the nonclinical personality perspective of psychopathy positions it as comprising three traits: boldness (e.g., interpersonal dominance), disinhibition (e.g., impulsivity), and meanness (e.g., lack of empathy; Patrick, Fowles, & Krueger, 2009). Nonetheless, debate over whether psychopathy is more properly classified as a personality trait or a behavioral disorder has continued for decades (Lilienfeld & Andrews, 1996), with arguments that the behavioral approach allows for false positives and the personality approach for false negatives (Lilienfeld, 1994). We follow previous organizational research (e.g., Landay, Harms, & Credé, 2017; Mathieu & Babiak, 2016b; Schütte et al., 2018) in viewing psychopathy as a constellation of personality traits rather than a clinical disorder. Moreover, because the base rate of *clinical* psychopathy is extremely low (Cleckley, 1950/2015; Hare, 1996), conceptualizing psychopathy from the nonclinical personality perspective allows us to consider individuals who demonstrate more moderate levels of some, although perhaps not all, of these traits. Accordingly, the trait-based view argues that individuals can vary in the extent to which they possess some or all of the aforementioned characterizations (Hall & Benning, 2006).

This conceptualization of trait is consistent with both antisocial personality disorder as described in the Diagnostic and Statistical Manual of Mental Disorders-IV (DSM-IV; American Psychiatric Association, 1994) and nonclinical measures of deviant personality such as the Hogan Development Survey (HDS; Hogan & Hogan, 2001). Derived from the DSM-IV, but explicitly designed as a subclinical instrument "to identify the personality characteristics underlying career derailment" (Hogan & Hogan, 2001, p. 41), the HDS positions psychopathy as one such career "derailer." Individuals high on psychopathy, or the less intimidating moniker "Mischievous" according to the HDS, are described as impulsive and manipulative, but can appear friendly and charming (Hogan & Hogan, 2009). These behaviors may vary across contexts, whereas those of a clinically diagnosed psychopath do not (Hogan & Hogan, 2009). Therefore, for the purposes of this chapter, we refrain from referring to individuals as "psychopaths" – which implies a clinical diagnosis – and instead discuss them in terms of possessing psychopathic tendencies or high levels of psychopathy.

Measurement

Not surprisingly, the disparate characterizations of psychopathy as both a clinical disorder and a personality trait have given rise to a proliferation of measurement instruments consisting of anywhere from two to four factors. In the widely regarded Psychopathy Checklist – Revised (PCL-R), Hare (2003) brought the two perspectives together by utilizing a two-factor structure. Factor 1 represents the personality approach through interpersonal and affective items such as superficial charm, shallow affect, and callousness (Hare, 2003). Factor 2 represents the behavioral approach through lifestyle and antisocial items such as being prone to boredom, poor control, over behavior, and impulsivity (Hare, 2003).

However, the Psychopathic Personality Inventory – Revised (PPI-R) comprises three factors (Lilienfeld & Widows, 2005). The first factor, labeled as fearless dominance, comprises interpersonal items such as reactions to fear, anxiety, and stress (Benning, Patrick, Blonigen, Hicks, & Iacono, 2005). The second, labeled as self-centered impulsivity, comprises behavioral items such as impulsivity, aggression, and control (Benning et al., 2005; Lilienfeld & Widows, 2005). The third factor, labeled as cold-heartedness, comprises lack of empathy and callousness, which is loaded separately from the previous two factors (Benning, Patrick, Hicks, Blonigen, & Krueger, 2003; Lilienfeld & Widows, 2005). Finally, there is some support for a four-factor model, in which Hare's two original factors are divided into separate interpersonal, affective, lifestyle, and antisocial factors (Hare & Neumann, 2009; Vitacco, Neumann, & Jackson, 2005). A number of studies have found the four-factor model to be a stronger predictor of violent behaviors in clinical and offender samples than the three-factor model (Hill, Neumann, & Rogers, 2004; Vitacco, Neumann, Caldwell, Leistico, & Van Rybroek, 2006; Vitacco et al., 2005).

Although the PPI-R is intended for use in both clinical and nonclinical samples (Lilienfeld & Widows, 2005), other self-report subclinical measures have been developed specifically for the workplace context. These include several measures based on the four-factor model, such as the B-Scan (Mathieu & Babiak, 2016b) and the Self-Report Psychopathy Scale III (Williams, Nathanson, & Paulhus, 2003). Other subclinical scales take a different approach, such as the Mischievous Scale of the HDS (Hogan & Hogan, 2009), which is based on antisocial personality disorder as described in the DSM-IV but explicitly avoids clinical content (Hogan & Hogan, 2001, 2009) as well as the Psychopathy Measure–Management Research Version (Boddy, 2011a), which appears to focus only on the interpersonal/affective factor (Jones & Hare, 2016).

Nonetheless, while numerous measurement instruments exist, scholars and clinicians generally agree that the hallmarks of psychopathy include interpersonal, affective, and behavioral tendencies such as impulsivity, superficial charm, and generally socially deviant behavior (e.g., Hare, 1998a; Lilienfeld & Widows, 2005). The appropriate choice of measurement in a given context is informed by both the population being examined (e.g., prisoners, executives, etc.) and the research question (e.g., associations of clinical psychopathy with violence vs associations of psychopathic tendencies and abusive supervision).

Consequences of Psychopathy at Work

Overall, psychopathic tendencies are typically viewed in a very negative light by organizational researchers (e.g., O'Boyle, Forsyth, Banks, & McDaniel, 2012; Spain, Harms, & LeBreton, 2014; Wu & LeBreton, 2011); not surprisingly, the overwhelming majority of research supports this notion. Psychopathic tendencies have been found to be negatively related to job performance (O'Boyle et al., 2012) and helping behaviors (Smith, Wallace, & Jordan, 2016), and positively related to counterproductive work behaviors (O'Boyle et al., 2012). In addition, individuals with antisocial personality disorder have higher probability levels of both trouble with a supervisor or colleague and being unemployed in the previous 12 months (Ettner, MacLean, & French, 2011).

In the leadership domain, psychopathic tendencies are negatively related to transformational leadership (Landay et al., 2017). Leader emergence and leader effectiveness, however, differ by gender, with a weak positive relationship for men but weak negative relationship for women (Landay et al., 2017). In terms of follower outcomes, psychopathic tendencies in supervisors are related negatively to employee job satisfaction (Mathieu & Babiak, 2016a; Sanecka, 2013; Volmer et al., 2016) and satisfaction with one's supervisor (Sanecka, 2013), and positively related to abusive supervision (Mathieu & Babiak, 2016a), bullying (Boddy, 2014), and employee turnover intentions (Mathieu & Babiak, 2016a).

Yet, psychopathic tendencies are not, as both research and popular press coverage may lead one to believe, uniformly negative in the workplace. These individuals' characteristic lack of both fear and sadness may well be beneficial in certain jobs or occupations (Dutton, 2012). In fact, combined with traits such as political skills, psychopathic tendencies can be quite functional in the workplace (Schütte et al., 2018). Moreover, in leadership positions, individuals with psychopathic tendencies tend to be perceived as more innovative, strategic, and effective (Babiak, Neumann, & Hare, 2010; Lilienfeld et al., 2012).

Finally, recent research has begun to examine the types of jobs or industries that individuals with psychopathic tendencies find attractive and/or in which they tend to excel. For example, psychopathic tendencies were positively correlated with vocational preferences for practical, hands-on work (i.e., trades; Jonason, Wee, Li, & Jackson, 2014). The authors also observed that "those high on psychopathy [...] prefer to work in jobs where they do not have to interact with others and have little supervision" (Jonason et al., 2014, p. 122). Further, psychopathic tendencies appear more prevalent among private sector employees and within the financial services sector as compared to public sector employees and emergency services workers (Furnham, Hyde, & Trickey, 2014) and the general community (Howe, Falkenbach, & Massey, 2014).

Finally, several studies of undergraduate students found that business students possess higher levels of psychopathic traits than psychology students (Hassall, Boduszek, & Dhingra, 2015; Wilson & McCarthy, 2011). Similarly, there is speculation that individuals with psychopathic personality tendencies prefer large financial, commercial, or government organizations. Individuals with elevated psychopathic tendencies are likely attracted to business environments (Schneider, 1987) because they provide them with opportunities to achieve prestige and power (Boddy, 2011b). Moreover, organizations undergoing extensive changes or those with flexible structures tend to attract individuals with elevated levels of psychopathy, as they are replete with opportunities to progress quickly through the ranks and usurp power (Babiak & Hare, 2006). Not surprisingly, some scholars have opined that part of the global financial crisis can be attributed to these so-called "corporate psychopaths" (Boddy, 2010, 2011b; Hare, 1999).

PSYCHOPATHY IN THE MILITARY

For the most part, research evidence to date illustrates a wide variety of negative effects of psychopathy and psychopathic tendencies on numerous outcomes, including well-being and performance. Yet, there are also suggestions that individuals with psychopathic tendencies might excel in certain jobs, industries, or situations. The attraction–selection–attrition (ASA) model in particular may shed light on why individuals with psychopathic tendencies may be attracted to, select into, and remain members of the military (Schneider, 1987).

The military represents a unique work environment in that the job – at least of soldiers in combat – is killing (Calhoun, 2002). Therefore, it seems rather obvious that psychopathy in a military context might become a desirable attribute. For instance, low anxiety is considered a hallmark of psychopathy (Cleckley, 1941), and evidence shows that bomb-disposal personnel experience fewer physical fear-related reactions than other soldiers or civilians (Cox, Hallam, O'Connor, & Rachman, 1983). In addition, psychopathy has been found to predict attitudes toward violence (Adebayo, Olawa, Ogunleye, & Ayeye, 2014) and correlates positively with heroism (Smith, Lilienfeld, Coffey, & Dabbs, 2013). These findings seem to support the idea that at least in the military context, psychopathy might not be such a bad trait to possess.

Typically, thoughts of the military evoke images of soldiers and combat. However, combat positions involve a relatively narrow set of tasks involving the use of specialized weapons and vehicles to carry out action against enemy forces as a well as leadership of such operations (Bureau of Labor Statistics (BLS), US Department of Labor, 2015). In the US military, only approximately 14% of enlisted personnel and 22% of officers are in combat roles (BLS, 2015). Yet, the military is a microcosm of society, requiring professions such as emergency responders (e.g., firemen), professionals (e.g., doctors), service workers (e.g., cooks), laborers (e.g., construction personnel), clergy (e.g., chaplains), and administrative workers in addition to combat service members (BLS, 2015). Thus, the vast majority of US military personnel serve in non-combat roles (BLS, 2015). As a caveat, any personnel present in the combat zone, regardless of their role, may be considered soldiers, as they are vulnerable to enemy attack (Brusher, 2007).

Therefore, the military setting is bifurcated, with potentially vastly different standards and expectations for performance in combat and non-combat environments, and correspondingly different effects on stress, performance, and well-being. An engineer on deployment in Iraq is subject to a distinct set of stressors (e.g., work–family conflict related to deployment and physical danger) from a clerk assigned to a stateside base (e.g., an abusive supervisor and working hours), yet both undoubtedly experience stress on the job. However, our discussion of the effects of psychopathy on stress and strain in the military that follows is limited to combat scenarios, as this aspect is most unique to the military environment. Given the similarity of non-combat military roles to those in more typical organizations, we urge interested readers to consult the growing literature on psychopathy in the general workplace.

Stress in the Military

Stress is obviously an undesirable outcome in its own right, and one that can also negatively impact the entire performance domain (Sonnentag & Frese, 2003), including task and contextual performance (i.e., organizational citizenship behaviors) as well as counterproductive work behaviors. Furthermore, Pflanz and Ogle (2006, p. 681) noted that "work stress is a significant occupational health hazard in the routine military work environment." Workplace stressors have been linked to violent behaviors such as aggression, hostility, and sabotage (Chen & Spector, 1992), which could have particularly frightening consequences in the military environment. In what follows, we consider two types of stress in the military context: psychological and physical. Psychological stress includes cognitive (e.g., decision making) and emotional stressors (e.g., fear; Brusher, 2007), whereas physical stress includes environmental (e.g., temperature) and individual physiological condition stressors (e.g., fatigue; Brusher, 2007).

Psychological Stress

Combat-related psychological stress is likely to affect individuals with high levels of psychopathic tendencies differently than individuals with low levels. However, research examining the effects of psychopathy on executive functions (e.g., reaction time and working memory) is markedly divided. That is, while some research suggests that individuals with high levels of psychopathy have improved executive function (Hansen, Johnsen, Thornton, Waage, & Thayer, 2007; Ishikawa, Raine, Lencz, Bihrle, & Lacasse, 2001), other research suggests that psychopaths' executive functioning does not differ compared to individuals with low levels of psychopathy (Hare, 1984). If individuals with psychopathic tendencies do in fact have some sort of improved or protected executive functioning, this could provide them an advantage in dealing with cognitive stressors in combat environments (e.g., information overload and ambiguous situations; Brusher, 2007). Thus, higher levels of psychopathic tendencies may protect individuals from psychological strain experienced in combat arenas. However, due to the noted lack of empathy and impulse control associated with psychopathic tendencies (e.g., Cleckley, 1941; Hare, 1998a), this seeming advantage could ultimately have negative consequences for those around them in the form of, for instance, overly aggressive actions.

Related to emotional stressors, research has shown that individuals with psychopathic tendencies lack both a startle reflex and the tendency to experience fear (e.g., Birbaumer et al., 2005; Levenston, Patrick, Bradley, & Lang, 2000). For instance, compared to non-psychopaths, male prisoners assessed as *clinically* psychopathic display an inhibited startle reflex in response to photographs depicting violent imagery such as mutilation or gruesome attacks on others (Levenston et al., 2000; Patrick, Bradley, & Lang, 1993). These characteristics may also cause individuals with psychopathic tendencies difficulty in learning to avoid punishment (Hare, 1998b; Patrick, 1994; Patrick et al., 1993). That is, "psychopaths show little fear in anticipation of an unpleasant or painful event" (Hare, 1998b, p. 107). Thus, the limited affective response of psychopaths seems to render them nearly immune to common emotional stressors in the military such as homesickness, divided loyalties, or crises of faith (Brusher, 2007). Undoubtedly, this could be construed as a positive byproduct of psychopathic personality tendencies among soldiers in combat. Specifically, such individuals might be seen as "super soldiers" who advance their mission against obstacles that typical soldiers would find daunting or even impossible.

However, soldiers' behavioral reactions to stressors (e.g., malingering and alcohol abuse) may be even more prevalent and pronounced (e.g., brutality, torture, and mutilation of human remains) among combat personnel (Brusher, 2007). Individuals with psychopathic tendencies may not naturally respond to stressors in this manner due to their inability to process emotions (i.e., cold-heartedness; Lilienfeld & Widows, 2005). However, they may be able to unduly influence already stressed fellow soldiers and encourage them to engage in such behaviors. For example, US Army Staff Sergeant Calvin Gibbs not only murdered Afghan civilians and took their body parts as trophies, but also exhorted members of his unit to do the same, earning them the moniker "kill team" (McGreal, 2011).

Thus, as suggested by the ASA model (Schneider, 1987), it is conceivable that individuals with high levels of psychopathy might actually prefer (and seek out) psychologically stressful combat situations as an ideal environment in which to indulge their violent tendencies without retribution and encourage their comrades in arms to do the same. Therefore, while they might themselves benefit from the reduced strain, the same benefit would not extend to those around them. Peripheral others (i.e., comrades) may be subject to heightened strain as a result of their colleagues' general disregard for cognitive, emotional, or physical harm.

Physical Stress

Military combat has long been recognized as a source of physical stress (e.g., Lazarus, Deese, & Osler, 1952; Milgram, Orenstein, & Zafrir, 1989). The question thus arises whether combat personnel with psychopathic tendencies are more resilient to these physical stressors. Research has shown that the brains of psychopathic individuals appear to differ from those of non-psychopaths (e.g., Anderson & Kiehl, 2012; Yang & Raine, 2009). Moreover, individuals with psychopathic tendencies experience lower heart rate and cortisol levels in response to stress (e.g., Hansen et al., 2007; Hare, Frazelle, & Cox, 1978; Ishikawa et al., 2001; O'Leary, Loney, & Eckel, 2007). Yet, despite the fact that individuals with psychopathic tendencies might *think* of and *perceive* stressors differently, it does not seem plausible that such differences would cause individuals high in psychopathy to *feel* physical stressors differently. That is, physical trauma (e.g., bullet wounds) should theoretically cause the same amount of physical injury to the body regardless of individuals' levels of psychopathic tendencies. However, no studies to date appear to have examined whether psychopaths are hardy against physical injury, extreme temperatures, illness, and the like.

Psychopathy and Current Military Issues

Gender

Issues of gender diversity are widely acknowledged in the traditionally male-dominated US military (e.g., Carey, 2015; Minsberg, 2015). However, the integration of women into all branches and roles of the armed forces has been a slow and contentious process. For instance, in 1990, women comprised 11% of active duty military personnel, a figure that increased just 4% by 2015 (Parker, Cilluffo, & Stepler, 2017). Female recruits face not just potential discrimination, harassment, and even sexual assault from men within the ranks (e.g., Reuters, 2017; Watson, 2016), but also increased risk of a variety of injuries due to fundamental differences in female physiology from that of males (Epstein, Fleischmann, Yanovich, & Heled, 2015; Springer & Ross, 2011). Thus, simply being female in the military presents numerous challenges for both female service members and their male comrades.

The consideration of psychopathy in this context adds additional layers of complexity. Although researchers have recently begun to acknowledge the existence of psychopathy and psychopathic tendencies in women, research to date has been limited (Cale & Lilienfeld, 2002; Kreis & Cooke, 2011). In addition to the aforementioned conceptual issues surrounding the definition of psychopathy, the examination of gender as it relates to psychopathy is further complicated by measurement issues. Specifically, the PCL-R, the most commonly used measure of clinical psychopathy, was developed and validated on male samples (e.g., Hare, 1980; Hare et al., 1990); therefore, it is unknown whether the measure is invariant across genders and thus appropriate for use among females (Lehmann & Ittel, 2012; Neumann, Schmitt, Carter, Embley, & Hare, 2012; Vitale & Newman, 2001). Moreover, the base rate of psychopathy in women appears lower than in men (Cale & Lilienfeld, 2002), although even this notion is somewhat contested (Warren et al., 2003).

Central to this debate is the growing understanding that psychopathic traits may manifest differently in women than in men (Forouzan & Cooke, 2005). For instance, one prototype model suggested that females with elevated psychopathic tendencies may be less aggressive and domineering, more manipulative and emotionally unstable, and display, *at least the appearance of*, more empathy and anxiety than their male counterparts (Kreis & Cooke, 2011). However, other scholars downplay gender differences (Neumann et al., 2012; Vitale & Newman, 2001). Nonetheless, given the very low rates of women joining the military (Parker et al., 2017), it is likely that women who are attracted to the military possess higher levels of psychopathic tendencies; that is, regardless of how these traits manifest, women may be attracted to the military because of the presence of like others (i.e., others high on psychopathic tendencies regardless of gender; Schneider, 1987).

Gender differences also come into play in response to stressors. Among active duty military personnel, women reported higher levels of occupational stress than men, and respondents with high levels of stress also reported decreased job performance (Hourani, Williams, & Kress, 2006). Research has found that males with psychopathic tendencies have lower baseline cortisol levels (Loney, Butler, Lima, Counts & Eckel, 2006) and do not demonstrate increased cortisol levels in response to stressors (O'Leary et al., 2007). That is, these individuals both appraise and experience stress differently. However, whether a similar effect exists in women with psychopathic tendencies is less established (O'Leary et al., 2007), although one study found support for a stress-induced cortisol response in women once the effects of their menstrual cycles were taken into account (O'Leary, Taylor, & Eckel, 2010).

Thus, the intersection of individuals with psychopathic tendencies in the military with existing gender challenges presents a fascinating, yet dangerous, tangle. In a male-dominated environment where aggression is encouraged, males with psychopathic tendencies may feel very little of the stress their comrades are experiencing (O'Leary et al., 2007, 2010). Accordingly, it is entirely plausible that males with these traits may be responsible for a disproportionate number of aggressive behaviors aimed at female comrades. For instance, numerous studies have found that in heterosexual couples, male psychopathy contributes to intimate partner violence (e.g., Chase, O'Leary, & Heyman, 2001; Fowler & Westen, 2011). Owing to the team-based nature of today's military, in which comrades may come to feel intimate with each other, this propensity could have negative consequences.

More specifically, males with psychopathic tendencies may see an opportunity to, under the guise of stress, indulge their worst instincts with potentially little or no punishment. Indeed, given the tendency for aggressive behaviors to appear "leader like" (Hogan, Curphy, & Hogan, 1994), especially in the military context, and the association between aggressive behaviors and emergence of leader among men (Landay et al., 2017), such males may actually be rewarded with promotions. Therefore, for men in the military, psychopathic tendencies may be personally beneficial because such contexts likely allow them to express their true personalities and attain hierarchical promotions; however, these traits may pose a threat to comrades lacking psychopathic tendencies, particularly females.

Females with psychopathic tendencies, on the other hand, may face a somewhat different situation in the military context. Specifically, females with psychopathic tendencies may find that such tendencies provide protection from the common negative military experiences of women (e.g., sexual assault; Reuters, 2017). That is, women with psychopathic tendencies may be less likely to suffer the consequences of being female in a male-dominated environment; therefore, they should experience fewer stressors and as a result would be more likely to be successful. However, females with psychopathic tendencies may be less likely to receive promotions, as such individuals are actually less likely to emerge as leaders than their similarly minded male counterparts (Landay et al., 2017).

Thus, for women in the military, psychopathic tendencies are likely quite beneficial from a stress-buffering perspective, but less so from a promotional and career-trajectory perspective. In other words, the possession of psychopathic tendencies by women in the military may be more of an equalizer – rather than an advantage, as it is for men – that enables them to defend against the distinct challenges that accrue to them simply due to their gender. In terms of their impact on their fellow comrades, we suspect that women with psychopathic tendencies would have less of a negative effect on peripheral others than men with psychopathic tendencies. For example, women in possession of these traits may be more aggressive than women without psychopathic tendencies, but no more so than their average male comrades in the military setting.

Leadership

Although leadership serves an important role in all organizations, in few contexts are the consequences of leadership so pronounced as in the military (Samuels, Foster, & Lindsay, 2010). The additional consideration of psychopathic tendencies in military leaders adds to the potential seriousness of leadership outcomes. When individuals with psychopathic tendencies serve as leaders, they may make poor decisions due to issues with communication, delegation, and trust (Rodriguez & Brown, 2016). Moreover, leaders can even serve as a source of stress for their subordinates (Schmidt et al., 2014). In fact, the consequences of leaders with psychopathic tendencies are seemingly so dire that some scholars even recommend that candidates for public leadership positions should be screened for the presence of psychopathy (Boddy, 2016).

The military environment places unique demands on its leaders. Nonetheless, little research has investigated how leadership in extreme settings differs from more routine contexts (Hannah, Campbell, & Matthews, 2010). The act of leadership requires uncertainty reduction, in which leaders reduce ambiguity for their subordinates through processes of framing, heedful interrelating, and adjusting (Baran & Scott, 2010). In situations with a high degree of risk, ambiguity, and physical danger, this may be a key skill for group survival (Baran & Scott, 2010). Thus, while psychopathy is considered an undesirable leadership trait in general (e.g., Babiak & Hare, 2006; Smith & Lilienfeld, 2013), it may be even more so in the military given the extremity of the environment.

Nonetheless, the implications of psychopathic personality on effectiveness of leadership in the military setting are less straightforward than one might expect. For example, recent meta-analytic research found psychopathic tendencies to be positively related to leader emergence, yet unrelated to leader effectiveness across a heterogeneous population of leaders (Landay et al., 2017). The equivocal findings relating psychopathic tendencies to leadership effectiveness may be rectified upon closer examination of the various dimensions of psychopathy and the implications of such on leadership effectiveness within the military context.

On one hand, military leaders with psychopathic tendencies should remain "cool, calm, and collected" during stressful or dangerous situations, allowing them to make more composed decisions that could save lives. Conversely, the trademark self-centered impulsivity (Lilienfeld & Widows, 2005) characteristic of individuals with psychopathic tendencies might provoke such individuals to take foolhardy chances with the lives of others, leading to more deaths instead of fewer. Finally, the cold-heartedness dimension (Lilienfeld & Widows, 2005) may allow the leader to have less empathy for the enemy, but this could also translate to less empathy for those being led, or even for innocent bystanders who could potentially become collateral damage (e.g., civilians, women, and children). Yet this very lack of empathy could be instrumental in continuing to lead and persevere in the face of critical injuries or losses. Taken together, it remains to be seen how psychopathy affects military leaders and their subordinates. There exists the potential for military leaders with psychopathic tendencies to be both largely effective and largely ineffective; their effectiveness will likely depend on the context with which they face as well as the dimension of psychopathy that manifests more prominently in their behavior.

Teams and Teamwork

The military has a unique organizational structure centered around teams. Small teams such as fire teams and squads make up larger teams such as platoons and companies (Powers, 2017), in which members are dependent on each other in life and death situations. This nested structure creates circumstances in which teams may be led both hierarchically (e.g., leaders of platoons outrank leaders of squads) and laterally (e.g., platoon sergeants and platoon leaders are approximately equal in rank; Mael & Alderks, 1993). This complex design reflects the longstanding importance of teamwork to the military (Salas, Bowers, & Cannon-Bowers, 1995).

Meta-analyses have found that both group cohesion (Beal, Cohen, Burke, & McLendon, 2003) and information sharing (Mesmer-Magnus & DeChurch, 2009) are positively related to team performance, whereas relationship conflict is negatively related to team performance (De Dreu & Weingart, 2003). However, research has shown that high levels of psychopathic tendencies are strongly negatively associated with perceptions of the ability to build and effectively manage a team (Babiak et al., 2010). Moreover, popular accounts emphasize the deliberate lack of interest in teamwork exhibited by those with psychopathic tendencies except in service of their own selfish motives (e.g., Babiak & Hare, 2006; Clarke, 2005).

Thus, the consideration of individuals with psychopathic tendencies in this context raises serious concerns. For instance, in a small team such as a fire squad, the presence of even one member with psychopathic tendencies could prove deadly for others due to that member's impulsivity or disregard for consequences (i.e., self-centered impulsivity; Lilienfeld & Widows, 2005). However, given the tendency of organizations to become increasingly homogenous as individuals churn through the ASA cycle (Schneider, 1987), it is entirely possible that military teams may contain multiple individuals with psychopathic tendencies.

Given that organizational research to date has focused on the adverse impacts of single individuals with psychopathic tendencies on outcomes such as leadership emergence or job performance (e.g., Landay et al., 2017; O'Boyle et al., 2012), it is difficult to conjecture how the presence of two or more such individuals might affect teamwork processes and outcomes. It is likely that team members with elevated levels of psychopathy may encourage each other's worst instincts; in this manner, their aberrant personality traits may increase group cohesiveness and functioning, although perhaps to the detriment of organization-level outcomes (e.g., torture and civilian causalities). On the other hand, team members with elevated levels of psychopathic tendencies may compete with one another for the distinction of "most ruthless"; accordingly, this would place comrades directly at odds, thereby disrupting team cohesion and team functioning. These opposing possibilities have yet to be rectified.

Turnover

Turnover is a major problem for the military. For instance, the US Army has close to 50% turnover every two years and brings on 60,000 to 80,000 new recruits each year (Lopez, 2015). At the officer level, greater investments in training (e.g., military academies and scholarships) tend to have the inverse effect on retention (Lopez, 2015). These types of conundrums add to the already astronomical costs of recruitment, where, for instance, the army is being forced to spend an additional $300 million simply to meet its 2017 soldier recruitment goal (Brook, 2017). This difficulty in retaining qualified troops is shared across all the branches of the service (Barno & Bensahel, 2015).

The ASA model (Schneider, 1987) provides one explanation for high turn over rates. Specifically, attraction suggests that individuals attempt to match themselves with their environments, and attrition suggests that individuals who find that they do not fit with their selected organization's environment will leave (Schneider, 1987). As noted previously, it has been speculated that individuals with psychopathic tendencies are attracted to organizations undergoing extensive amounts of change, with the logic that this type of environment allows less oversight for individuals seeking to rise quickly through the ranks (Babiak & Hare, 2006).

This line of reasoning might suggest that individuals with psychopathic tendencies may be willing to remain in the military as the workforce undergoes routine change. This is especially concerning because the higher retention of individuals with psychopathic personality characteristics may come at the expense of higher attrition of individuals lacking these aberrant characteristics (Schneider, 1987). In support, research suggests that supervisors' psychopathic tendencies are positively correlated with subordinates' turnover intentions (Mathieu & Babiak, 2015, 2016a). Further, many popular accounts of co-workers or bosses with psychopathic tendencies note the difficulty in remaining in their immediate proximity and attribute substantial turnover to these few toxic individuals (e.g., Babiak & Hare, 2006; Clarke, 2005; Hare, 1999).

However, given their impulsivity, individuals with psychopathic tendencies may be just as likely, or even more likely, to exit the military than their comrades. Indeed, evidence suggests that personality disorders in marines predicted both voluntary separation and lack of recommendation for re-enlistment following their first term of duty (Schmied, Highfill-McRoy, & Larson, 2012). Some might argue that voluntary turnover of individuals with psychopathic tendencies is beneficial, and thus not of great concern for the military. Yet, their characteristic charm and cool self-confidence may enable individuals with psychopathic tendencies to influence their comrades to follow suit. Thus, on the one hand, individuals with psychopathic tendencies may be more inclined to remain with the military, as such a setting affords them opportunities to capitalize on the constant turnover among personnel; however, their staying may cause others in their wake to quit. On the other hand, individuals with psychopathic tendencies may be more likely to quit due to their impulsivity, but may also influence others to follow suit. Regardless, it appears that the presence of individuals with psychopathic tendencies in the military is likely to drive continued turnover.

Post-traumatic Stress Disorder

Along with emergency responders such as police and firefighters, soldiers are most likely to experience traumatic stressors, which "are single events such as the exposure to disasters, major accidents, or extremely dangerous activities" (Sonnentag & Frese, 2003, p. 455). Not surprisingly, the number of traumatic events an individual is exposed to, as well as their intensity, is positively correlated with the severity of PTSD symptoms (Hecker, Hermenau, Maedl, Schauer, & Elbert, 2013; Lauterbach & Vrana, 2001). Traumatic stressors can have long-term consequences, as soldiers may commit aggressive crimes in response to interpersonal stress even years after initial exposure to such stressors (Fastovtsov, 2011). The findings regarding appetitive aggression, defined "as perceiving aggressive behavior towards others as positive and fascinating even without gaining any external benefit" (Hecker, Hermenau, Maedl, Elbert, & Schauer, 2012, p. 245), are even more alarming. Appetitive aggression is negatively correlated with the severity of PTSD symptoms and can actually have a buffering effect on the development of PTSD (Hecker et al., 2013).

Given the hallmark traits of psychopathy (e.g., cold-heartedness; Lilienfeld & Widows, 2005), one might think that such individuals would be less vulnerable to PTSD. However, some research has found psychopathic tendencies and PTSD to be correlated *positively*. For example, in a group of veterans seeking help with substance abuse, those suffering PTSD had significantly higher scores on the Psychopathic Deviate Scale of the Minnesota Multiphasic Personality Inventory. The positive correlation between psychopathic tendencies and PTSD has also been documented within neurological research. Specifically, Mazza et al. (2015) found that individuals with PTSD have impaired emotional, but not cognitive, empathy. This aligns with psychopaths who lack emotion and empathy in a way that has been described as knowing "the words but not the music; the denotative meaning of words and phrase may be intact, but the connotative emotional or motivational component is lost" (Johns & Quay, 1962, p. 217). Thus, although the causal order is unclear, there appears to be some positive association between psychopathic tendencies and PTSD.

Conversely, other research lends credence to the possibility that psychopathic tendencies are inversely related to PTSD. For example, studies have found that the interpersonal factor of psychopathy attenuates the effect of exposure to trauma and post-traumatic stress (Anestis, Harrop, Green, & Anestis, 2017; Sellbom, 2015; Willemsen, De Ganck, & Verhaeghe, 2012) likely due to the psychopath's characteristic lack of emotion and anxiety. In addition, feelings of guilt and shame often lead to the emergence of PTSD symptoms (Nazarov et al., 2015). However, psychopaths are unlikely to experience such emotions. Therefore, individuals with high levels of psychopathic tendencies might prove more immune to the types of stressors that result in PTSD. If so, this seemingly undesirable individual characteristic might stand to benefit military personnel.

Adding further confusion to the PTSD–psychopathy relationship, recent research has concluded that severity of PTSD symptoms has no relation to psychopathic tendencies (Gobin, Reddy, Zlotnick, & Johnson, 2015). Thus, it is challenging to definitively state whether and how psychopathy and PTSD may be related. However, given the prevalence of PTSD in the military, which is as high as 17% (Richardson, Frueh, & Acierno, 2010), all concerns related to PTSD warrant further examination.

Suicide

Lastly, the issue of suicide in the military unfortunately cannot be avoided. Suicide rates among active duty US military personnel have been at alarmingly high levels for the past decade, with 265 such deaths in 2016 alone (Zoroya, 2016). The risk does not abate after active service, as according to the U.S. Department of Veterans Affairs (2016), veterans are at a 21% higher risk of suicide than civilians. In addition, there is an established connection between stress and mental illness specifically in military personnel (Pflanz, 2001, 2002); relatedly, depression has been positively associated with suicidal ideation in a military sample (Nosratabadi & Halvaiepour, 2016).

In the interpersonal theory of suicide, researchers have argued that two interpersonal constructs or states – thwarted belongingness and perceived burdensomeness – contribute to suicidal desire (Granato, Smith, & Selwayn, 2015; Van Orden et al., 2010). This is separate from ability to commit suicide, which comprises a lack of fear of death and an ability to tolerate physical pain (Van Orden et al., 2010). These ability attributes are more likely to be acquired by men due to masculine gender norms that emphasize traits such as emotional stoicism and aggression (Granato et al., 2015). This finding is concerning, as the vast majority of US military service members are males (Department of Defense (DoD), 2015), and thus likely at greater risk of suicide simply as a function of their biological gender. Further fueling these concerns, psychopathy is more prevalent in men (e.g., Cale & Lilienfeld, 2002; Harms, 2016).

Yet, very little research has examined the intersection of psychopathy or psychopathic tendencies and suicide in a military context. However, given that psychopathy and narcissism correlate somewhat highly ($r = 0.50$; Paulhus & Williams, 2002), recent research examining the effects of the other dark triad traits on suicide may provide valuable insight. Specifically, in a US Army sample, respondents who reported detailed plans yet low desire for suicide scored significantly higher on self-report assessments of both antisocial personality disorder and narcissism (Chu, Buchman-Schmitt, Joiner, & Rudd, 2017). This result aligns with Cleckley's (1950/2015) assertion that, though psychopaths possess a relative immunity to suicide, they are also prone to offering threats and plans for suicide as a method of attracting attention.

Another research has disputed this assessment of psychopathic tendencies and suicide, instead finding differing results between the interpersonal and lifestyle factors of psychopathy. That is, suicide is positively related to the lifestyle factor (Anestis et al., 2016) but negatively related to the interpersonal factor (Anestis et al., 2016; Lohner & Konrad, 2006). Thus, impulsivity and poor control over behavior (i.e., lifestyle factor) may point psychopaths or those with psychopathic tendencies toward suicide, even as a grandiose sense of self-worth and inability to accept responsibility for their actions (i.e., interpersonal factor) turns them away from suicide. This aligns with the finding that outwardly directed aggression is associated with suicide attempts but not with suicidal ideation (Swogger, Van Orden, & Conner, 2014). In addition, weak inhibition control and high sensitivity to threats align with the hallmark features of psychopathy (i.e., impulsivity and lack of remorse) and both separately and interactively predict risk of suicide (Venables et al., 2015).

Therefore, given the scant existing evidence and opposing findings, it is difficult to conclude whether psychopaths in the military will display typical levels of suicide. What is especially concerning within the military context is that the risk of individual suicide attempts increases as the number of previous suicide attempts within a soldier's unit increases (Ursano et al., 2017). Thus, even if psychopaths are unlikely to carry out suicide actually (Cleckley, 1950/2015), false threats of suicide by individuals with psychopathic tendencies will be taken seriously. That is, such individuals could easily manipulate concern about well-being for their own ends, leading to unnecessary stress for their comrades as well as waste of mental health resources.

CONCLUSION

In the present chapter, we examined the literature pertaining to the effects of individuals with psychopathic tendencies on stress and well-being in the military. We identified a number of areas unique to the military context in which psychopathic tendencies may have varying effects on the individuals in possession of these traits as well as those with whom they interact. These included psychological and physical stress in combat environments as well as issues concerning gender, leadership, teamwork, turnover, PTSD, and suicide. Our discussion of the existing literature suggests that consequences of psychopathic tendencies are neither uniformly positive nor negative but rather depend greatly on the given situation and the outcomes under consideration. We hope that this review helps stimulate the future research in this area.

REFERENCES

Adebayo, S. O., Olawa, B. D., Ogunleye, A. J., & Ayeye, F. (2014). Influence of psychopathy and cultic disposition on attitude toward violence among students of tertiary institutions in Ekiti State. *Asian Social Science*, *10*, 258–264.

American Psychiatric Association. (1994). *Diagnostic and statistical manual of mental disorders* (4th ed.). Washington, DC: American Psychiatric Association.

Anderson, N. E., & Kiehl, K. A. (2012). The psychopath magnetized: Insights from brain imaging. *Trends in Cognitive Sciences*, *16*, 52–60.

Anestis, J. C., Anestis, M. D., Rufino, K. A., Cramer, R. J., Miller, H., Khazem, L. R., & Joiner, T. E. (2016). Understanding the relationship between suicidality and psychopathy: An examination of the interpersonal-psychological theory of suicidal behavior. *Archives of Suicide Research*, *20*, 349–368.

Anestis, J. C., Green, B. A., Arnau, R. C., & Anestis, M. D. (in press). Psychopathic personality traits in the military: An examination of the Levenson Self-Report Psychopathy Scales in a novel sample. *Assessment*. https://doi.org/10.1177/1073191117719511

Anestis, J. C., Harrop, T. M., Green, B. A., & Anestis, M. D. (2017). Psychopathic personality traits as protective factors against the development of post-traumatic stress disorder symptoms in a sample of national guard combat veterans. *Journal of Psychopathology and Behavioral Assessment*, *2*, 220–229.

Babiak, P., & Hare, R. D. (2006). *Snakes in suits: When psychopaths go to work*. New York, NY: Regan Books.

Babiak, P., Neumann, C. S., & Hare, R. D. (2010). Corporate psychopathy: Talking the walk. *Behavioral Sciences & the Law*, *28*, 174–193.

Baran, B. E., & Scott, C. W. (2010). Organizing ambiguity: A grounded theory of leadership and sensemaking within dangerous contexts. *Military Psychology*, *22*, S42–S69.

Barno, D., & Bensahel, N. (2015, November 5). Can the U.S. military halt its brain drain? *The Atlantic*. Retrieved from https://www.theatlantic.com/politics/archive/2015/11/us-military-tries-halt-brain-drain/413965/. Accessed on August 18, 2017.

Beal, D. J., Cohen, R. R., Burke, M. J., & McLendon, C. L. (2003). Cohesion and performance in groups: A meta-analytic clarification of construct relations. *Journal of Applied Psychology*, *88*, 989–1004.

Benning, S. D., Patrick, C. J., Blonigen, D. M., Hicks, B. M., & Iacono, W. G. (2005). Estimating facets of psychopathy from normal personality traits: A step toward community epidemiological investigations. *Assessment*, *12*, 3–18.

Benning, S. D., Patrick, C. J., Hicks, B. M., Blonigen, D. M., & Krueger, R. F. (2003). Factor structure of the psychopathic personality inventory: Validity and implications for clinical assessment. *Psychological Assessment*, *15*, 340–350.

Birbaumer, N., Veit, R., Lotze, M., Erb, M., Hermann, C., Grodd, W., & Flor, H. (2005). Deficient fear conditioning in psychopathy: A functional magnetic resonance imaging study. *Archives of General Psychiatry*, *62*, 799–805.

Boddy, C. R. (2010). Corporate psychopaths and organizational type. *Journal of Public Affairs*, *10*, 300–312.

Boddy, C. R. (2011a). Corporate psychopaths, bullying and unfair supervision in the workplace. *Journal of Business Ethics*, *100*, 367–379.

Boddy, C. R. (2011b). The corporate psychopaths theory of the global financial crisis. *Journal of Business Ethics*, *102*, 255–259.

Boddy, C. R. (2014). Corporate psychopaths, conflict, employee affective well-being and counterproductive work behaviour. *Journal of Business Ethics*, *121*, 107–121.

Boddy, C. R. (2016). Psychopathy screening for public leadership. *International Journal of Public Leadership*, *12*, 254–274.

Bowling, N. A., & Eschleman, K. J. (2010). Employee personality as a moderator of the relationships between work stressors and counterproductive work behavior. *Journal of Occupational Health Psychology*, *15*, 91–103.

Brook, T. V. (2017, February 14). Army to spend $300 million on bonuses and ads to get 6,000 more recruits. *USA Today.* Retrieved from https://www.usatoday.com/story/news/politics/2017/02/12/army-spend-300-million-bonuses-and-ads-get-6000-more-recruits/97757094/. Accessed on July 1, 2017.

Brusher, E. A. (2007). Combat and operational stress control. *International Journal of Emergency Mental Health*, *9*, 111–122.

Bureau of Labor Statistics (BLS), U.S. Department of Labor. (2015). *Occupational outlook handbook: Military careers*. Retrieved from https://www.bls.gov/ooh/military/military-careers.htm. Accessed on January 30, 2017.

Cale, E. M., & Lilienfeld, S. O. (2002). Sex differences in psychopathy and antisocial personality disorder: A review and integration. *Clinical Psychology Review*, *22*, 1179–1207.

Calhoun, L. (2002). The phenomenology of paid killing. *The International Journal of Human Rights*, *6*, 1–18.

Carey, B. (2015, May 24). While at war, female soldiers fight to belong. *The New York Times*. Retrieved from https://www.nytimes.com/2015/05/25/health/while-at-war-female-soldiers-fight-to-belong.html. Accessed on August 14, 2017.

Chase, K. A., O'Leary, K. D., & Heyman, R. E. (2001). Categorizing partner-violent men within the reactive–proactive typology model. *Journal of Consulting and Clinical Psychology*, *69*, 567–572.

Chen, P. Y., & Spector, P. E. (1992). Relationships of work stressors with aggression, withdrawal, theft and substance use: An exploratory study. *Journal of Occupational and Organizational Psychology*, *65*, 177–184.

Chu, C., Buchman-Schmitt, J. M., Joiner, T. E., & Rudd, M. D. (2017). Personality disorder symptoms and suicidality: Low desire and high plans for suicide in military inpatients and outpatients. *Journal of Personality Disorders*, *31*, 145–155.

Clarke, J. (2005). *Working with monsters: How to identify and protect yourself from the workplace psychopath.* Sydney, Australia: Random House.

Cleckley, H. (1941). *The mask of sanity: An attempt to reinterpret the so-called psychopathic personality.* St. Louis, MO: C. V. Mosby.

Cleckley, H. (1950/2015). *The mask of sanity: An attempt to reinterpret the so-called psychopathic personality* (2nd ed.). St. Louis, MO: C. V. Mosby.

Cox, D., Hallam, R., O'Connor, K., & Rachman, S. (1983). An experimental analysis of fearlessness and courage. *British Journal of Psychology*, *74*, 107–117.

De Dreu, C. K., & Weingart, L. R. (2003). Task versus relationship conflict, team performance, and team member satisfaction: A meta-analysis. *Journal of Applied Psychology*, *88*, 741–749.

Department of Defense (DoD). (2015). *2015 demographics: Profile of the military community*. Retrieved from http://download.militaryonesource.mil/12038/MOS/Reports/2015-Demographics-Report.pdf. Accessed on June 30, 2017.

Dutton, K. (2012). *The wisdom of psychopaths: What saints, spies, and serial killers can teach us.* New York, NY: Farrar, Straus and Giroux.

Epstein, Y., Fleischmann, C., Yanovich, R., & Heled, Y. (2015). Physiological and medical aspects that put women soldiers at increased risk for overuse injuries. *The Journal of Strength & Conditioning Research*, *29*, S107–S110.

Ettner, S. L., MacLean, J. C., & French, M. T. (2011). Does having a dysfunctional personality hurt your career? Axis II personality disorders and labor market outcomes. *Industrial Relations: A Journal of Economy and Society*, *50*, 149–173.

Fastovtsov, G. A. (2011). Characteristics of stress-induced mental disorders in combatants who have committed criminal actions. *Neuroscience and Behavioral Physiology*, *41*, 267–271.

Forouzan, E., & Cooke, D. J. (2005). Figuring out la femme fatale: Conceptual and assessment issues concerning psychopathy in females. *Behavioral Sciences & the Law*, *23*, 765–778.

Fowler, K. A., & Westen, D. (2011). Subtyping male perpetrators of intimate partner violence. *Journal of Interpersonal Violence*, *26*, 607–639.

Furnham, A., Hyde, G., & Trickey, G. (2014). Do your dark side traits fit? Dysfunctional personalities in different work sectors. *Applied Psychology*, *63*, 589–606.

Gobin, R. L., Reddy, M. K., Zlotnick, C., & Johnson, J. E. (2015). Lifetime trauma victimization and PTSD in relation to psychopathy and antisocial personality disorder in a sample of incarcerated women and men. *International Journal of Prisoner Health*, *11*, 64–74.

Granato, S. L., Smith, P. N., & Selwyn, C. N. (2015). Acquired capability and masculine gender norm adherence: Potential pathways to higher rates of male suicide. *Psychology of Men & Masculinity*, *16*, 246–253.

Grossman, D. (2014). *On killing: The psychological cost of learning to kill in war and society* (Rev. ed.). New York, NY: Open Road Integrated Media.

Hall, J. R., & Benning, S. D. (2006). The "successful" psychopath. In Patrick, C. J. (Ed.), *Handbook of psychopathy* (pp. 459–478). New York, NY: The Guilford Press.

Hannah, S. T., Campbell, D. J., & Matthews, M. D. (2010). Advancing a research agenda for leadership in dangerous contexts. *Military Psychology*, *22*, S157–S189.

Hansen, A. L., Johnsen, B. H., Thornton, D., Waage, L., & Thayer, J. F. (2007). Facets of psychopathy, heart rate variability and cognitive function. *Journal of Personality Disorders*, *21*, 568–582.

Hare, R. D. (1980). A research scale for the assessment of psychopathy in criminal populations. *Personality and Individual Differences*, *1*, 111–119.

Hare, R. D. (1984). Performance of psychopaths on cognitive tasks related to frontal lobe function. *Journal of Abnormal Psychology*, *93*, 133–140.

Hare, R. D. (1996). Psychopathy: A clinical construct whose time has come. *Criminal Justice and Behavior*, *23*, 25–54.

Hare, R. D. (1998a). The Hare PCL-R: Some issues concerning its use and misuse. *Legal and Criminological Psychology*, *3*, 99–119.

Hare, R. D. (1998b). Psychopathy, affect and behavior. In D. J. Cooke, A. E. Forth, & R. D. Hare (Eds.), *Psychopathy: Theory, research and implications for society* (pp. 105–137). Dordrecht: Springer.

Hare, R. D. (1999). *Without conscience: The disturbing world of the psychopaths among us*. New York, NY: The Guilford Press.

Hare, R. D. (2003). *The psychopathy checklist* (Revised). Ontario, Canada: Multi-Health Systems.

Hare, R. D., Frazelle, J., & Cox, D. N. (1978). Psychopathy and physiological responses to threat of an aversive stimulus. *Psychophysiology*, *15*, 165–172.

Hare, R. D., Harpur, T. J., Hakstian, A. R., Forth, A. E., Hart, S. D., & Newman, J. P. (1990). The revised psychopathy checklist: Reliability and factor structure. *Psychological Assessment: A Journal of Consulting and Clinical Psychology*, *2*, 338–341.

Hare, R. D., & Neumann, C. S. (2009). Psychopathy and its measurement. In P. J. Corr & G. Matthews (Eds.), *Cambridge handbook of personality psychology* (pp. 660–686). New York, NY: Cambridge University Press.

Harms, P. D. (2016). When high potential women go bad. *Talent Quarterly*, *12*, 49–51.

Harms, P. D., Krasikova, D. V., Vanhove, A. J., Herian, M. N., & Lester, P. B. (2013). Stress and emotional well-being in military organizations. In P. L. Perrewé, C. C. Rosen, & J. R. B. Halbesleben (Eds.), *Research in occupational stress and well-being* (Vol. 11, pp. 103–132). Bingley: Emerald Group Publishing.

Hassall, J., Boduszek, D., & Dhingra, K. (2015). Psychopathic traits of business and psychology students and their relationship to academic success. *Personality and Individual Differences, 82*, 227–231.

Hecker, T., Hermenau, K., Maedl, A., Elbert, T., & Schauer, M. (2012). Appetitive aggression in former combatants – Derived from the ongoing conflict in DR Congo. *International Journal of Law and Psychiatry, 35*, 244–249.

Hecker, T., Hermenau, K., Maedl, A., Schauer, M., & Elbert, T. (2013). Aggression inoculates against PTSD symptom severity – Insights from armed groups in the eastern DR Congo. *European Journal of Psychotraumatology, 4*, 1–9.

Hill, C. D., Neumann, C. S., & Rogers, R. (2004). Confirmatory factor analysis of the psychopathy checklist: Screening version in offenders with Axis I disorders. *Psychological Assessment, 16*, 90–95.

Hogan, R., Curphy, G. J., & Hogan, J. (1994). What we know about leadership: Effectiveness and personality. *American Psychologist, 49*, 493–504.

Hogan, R., & Hogan, J. (2001). Assessing leadership: A view from the dark side. *International Journal of Selection and Assessment, 9*, 40–51.

Hogan, R., & Hogan, J. (2009). *Hogan development survey manual.* Tulsa, OK: Hogan Assessment Systems.

Hourani, L. L., Williams, T. V., & Kress, A. M. (2006). Stress, mental health, and job performance among active duty military personnel: Findings from the 2002 Department of Defense Health-Related Behaviors Survey. *Military Medicine, 171*, 849.

Howe, J., Falkenbach, D., & Massey, C. (2014). The relationship among psychopathy, emotional intelligence, and professional success in finance. *International Journal of Forensic Mental Health, 13*, 337–347.

Ishikawa, S. S., Raine, A., Lencz, T., Bihrle, S., & Lacasse, L. (2001). Autonomic stress reactivity and executive functions in successful and unsuccessful criminal psychopaths from the community. *Journal of Abnormal Psychology, 110*, 423–432.

Jex, S. M., & Bliese, P. D. (1999). Efficacy beliefs as a moderator of the impact of work-related stressors: A multilevel study. *Journal of Applied Psychology, 84*, 349–361.

Johns, J. H., & Quay, H. C. (1962). The effect of social reward on verbal conditioning in psychopathic and neurotic military offenders. *Journal of Consulting Psychology, 26*, 217–220.

Jonason, P. K., Wee, S., Li, N. P., & Jackson, C. (2014). Occupational niches and the dark triad traits. *Personality and Individual Differences, 69*, 119–123.

Jones, D. N., & Hare, R. D. (2016). The mismeasure of psychopathy: A commentary on Boddy's PM-MRV. *Journal of Business Ethics, 138*, 579–588.

Kreis, M. K., & Cooke, D. J. (2011). Capturing the psychopathic female: A prototypicality analysis of the Comprehensive Assessment of Psychopathic Personality (CAPP) across gender. *Behavioral Sciences & the Law, 29*, 634–648.

Landay, K., Harms, P. D., & Credé, M. (2017, June). *Are we serving the dark lords? A meta-analysis of psychopathy and leadership.* Poster presented at the 5th biennial meeting of Association for Research in Personality, Sacramento, CA.

Lauterbach, D., & Vrana, S. (2001). The relationship among personality variables, exposure to traumatic events, and severity of posttraumatic stress symptoms. *Journal of Traumatic Stress, 14*, 29–45.

Lazarus, R. S., Deese, J., & Osler, S. F. (1952). The effects of psychological stress upon performance. *Psychological Bulletin, 49*, 293–317.

Lehmann, A., & Ittel, A. (2012). Aggressive behavior and measurement of psychopathy in female inmates of German prisons – A preliminary study. *International Journal of Law and Psychiatry, 35*, 190–197.

Levenston, G. K., Patrick, C. J., Bradley, M. M., & Lang, P. J. (2000). The psychopath as observer: Emotion and attention in picture processing. *Journal of Abnormal Psychology, 109*, 373–385.

Lilienfeld, S. O. (1994). Conceptual problems in the assessment of psychopathy. *Clinical Psychology Review, 14*, 17–38.

Lilienfeld, S. O., & Andrews, B. P. (1996). Development and preliminary validation of a self-report measure of psychopathic personality traits in noncriminal population. *Journal of Personality Assessment, 66*, 488–524.

Lilienfeld, S. O., Waldman, I. D., Landfield, K., Watts, A. L., Rubenzer, S., & Faschingbauer, T. R. (2012). Fearless dominance and the US presidency: Implications of psychopathic personality traits for successful and unsuccessful political leadership. *Journal of Personality and Social Psychology*, *103*, 489–505.

Lilienfeld, S. O., & Widows, M. R. (2005). *The psychopathic personality inventory-revised (PPI-R): Professional manual*. Lutz, FL: Psychological Assessment Resources.

Liu, C., Liu, Y., Mills, M. J., & Fan, J. (2013). Job stressors, job performance, job dedication, and the moderating effect of conscientiousness: A mixed-method approach. *International Journal of Stress Management*, *20*, 336–363.

Lohner, J., & Konrad, N. (2006). Deliberate self-harm and suicide attempt in custody: Distinguishing features in male inmates' self-injurious behavior. *International Journal of Law and Psychiatry*, *29*, 370–385.

Loney, B. R., Butler, M. A., Lima, E. N., Counts, C. A., & Eckel, L. A. (2006). The relation between salivary cortisol, callous-unemotional traits, and conduct problems in an adolescent non-referred sample. *Journal of Child Psychology and Psychiatry*, *47*, 30–36.

Lopez, C. T. (2015, June 26). To become 'force of the future,' Army must fix personnel churn. *U.S. Army*. Retrieved from https://www.army.mil/article/151308. Accessed on July 1, 2016.

Mael, F. A., & Alderks, C. E. (1993). Leadership team cohesion and subordinate work unit morale and performance. *Military Psychology*, *5*, 141–158.

Mathieu, C., & Babiak, P. (2015). Tell me who you are, I'll tell you how you lead: Beyond the full-range leadership model, the role of corporate psychopathy on employee attitudes. *Personality and Individual Differences*, *87*, 8–12.

Mathieu, C., & Babiak, P. (2016a). Corporate psychopathy and abusive supervision: Their influence on employees' job satisfaction and turnover intentions. *Personality and Individual Differences*, *91*, 102–106.

Mathieu, C., & Babiak, P. (2016b). Validating the B-scan self: A self-report measure of psychopathy in the workplace. *International Journal of Selection and Assessment*, *24*, 272–284.

Mazza, M., Tempesta, D., Pino, M. C., Nigri, A., Catalucci, A., Guadagni, V., … Ferrara, M. (2015). Neural activity related to cognitive and emotional empathy in post-traumatic stress disorder. *Behavioural Brain Research*, *282*, 37–45.

McGreal, C. (2011, November 10). 'Kill team' US platoon commander guilty of Afghan murders. *The Guardian*. Retrieved from https://www.theguardian.com/world/2011/nov/11/kill-team-calvin-gibbs-convicted. Accessed on January 8, 2018.

Mesmer-Magnus, J. R., & DeChurch, L. A. (2009). Information sharing and team performance: A meta-analysis. *Journal of Applied Psychology*, *94*, 535–546.

Milgram, N. A., Orenstein, R., & Zafrir, E. (1989). Stressors, personal resources, and social supports in military performance during wartime. *Military Psychology*, *1*, 185–199.

Minsberg, T. (2015, May 24). Women describe their struggles with gender roles in military. *The New York Times*. Retrieved from https://www.nytimes.com/2015/05/25/health/women-describe-their-struggles-with-gender-roles-in-military.html. Accessed on August 14, 2017.

Nazarov, A., Jetly, R., McNeely, H., Kiang, M., Lanius, R., & McKinnon, M. C. (2015). Role of morality in the experience of guilt and shame within the armed forces. *Acta Psychiatrica Scandinavica*, *132*, 4–19.

Neumann, C. S., Schmitt, D. S., Carter, R., Embley, I., & Hare, R. D. (2012). Psychopathic traits in females and males across the globe. *Behavioral Sciences & the Law*, *30*, 557–574.

Nosratabadi, M., & Halvaiepour, Z. (2016). A structural equation modeling of the relationships between depression, drug abuse, and social support with suicidal ideation among soldiers in Iran in 2015. *Journal of Research in Health Sciences*, *16*, 212–216.

O'Boyle, E. H., Jr, Forsyth, D. R., Banks, G. C., & McDaniel, M. A. (2012). A meta-analysis of the dark triad and work behavior: A social exchange perspective. *Journal of Applied Psychology*, *97*, 557–579.

O'Leary, M. M., Loney, B. R., & Eckel, L. A. (2007). Gender differences in the association between psychopathic personality traits and cortisol response to induced stress. *Psychoneuroendocrinology*, *32*, 183–191.

O'Leary, M. M., Taylor, J., & Eckel, L. (2010). Psychopathic personality traits and cortisol response to stress: The role of sex, type of stressor, and menstrual phase. *Hormones and Behavior*, *58*, 250–256.

Orasanu, J. M., & Backer, P. (1996). Stress and military performance. In J. E. Driskell & E. Salas (Eds.), *Stress and human performance* (pp. 89–125). Hillsdale, NJ: Lawrence Erlbaum.

Parker, K., Cilluffo, A., & Stepler, R. (2017, April 13). *6 facts about the U.S. military and its changing demographics*. Pew Research Center. Retrieved from http://www.pewresearch.org/fact-tank/2017/04/13/6-facts-about-the-u-s-military-and-its-changing-demographics/. Accessed on August 14, 2017.

Patrick, C. J. (1994). Emotion and psychopathy: Startling new insights. *Psychophysiology*, *31*, 319–330.

Patrick, C. J., Bradley, M. M., & Lang, P. J. (1993). Emotion in the criminal psychopath: Startle reflex modulation. *Journal of Abnormal Psychology*, *102*, 82–92.

Patrick, C. J., Fowles, D. C., & Krueger, R. F. (2009). Triarchic conceptualization of psychopathy: Developmental origins of disinhibition, boldness, and meanness. *Development and Psychopathology*, *21*, 913–938.

Paulhus, D. L., & Williams, K. M. (2002). The dark triad of personality: Narcissism, Machiavellianism, and psychopathy. *Journal of Research in Personality*, *36*, 556–563.

Pflanz, S. (2001). Occupational stress and psychiatric illness in the military: Investigation of the relationship between occupational stress and mental illness among military mental health patients. *Military Medicine*, *166*, 457–462.

Pflanz, S. (2002). Work stress in the military: Prevalence, causes, and relationship to emotional health. *Military Medicine*, *167*, 877–882.

Pflanz, S. E., & Ogle, A. D. (2006). Job stress, depression, work performance, and perceptions of supervisors in military personnel. *Military Medicine*, *171*, 861–865.

Philpott, T. (2014, September 20). Military update: 80,000 vets with PTSD could gain discharge upgrades. *The Times of Trenton*. Retrieved from http://www.nj.com/mercer/index.ssf/2014/09/military_update_80000_vets_with_ptsd_could_gain_discharge_upgrades.html. Accessed on January 27, 2017.

Powers, R. (2017, October 13). How the U.S. Army is organized? *The Balance*. Retrieved from https://www.thebalance.com/u-s-army-military-organization-from-squad-to-corps-4053660. Accessed on January 16, 2018.

Reidy, D. E., Shelley-Tremblay, J. F., & Lilienfeld, S. O. (2011). Psychopathy, reactive aggression, and precarious proclamations: A review of behavioral, cognitive, and biological research. *Aggression and Violent Behavior*, *16*, 512–524.

Reuters. (2017, May 1). *Sexual assault reports in U.S. military reach record high: Pentagon*. Retrieved from http://www.nbcnews.com/news/us-news/sexual-assault-reports-u-s-military-reach-record-high-pentagon-n753566. Accessed on August 14, 2017.

Richardson, L. K., Frueh, B. C., & Acierno, R. (2010). Prevalence estimates of combat-related post-traumatic stress disorder: Critical review. *Australian & New Zealand Journal of Psychiatry*, *44*, 4–19.

Rodriguez, A., & Brown, A. (2016). Conceptualizing leadership psychosis: The Department of Veteran Affairs scandal. *International Journal of Public Leadership*, *12*, 14–31.

Salas, E., Bowers, C. A., & Cannon-Bowers, J. A. (1995). Military team research: 10 years of progress. *Military Psychology*, *7*, 55–75.

Samuels, S. M., Foster, C. A., & Lindsay, D. R. (2010). Freefall, self-efficacy, and leading in dangerous contexts. *Military Psychology*, *22*, S117–S136.

Sanecka, E. (2013). The effects of supervisor's subclinical psychopathy on subordinates organizational commitment, job satisfaction and satisfaction with supervisor. *The Journal of Education, Culture, and Society*, *2*, 172–191.

Schmidt, B., Loerbroks, A., Herr, R., Litaker, D., Wilson, M., Kastner, M., & Fischer, J. (2014). Psychosocial resources and the relationship between transformational leadership and employees' psychological strain. *Work*, *49*, 315–324.

Schmied, E. A., Highfill-McRoy, R. M., & Larson, G. E. (2012). Mental health and turnover following an initial term of military service. *Military Medicine, 177*(7), 776–772.

Schneider, B. (1987). The people make the place. *Personnel Psychology*, *40*, 437–453.

Schütte, N., Blickle, G., Frieder, R. E., Wihler, A., Schnitzler, F., Heupel, J., & Zettler, I. (2018). The role of interpersonal influence in counterbalancing psychopathic personality trait facets at work. *Journal of Management*. *44*, 1338–1368. doi: 0149206315607967.

Sellbom, M. (2015). Elucidating the complex associations between psychopathy and post-traumatic stress disorder from the perspective of trait negative affectivity. *International Journal of Forensic Mental Health*, *14*, 85–92.

Sinclair, R. R., & Tucker, J. S. (2006). Stress-CARE: An integrated model of individual differences in soldier performance under stress. In T. W. Britt, C. A. Castro, & A. B. Adler (Eds.), *Military life: The psychology of serving in peace and combat* (Vol. 1, pp. 202–231). Westport, CT: Praeger Security International.

Skeem, J. L., Polaschek, D. L., Patrick, C. J., & Lilienfeld, S. O. (2011). Psychopathic personality: Bridging the gap between scientific evidence and public policy. *Psychological Science in the Public Interest*, *12*, 95–162.

Smith, S. F., & Lilienfeld, S. O. (2013). Psychopathy in the workplace: The knowns and unknowns. *Aggression and Violent Behavior*, *18*, 204–218.

Smith, S. F., Lilienfeld, S. O., Coffey, K., & Dabbs, J. M. (2013). Are psychopaths and heroes twigs off the same branch? Evidence from college, community, and presidential samples. *Journal of Research in Personality*, *47*, 634–646.

Smith, M. B., Wallace, J. C., & Jordan, P. (2016). When the dark ones become darker: How promotion focus moderates the effects of the dark triad on supervisor performance ratings. *Journal of Organizational Behavior*, *37*, 236–254.

Sonnentag, S., & Frese, M. (2003). Stress in organizations. In W. C. Borman, D. R. Ilgen, & R. J. Klimoski (Eds.), *Handbook of psychology* (pp. 453–491). Hoboken, NJ: John Wiley.

Spain, S. M., Harms, P., & LeBreton, J. M. (2014). The dark side of personality at work. *Journal of Organizational Behavior*, *35*, S41–S60.

Springer, B. A., & Ross, A. E. (2011). *Musculoskeletal injuries in military women*. Borden Institute Monograph Series. Fort Detrick, MD: Borden Institute.

Swogger, M. T., Van Orden, K. A., & Conner, K. R. (2014). The relationship of outwardly directed aggression to suicidal ideation and suicide attempts across two high-risk samples. *Psychology of Violence*, *4*, 184–195.

Ursano, R. J., Kessler, R. C., Naifeh, J. A., Mash, H. H., Fullerton, C. S., Bliese, P. D., … Stein, M. B. (2017). Risk of suicide attempt among soldiers in army units with a history of suicide attempts. *JAMA Psychiatry*, *74*, 924–931.

U.S. Department of Veterans Affairs. (2016). *VA suicide prevention program: Facts about veteran suicide*. Retrieved from https://www.va.gov/opa/publications/factsheets/Suicide_Prevention_FactSheet_New_VA_Stats_070616_1400.pdf. Accessed on June 29, 2017.

Van Orden, K. A., Witte, T. K., Cukrowicz, K. C., Braithwaite, S. R., Selby, E. A., & Joiner, T. E., Jr. (2010). The interpersonal theory of suicide. *Psychological Review*, *117*, 575–600.

Venables, N. C., Sellbom, M., Sourander, A., Kendler, K. S., Joiner, T. E., Drislane, L. E., … Patrick, C. J. (2015). Separate and interactive contributions of weak inhibitory control and threat sensitivity to prediction of suicide risk. *Psychiatry Research*, *226*, 461–466.

Vitacco, M. J., Neumann, C. S., Caldwell, M. F., Leistico, A. M., & Van Rybroek, G. J. (2006). Testing factor models of the psychopathy checklist: Youth version and their association with instrumental aggression. *Journal of Personality Assessment*, *87*, 74–83.

Vitacco, M. J., Neumann, C. S., & Jackson, R. L. (2005). Testing a four-factor model of psychopathy and its association with ethnicity, gender, intelligence, and violence. *Journal of Consulting and Clinical Psychology*, *73*, 466–476.

Vitale, J. E., & Newman, J. P. (2001). Using the psychopathy checklist-revised with female samples: Reliability, validity, and implications for clinical utility. *Clinical Psychology: Science and Practice*, *8*, 117–132.

Volmer, J., Koch, I. K., & Göritz, A. S. (2016). The bright and dark sides of leaders' dark triad traits: Effects on subordinates' career success and well-being. *Personality and Individual Differences*, *101*, 413–418.

Walker, D., & Bourgeois, J. (2007). The management of fitness for duty in the United States military. In A. Felthous & H. Saß (Eds.), *International handbook on psychopathic disorders and the law: Laws and policies* (Vol. II, pp. 113–123). West Sussex: John Wiley.

Warren, J. I., Burnette, M. L., South, S. C., Chauhan, P., Bale, R., Friend, R., & Van Patten, I. (2003). Psychopathy in women: Structural modeling and comorbidity. *International Journal of Law and Psychiatry*, *26*, 223–242.

Watson, J. (2016, February 12). Army pays woman $820,000 to settle sexual harassment case. *Military.com*. Retrieved from http://www.military.com/daily-news/2016/02/12/army-pays-woman-820-000-settle-sexual-harassment-case.html

Westman, M. (1990). The relationship between stress and performance: The moderating effect of hardiness. *Human Performance*, *3*, 141–155.

Williams, K. M., Nathanson, C., & Paulhus, D. L. (2003, August 7–10). *Structure and validity of the self-report psychopathy scale-III in normal populations*, Toronto, Canada: *American Psychological Association*.

Willemsen, J., De Ganck, J., & Verhaeghe, P. (2012). Psychopathy, traumatic exposure, and lifetime posttraumatic stress. *International Journal of Offender Therapy and Comparative Criminology*, *56*, 505–524.

Wilson, M. S., & McCarthy, K. (2011). Greed is good? Student disciplinary choice and self-reported psychopathy. *Personality and Individual Differences*, *51*, 873–876.

Wu, Y. C. (2011). Job stress and job performance among employees in the Taiwanese finance sector: The role of emotional intelligence. *Social Behavior and Personality: An International Journal*, *39*, 21–31.

Wu, J., & Lebreton, J. M. (2011). Reconsidering the dispositional basis of counterproductive work behavior: The role of aberrant personality. *Personnel Psychology*, *64*, 593–626.

Yang, Y., & Raine, A. (2009). Prefrontal structural and functional brain imaging findings in antisocial, violent, and psychopathic individuals: A meta-analysis. *Psychiatry Research: Neuroimaging*, *174*, 81–88.

Zoroya, G. (2016, April 1). U.S. military suicides remain high for 7th year. *USA Today*. Retrieved from https://www.usatoday.com/story/news/nation/2016/04/01/us-military-suicides-remain-stubbornly-high/82518278/. Accessed on June 30, 2017.

MEASURING JOB PERFORMANCE IN THE ARMY: INSIGHTS FROM EVIDENCE ON CIVILIAN STRESS AND HEALTH

Stacy Ann Hawkins, Loryana L. Vie, Pedro S. A. Wolf, Paul B. Lester, Kerry S. Whittaker, Jacob N. Hawkins and Alycia L. Perez

ABSTRACT

Job performance in the US Army is a complex construct, in part because of the stressors that soldiers face, both day-to-day and during deployment. This chapter critically reviews job performance, and the connections between performance and stress and health, discussing how findings may also be relevant within the specific context of the Army. We review established conceptualizations and metrics of job performance within the Army as well as the civilian sector. Then, we discuss the existing research on the associations between performance and stress, physical health, health behaviors, and mental health. Considering these findings, we discuss lessons learned for Army performance metrics, recommending that stress- and health-related issues be incorporated into unit and leader performance metrics, with two critical caveats: (1) data are aggregated at a company level and (2) non-reactive measures are used. Finally, we discuss how existing data repositories can facilitate future research and note potential constraints of using secondary data.

Keywords: Job performance; stress; physical health; mental health; Army; military

Occupational Stress and Well-being in Military Contexts
Research in Occupational Stress and Well-being, Volume 16, 49–68
Copyright © 2018 by Emerald Publishing Limited
All rights of reproduction in any form reserved
ISSN: 1479-3555/doi:10.1108/S1479-355520180000016004

Job performance in the US Army is a complex construct, in part because of the wide variety of job tasks and occupations across the institution. Soldiers are required to complete a broad range of activities, including administrative tasks, physical labor, and dangerous work related to firearms and explosives. While deployment inarguably poses the most dangerous and complex risks and challenges, researchers are seeing high levels of stress and performance challenges even among those not serving on combat deployment, simply because of the demanding nature and the sensitivity of the military's goals and missions (Hourani, Williams, & Kress, 2006). Consequently, job performance in the Army may be more critical than within the civilian sector because incomplete or incorrect job performance can have life-changing and life-threatening consequences for individual soldiers, their units, and even their families.

With such critical repercussions for compromised performance, understanding the predictors of successful and unsuccessful job performance is particularly important within the Army. Personnel stress and health are some of these critical predictors, as indicated by a breadth of both military and civilian literature (Arshadi & Damiri, 2013; Hourani et al., 2006; Park, 2007). Health and stress are particularly relevant within the Army context, as there are many physical and emotional demands that can lead to compromised health and increased stress for American soldiers, including combat exposure and deployment (e.g., Hoge, Auchterlonie, & Milliken, 2006; Tanielian et al., 2008), separation from families (Hourani et al., 2006), and physically demanding training (Kaufman, Brodine, & Shaffer, 2000; Lauder, Baker, Smith, & Lincoln, 2000).

STRESS AND HEALTH

By the very nature of their service, soldiers are a population that may experience stress at higher rates than the general population and face unique stressors not often encountered in civilian life. For soldiers and civilians alike, prolonged stress exposure, as well as acute or traumatic stressors, can have a broad-reaching impact on one's physical and mental health, social life, and job performance. To understand better the effects of stress on physical health, mental health, and job performance, it is necessary to have a fundamental understanding of both physiology and psychology of stress.

The simplest definition of stress is "the nonspecific response of the body to a demand" (Selye, 1956, p. 55). However, this view of stress is often seen as too simplistic. In the decades of research that have followed, scientists have begun to unravel the nuances of stress; some positive (eustress – a joyful event) and some negative (distress – an event that is unwanted), which has led to a deeper understanding and a more encompassing definition of the concept of stress. Stress is a biopsychosocial process that occurs when an individual encounters a situation or event that he or she perceives as being beyond their ability to cope or adapt. This view of stress highlights the importance of perception and appraisal, coping skills, physical and social resources and not just the autonomic physiological response of the human body. The physiological changes in the human body in response to stress are more objectively measureable and for this reason have been more often studied; however, each aspect of the stress response can have a profound and unique impact on an individual's overall health. When it comes to the impact of stress on mental health, well-being, and job performance in particular, the effects of stress appraisal, perception, and coping are critical.

An individual's physical health can have an impact on their work and performance, and stress has been shown to impact physical health in many ways. On a physiological level, when presented with a stressor, the sympathetic nervous system takes over and produces what is colloquially called the "fight-or-flight" response (releasing epinephrine and norepinephrine, raising heart rate and blood pressure, diverting energy to deal with the immediate threat, and triggering release of cortisol to maintain a heightened state of alertness until the stressor is over). Although these stress hormones play an important, even beneficial role in the short term, when an individual is chronically exposed to stressors, the consequences can be quite damaging. In a poll conducted by the American Psychological Association (2017), 80% of respondents reported experiencing at least one symptom of stress (either physical or emotional) during the last month. Researchers estimate that as many as 60–80% of visits to primary care physicians are in some part stress-related (Nerurkar, Bitton, Davis, Phillips, & Yeh, 2013).

As with physical health, stress has a profound impact on mental health and well-being. Many of the stressors of modern life are psychological in nature; demands on time or resources can be just as potent stressors as threats to physical safety. The link between stress and psychological health might seem more intuitive, especially given that "being stressed out" has become such a common refrain for the average American. Just as stress produces physiological symptoms, psychological symptoms of stress can also be quite detrimental. Stress can lead to feelings of anxiety, irritability, anger, depression, and mood swings. Stress hormones have even been shown to elicit structural changes and alter the neurochemical environment of the brain, and these changes have been linked to depression (McEwen, 2005). Extreme or traumatic stressors can lead to psychiatric disorders, such as post-traumatic stress disorder and acute stress disorder. These disorders can be debilitating, as many individuals withdraw and become avoidant while suffering from symptoms of extreme anxiety, fear, hyper arousal, and flashbacks of the trauma.

Stress also affects mental health by changing the ways individuals interact with their environments. Maintaining social support, strong social networks, and engaging in healthy lifestyle choices (such as good sleep practices, regular exercise, and eating a healthy diet) are all ways to lessen the negative effects of stress on an individual's health. Many of these techniques are in fact positive coping styles that people actively employ to deal with stressful situations. However, people can become overwhelmed by a stressor or lack appropriate coping strategies for certain stressful situations, which can lead to poor mental health. People often experience cognitive impairments as a result of stress, becoming more prone to making mistakes or forgetting important details or information. These cognitive impairments can, in and of themselves, be stressful, causing a cycle of stress that perpetuates and results in continued poor health outcomes.

CHAPTER OVERVIEW

This chapter critically examines the measurement and concept of job performance and the connections between performance, stress, and health within the context of the Army. First, we describe the current formal and semiformal job performance measures used by the Army. We focus on the performance and review processes and documentation for Army leaders (i.e., corporals and above). Understanding the established method and metrics provides a foundation of knowledge that can help us better understand how the Army might correspond with or diverge from the general research on performance, stress, and health. Then, we review established conceptualizations and metrics of job performance within the civilian sector, focusing on broad indicators and definitions of performance. This review provides a context for understanding how job performance is related to stress and health within the unique and widely varying settings of the Army, and serves as a comparison to the Army's methods of performance evaluation.

The next section reviews associations between performance and stress, physical health, health behaviors, and mental health. We describe literature primarily within the civilian sector, and, as it is available, within the military community. Through this review, we identify the types, features, and measures of job performance that are most commonly and most strongly related to employee health and stress. Following the review of performance, stress, and health, we discuss lessons learned for Army performance metrics, especially within the context of stress and health. We describe potential strategies for improving measurement of job performance by incorporating stress and health indicators. Finally, we describe emerging opportunities for research on job performance, stress, and health in the military. We discuss key considerations and strategies for measuring performance, stress, and health, and address the constraints of using secondary data.

JOB PERFORMANCE METRICS WITHIN THE ARMY

Excellent performance and leadership are hallmarks of the US Army, and the organization stakes much of its reputation on developing outstanding leaders at all levels. As part of leader development, the Army has created several formal and semiformal tools that assess job performance. Since the Army places so much emphasis on leader development, and because the Army views all individuals past the rank of corporal as a leader (regardless of whether or not a particular soldier is in a formal leadership role), much of the focus in this section will be on those job performance measures that are geared toward leadership development.

Formal Job Performance Measures

Formal job performance feedback begins early in a soldier's career (e.g., in basic combat training) and is designed to be developmental, be it to promote positive work behaviors, or to address job performance shortcomings, or both. During feedback and performance evaluation sessions, a plan of action to modify or sustain a soldier's job performance is made, and includes specific rater responsibilities for implementing the plan of action, and later feedback sessions reassess performance based on the plan. The products of feedback and performance evaluation sessions weigh heavily in promotion and award recommendations, and thus are critical for soldiers' development and success throughout their careers.

In addition to feedback sessions, performance raters complete Officer Evaluation Reports (OER) and Non-Commissioned Officer Evaluation Reports (NCOER) – formal annual performance evaluations. The Army's evaluation process serves a dual purpose. Like developmental counseling, receiving an OER or NCOER is a developmental process, yet it also permanently documents a leader's job performance over the course of a year. The OER and NCOER forms are similar, yet distinct. The OER form calls for information about the rated commissioned officer in the areas of character, presence, intellect, leadership, development, and achievements. In contrast, the NCOER form calls for information about the rated non-commissioned officer (NCO) in the areas of supporting the Army values, competence, physical fitness and military bearing, leadership, training, and responsibility and accountability. These differences are primarily attributable to the differing missions of the officer and NCO corps.

An OER or NCOER is completed by two leaders: the rater, typically an immediate supervisor, and a senior rater, typically a leader two levels above the leader being rated. Raters and senior raters have slightly different options on the OER and NCOER forms in order to help limit positive evaluation inflation. On an OER, raters may deem a leader's performance as excels, proficient, capable, or unsatisfactory, while senior raters may select most qualified, highly qualified, qualified, not qualified. The NCOER is somewhat similar, with raters selecting far exceed standard, exceed standard, met standard, and did not meet standard, while senior rater block check options mirror those of the OER.

Both OERs and NCOERs allow for either bullet comments or longer narratives that describe a leader's performance; however, it became apparent on earlier versions of the forms that promotion and selection boards placed special emphasis on evaluation blocking because, quite simply, it served as an easier and faster metric to gauge performance. With this in mind, the Army further instituted caps on the percentage of leaders a rater or senior rater can mark in the highest performance categories. These caps are typically set at less than 50%, and these are calculated based on all evaluations completed by an individual rater or senior rater. Policies to limit evaluation inflation appear to be working, as most raters and senior raters maintain a "top block" profile of approximately 33%. Thus, receiving an OER with the highest blocking from both rater and senior rater makes the OER more impactful for a leader's career and serves as an important indicator of promotion and selection to key leadership assignments, although the basis for the ratings differs based on what job the soldier performs.

Semi-formal Job Performance Measures

Along with formal ratings and feedback, one of the most important forms of semi-formal performance evaluation is the multi-source assessment and feedback system or MSAF. The MSAF is a 360° performance feedback system that seeks feedback on a leader's performance from senior leaders, subordinates, and peers. There are multiple versions of the MSAF depending on the type of feedback needed (e.g., leader performance and unit performance). Along with the anonymized feedback, the MSAF website contains a wealth of training and coaching material that assists the leader in interpreting the feedback and improving her performance. Notably, the MSAF is not able to be used as official performance criteria because of the reliance on anonymous responses.

Whereas the majority of Army performance evaluations are formalized in *how* they rate soldiers, there are very few formalized systems that guide on what criteria Soldiers are rated. This is somewhat different from the civilian sector, discussed below. However, the Army has several semi-formal job performance measures that describe organizational performance and climate more specifically, which serve as indicators of a leader's performance. Recently appointed unit commanders receive feedback via the Defense Equal Opportunity Management Institute's Organizational Climate Survey (DEOCS), a 56-item survey focused on organizational climate (e.g., organizational performance, cohesion, and inclusion), equal opportunity concerns (e.g., diversity management and perceptions of discrimination), and sexual assault/sexual harassment within the workplace; local commanders can also include up to 10 locally developed questions.

JOB PERFORMANCE METRICS IN THE CIVILIAN SECTOR

Research on job performance within the civilian sector reveals many different ways to assess performance. Below, we review literature pertaining to the measurement of job performance within the civilian sector, which provides context and comparison for the processes used by the Army, as well as the connections between job performance, stress, and health.

As in the military, civilian job performance is most commonly measured using supervisor- or self-rated performance surveys. Research on job performance also assesses performance by tracking presenteeism (i.e., attending work while ill and not performing at usual levels) and absenteeism (Merrill et al., 2013; Sears, Shi, Coberley, & Pope, 2013). However, using metrics with more specific criteria can provide a more detailed understanding of job performance and how factors impact performance. For example, Barrick and Mount (1991) separated job performance into three aspects: job proficiency, training proficiency, and personnel data. Job proficiency consisted of performance ratings and productivity data, whereas measures of training proficiency utilized training performance ratings and additional training productivity data (e.g., time taken to complete training; Barrick & Mount, 1991). Personnel data consisted of information regarding salary, turnover, tenure, and position changes (Barrick & Mount, 1991).

Another approach to deconstructing job performance is by considering task performance and contextual performance as conceptually distinct elements of performance (Borman & Motowidlo, 1997; Motowidlo & Van Scotter, 1994). Broadly speaking, task performance refers to any employee behavior that directly supports an organization's product or goal. Motowidlo and Van Scotter (1994) break task performance into two categories: (1) an employee's activity or action that directly converts materials into product and (2) actions that help to maintain and replenish the materials of the organization. Task performance may include selling products, operating machinery, coordinating an operation, or supervising staff. In contrast, contextual performance does not relate specifically to the primary goals of the organization. Instead, it serves to support the social, psychological, and organizational environments of a company (Borman & Motowidlo, 1997; Motowidlo & Van Scotter, 1994). Contextual behavior includes volunteering for informal tasks, demonstrating persistent enthusiasm, cooperation and helpfulness, abiding by a company's rules and procedures despite personal inconvenience, and maintaining support and advocacy for the organization. Contextual performance encompasses some of the subtler facets of job performance, including organizational citizenship (Organ, 1988), organizational spontaneity (George & Brief, 1992), and pro-social organizational behavior (Brief & Motowidlo, 1986). Motowidlo and Van Scotter (1994) examined task and contextual performance as independent contributors to job performance and found that work experience is more highly correlated with task performance than contextual performance. This suggests that employees with more work experience are likely to have higher levels of task performance. A different pattern is evident for personality characteristics, which are more strongly associated with contextual performance than task performance (Borman & Motowidlo, 1997; Motowidlo & Van Scotter, 1994). Thus, while work experience can impact task performance, personality may be more likely to influence contextual performance.

Connections between Army and Civilian Metrics

It is not surprising that there are several parallels between how the Army evaluates job performance and the academic literature of job performance metrics implemented in the civilian sector. For instance, the OERs and NCOERs include clear measures of task performance, such as measures of significant duties, responsibilities, performance objectives, and significant contributions. The OERs and NCOERs also contain measures of contextual performance, with metrics on leadership, support of Army values, and responsibility. Likewise, the MSAF incorporates task and contextual performance by providing feedback across several performance disciplines. The developmental counseling form, utilized to promote positive work behaviors and to address job performance shortcomings, and the DEOCS items (e.g., organizational performance, cohesion, inclusion, and diversity management) are additional measures of contextual performance that allow the Army to form a more comprehensive view of their personnel and operations.

STRESS, HEALTH, AND JOB PERFORMANCE

With a clearer understanding of how job performance is commonly measured in the civilian sector and in the Army, we turn to the intersection of job performance, stress, and health. As previously discussed, stress is an important natural response process that can have far-reaching positive *and* negative effects on individuals. In this section, we review the existing research evidence that links job performance and stress, physical health, health behaviors, and mental health. These findings demonstrate how and under what circumstances, performance, stress, and health are interconnected. There is a dearth of evidence within the military about the role of stress on health and performance, so we rely heavily on civilian research and discuss the potential connections for Army soldiers based on civilian work.

Performance and Stress

Although stress can have a number of deleterious effects on health, cognition, and performance, it is a critical component of life. Aside from the physiological necessity of the stress response allowing our bodies to adapt to and survive in a variety of situations, the right amount of stress can actually be beneficial. Moderate amounts of stress can improve performance and motivation. The heightened level of arousal produced by the stress response can be directed into increased vigilance for a task at hand. Early research in the field suggests that the relationship between stress and performance follows the pattern of an inverted U-shape (Anderson, 1976; Yerkes & Dodson, 1908). If there is too little stress or too much stress, an individual's performance will likely be compromised, but under moderate amounts of stress, an individual's performance reaches its optimum level (known as the Yerkes–Dodson effect). However, the effects of stress on performance are complex, and research suggests that stress may only enhance performance on tasks that are well rehearsed; performance on novel tasks often suffers when an individual is under stress (Janis & Mann, 1977; Spence & Spence, 1966). Other research in the area of stress and performance suggests that exposure to a stressor (particularly one that is unpredictable and uncontrollable) results in performance deficits on a number of types of tasks (Cohen, 1980; Glass & Singer, 1972). Still others in the field criticize the idea of a curvilinear relationship between stress and performance for confounding stress with arousal, and suggest that increased arousal and not stress is responsible for any enhancement in task performance (Stanley & Burrows, 1987; Westman & Eden, 1996).

Understanding the impact of stress on performance has important implications for the workplace. Stress can have a tangible impact on employee's health, job performance, and success in the military, government, and private sectors. In general, greater stress has been associated with decreased job performance, and this association has been observed in studies assessing job performance using a variety of methods from self-reports (e.g., Arshadi & Damiri, 2013; Kazmi, Amjad, & Khan, 2008) to peer-ratings (e.g., Motowidlo, Packard, & Manning, 1986), and objective measures (e.g., Jamal, 2011). A study of 286 employees of an Iranian National Drilling company, for example, reported a significant, negative correlation between self-ratings of job stress and job performance (Arshadi & Damiri, 2013). In addition, a study of 171 nurses found that subjective stress was negatively correlated with six out of seven performance measures rated by a supervisor or a co-worker (Motowidlo et al., 1986). Similarly, a study of employees in Malaysia ($N = 305$) and Pakistan ($N = 325$) observed a negative linear relationship between subjective stress and objective job performance measures derived from business information contained in company files (Jamal, 2011).

For the most part, research on employees has yielded limited evidence of the hypothesized inverse U-shaped association between stress and performance (Yerkes & Dodson, 1908). A study of stress and job performance among nurses, however, did find a U-shaped association – but in the opposite direction – such that nurses who reported moderate levels of job stress believed that they performed their jobs less well than did those who reported low or high levels of job stress (AbuAlRub, 2004). A review of the literature, however, suggests that the failure to support the U-shaped hypothesis may be because of three critical research design limitations in the current literature (Muse, Harris, & Feild, 2003). First, research may not adequately identify or study individuals reporting low stress. Second, the negative connotation of stress may lead people to consistently under-report their stress levels (as an artifact of social desirability). Third, there may be a contextual range restriction on stress; the situations being studied may not elicit a broad enough range of responses to see a U-shaped relationship, if one exists. It remains to be seen whether rigorous studies that address the specified limitations will yield more support for the hypothesized inverse U-shape association between stress and job performance.

Job Stress and Performance

In addition to studies that have examined broad measures of job stress, a number of researchers have also examined whether specific aspects of job stress are associated with job performance. One study, for example, found that role conflict and role ambiguity (potential indicators of job stress) were negatively associated with job performance (Babin & Boles, 1996). Another study examined three dimensions of job stress – workload, emotional demands, and work/home conflict – and their associations with in-role and extra-role job performance (Bakker, Demerouti, & Verbeke, 2004). Although the job stress measures were not significantly related to in-role job performance, workload was significantly and positively correlated with extra-role job performance (Bakker et al., 2004).

Researchers have also applied meta-analytic techniques to better understand which aspects of job stress most consistently and directly relate to job performance. One meta-analysis, for example, statistically combined 169 samples and examined seven work-related stressors: role ambiguity, role conflict, role overload, job insecurity, work–family conflict, environmental uncertainty, and situational constraints (Gilboa, Shirom, Fried, & Cooper, 2008). The researchers observed a negative correlation between each of the seven stressors and job performance. In addition, role ambiguity and situational constraints were the stressors most strongly related negatively to performance. Two additional meta-analyses also revealed negative relationships between role ambiguity and job performance (Abramis, 1994; Tubre & Collins, 2000). Tubre and Collins (2000) also found only a negligible relationship between role conflict and job performance. These findings suggest that Army soldiers experiencing role ambiguity, role conflict, and situational constraints may also have compromised performance. These job stress factors may be especially likely to arise during high-demand situations such as training and deployment; however, research has not yet examined these potential connections. One avenue that should also be examined is the potential differential impact of job stress on performance of civilian and military personnel, and in different contexts. For example, it may be that these stressors have a similar effect on civilians and soldiers in "every day" situations, but vastly different effects on soldiers in training and combat situations.

Factors Influencing the Relationship between Stress and Job Performance

Researchers have examined a number of other moderators and mediators of the link between stress and job performance. Tubre and Collins (2000), for example, also found that job type moderates the association between role ambiguity and job performance. Specifically, the true score correlation between role ambiguity and job performance was greater for employees in professional, technical, and managerial jobs than for employees in clerical and sales or service jobs. In addition, another study found that organization-based self-esteem (OBSE) significantly moderated the relationship between job stress and job performance (Arshadi & Damiri, 2013). Employees with low OBSE may cope more passively with negative stimuli at the workplace, such as through increased absences and lower commitment and intrinsic motivation, which may result in decreased job performance (Arshadi & Damiri, 2013).

In addition to identifying key moderators of the stress and job performance association, researchers have also been in search of key factors that may mediate this relationship. One study, for example, found that depression mediates the negative association between stress and job performance (Motowidlo et al., 1986). Another study showed that greater self-reports of job demands (modeled as a latent measure) were associated with more exhaustion, which was associated with decreased in-role performance (Bakker et al., 2004). In addition, the path model revealed that job demands had a positive and direct effect on in-role performance such that greater self-rated job demands were associated with greater colleague-rated in-role performance (Bakker et al., 2004).

Performance and Physical Health

Another important factor in the relationship between stress and job performance is physical health, which may be of particular relevance to soldiers, given the physically demanding nature of their jobs. A number of links between stress and physical health have been identified clearly in the scientific literature. Chronic or persistently elevated levels of stress hormones have been shown to cause systemic inflammation and increase susceptibility to infections. Stress also has a profound impact on cardiovascular health. As noted earlier, stress hormones increase heart rate and blood pressure; stressors can trigger a cardiac event in patients with cardiovascular disease. Stress can also impact health behaviors, increasing the likelihood that an individual will engage in potentially harmful health behaviors such as cigarette smoking, eating junk food, and drinking alcohol to excess.

Given the impact stress has on physical health, and the consistent associations observed between stress and job performance, it is important to understand how physical health may also be related to performance at the workplace. Indeed, across a number of occupations (e.g., health care, insurance, and finance), chronic health conditions have been associated with decreased work performance and increased presenteeism. Obesity, in particular, has been linked with decreased job performance (Burton, Conti, Chen, Schultz, & Edington, 1999; Merrill et al., 2012, 2013), and diabetes has been linked to reduced productivity both cross-sectionally and over time (Burton et al., 1999; Gandy, Coberley, Pope, & Rula, 2014). Other studies have examined a spectrum of chronic conditions (e.g., high blood pressure, high cholesterol, diabetes, depression, heart attack, asthma, and pain) and observed links to decreased job performance and greater presenteeism (Burton, Pransky, Conti, Chen, & Edington, 2004; Collins, Karasek, & Costas, 2005; Frey, Osteen, Berglund, Junnett, & Ko, 2015; Merrill et al., 2012, 2013). Collins et al. (2005), for example, found that reporting a primary chronic health condition was associated with an 18% to 36% decrease in the ability to function at work. In addition, having a greater number of chronic health conditions has been associated with a decrease in overall productivity (Burton et al., 1999). Other chronic – and even acute – conditions may be of particular relevance for soldiers as they may be more likely to experience injury and physical health problems.

Performance and Health Behaviors

In order to identify potential intervention opportunities, a number of studies have examined associations between health behaviors (risk or protective) and job performance. Greater job performance has been linked with eating a healthy diet, consuming more fruits and vegetables, and exercising more (LeCheminant, Merrill, & Masterson, 2015; Merchant et al., 2014; Merrill et al., 2013). In addition, not eating a healthy diet, consuming fewer fruits and vegetables, and exercising less has been associated with a greater likelihood of being in the top quintile on presenteeism, while not smoking was associated with a lower likelihood of being in that group (Merrill et al., 2012). Along with this, a study of over 1,000 Taiwanese employees found that health behaviors mediated the association between organizational health culture and self-rated job performance (Lin & Lin, 2014). Extending this work to employer-sponsored interventions, studies show that employers who implement physical activity interventions can improve both the health of their personnel and simultaneously improve worksite productivity and outcomes (Conn, Hafdahl, Cooper, Brown, & Lusk, 2009).

Longitudinal studies provide an opportunity to assess the extent to which changes in health behaviors are associated with changes in job performance. For example, a three-year longitudinal study showed that greater health risks were related to decreased job productivity at baseline, and increasing health risks over time were related to decreased job productivity at subsequent measurement periods (Grossmeier, Mangen, Terry, & Haglund-Howieson, 2015). In another study, however, changes in well-being over two years predicted changes in job performance and presenteeism better than changes in health risk behaviors did (Gandy,

Coberley, Pope, & Rula, 2016). Thus, there may be other important factors to consider that play a role in the connection between physical health behaviors and job performance.

Performance and Mental Health

In light of the many ways in which stress impacts people's mental health and their interactions with their environment, it is also important to consider the extent to which mental health may relate to performance in the workplace. Higher psychological distress, in general, has been consistently linked with compromised job performance. For example, a study of over 60,000 employees in varied occupations found that higher psychological distress was associated with increased presenteeism across eight occupation types (i.e., executive, professional, technical, sales, clerical, service, precision production, and operator and laborer; Hilton, Scuffham, Sheridan, Cleary, & Whiteford, 2008). In addition, a smaller study of emergency service workers in Germany ($N = 87$) found that psychosomatic complaints were associated with decreased task performance both concurrently and when psychosomatic complaints were measured at the end of the workweek (i.e., Thursday or Friday evening) before task performance was assessed at the beginning of the following workweek (Fritz & Sonnentag, 2005). Another study of telephone customer service agents also found that high general distress was associated with failing to meet the company's productivity standard (Burton et al., 1999).

Depression may be one of the psychiatric disorders most studied in relation to job performance. Stewart, Ricci, Chee, Hahn, and Morganstein (2003) estimated that US workers with depression cost employers $35.73 billion per year in presenteeism, which is $26.56 billion more than the estimated cost of presenteeism among employees without depression. Indeed, across studies, there is a clear pattern that depression has a negative impact on employee performance (e.g., Lerner & Henke, 2008). Jain et al. (2013), for example, found that as depression severity increases, work productivity decreases, even after controlling for potential confounders such as demographic characteristics, type of employment, education level, and use of antidepressants. These findings are echoed by a study that demonstrated that individuals with depression reported more presenteeism than those without depression (4.6 hours per week compared to 1.1 hours per week, respectively; Stewart et al., 2003). Furthermore, employees with a clinical diagnosis of depression were less productive than employees in a healthy control group (Lerner et al., 2004). Depression may have long-lasting effects on job performance; Adler et al. (2006) found that even employees demonstrating clinical improvement of their depression remained consistently below control groups in terms of job performance. Although research indicates that some soldiers experience mental health issues, such as depression and post-traumatic stress disorder, there is no current evidence regarding the impact of these mental health conditions on job performance metrics.

Comparative Impact of Physical and Mental Health

While it is clear that physical health and mental health each exhibit a negative impact on job performance, it is important to also consider the relative importance of each health domain to job performance. Among studies that examined a combination of physical and mental conditions, mental health conditions consistently demonstrated stronger associations with job performance. For instance, in a sample of Reserve Officer Training Corps cadets, psychological strain was more highly correlated with objective job performance ratings (by trained assessors) than was physical strain (Lang, Thomas, Bliese, & Adler, 2007). In addition, Collins et al. (2005) found that depression, anxiety, and emotional disorders were associated with more work impairment than any physical condition studied. Similarly, a study of financial service employees found that depression demonstrated stronger associations with work limitations in time management (odds ratio [OR] = 2.05) and overall output (OR = 2.24), compared to the associations between any of the physical conditions examined and work limitations and overall output (Burton et al., 2004). A population-based study conducted in the Netherlands found that self-rated poor general health, as well as reporting two or more chronic conditions, was associated with low job performance (Van den Heuvel, Geuskens, Hooftman, Koppes, & Van den Bossche, 2010). Multivariate analyses examining the type of health condition revealed that psychological complaints or disorders were most strongly associated with low performance at work. In fact, of the 11 physical conditions examined, only musculoskeletal complaints were significantly associated with increased odds of low work performance (Van den Heuvel et al., 2010).

Ultimately, stress, physical health, health behaviors, and mental health are all important correlates of job performance. Mental health issues, in particular, may compromise job performance among employees. Additional research and evaluation efforts should continue to examine the extent to which different aspects of stress and health impact job performance. Importantly, additional research should examine these issues within a military context, given the particularly stressful nature of soldiers' jobs and the serious consequences of compromised performance within this context.

LESSONS LEARNED FOR ARMY JOB PERFORMANCE METRICS

Measurement is a cornerstone of a well-functioning army, and the Army gathers an enormous amount of data on its soldiers, missions, allies, and enemies. Further, all of these data can be integrated to help inform military strategy, logistics, and policies, including soldier performance. We know that experiencing stress and compromised physical or mental health can have negative effects on job performance. For the Army, these connections are especially critical, as soldiers are often in stressful and demanding situations, where performance can have life-or-death consequences. Given this, it may be beneficial for the Army to utilize stress- and health-related metrics as indicators of job performance.

However, using health and performance metrics could have consequences, which include the metric itself becoming a driving force behind soldiers' health behaviors. For example, career soldiers can be extremely competitive, and any metric used to assess job performance could easily become a motivating factor for their behavior. This can have positive effects (e.g., better overall performance), but also has the potential to become a corrupting influence (e.g., soldiers avoiding medical care for acute or chronic health issues).

One approach that minimizes the impact of metrics on the processes they measure is to avoid using stress- and health-related issues as indicators of an individual soldier's performance, and instead aggregate soldiers' data at a company-level to serve as an indicator of unit and leader performance. With this approach, the information of each individual soldier within a company would be considered in aggregate as an indicator of leadership performance. An aggregated approach would not put undue pressure on any individual soldier with stress or health problems, but would provide visibility on units in which there are significant concerns (e.g., those companies more than one standard deviation above the mean value of all companies). Focusing on company-level metrics allows for enough soldiers to calculate psychometrically stable estimates, while also limiting the aggregation to meaningful groups (e.g., units that regularly interact together and know their leaders).

The second approach is to use non-reactive measurement strategies, or those that do not involve direct contact with individuals (Webb, Campbell, Schwartz, & Sechrest, 1999). Asking soldiers or leaders to report directly stress and health issues would likely result in compromised metrics, as soldiers would inaccurately report problems in order to appear better performing; in other words, a self-presentation bias might lead to under-reporting of health issues. Instead, non-reactive measures, such as data that are routinely collected (e.g., administrative data and annual physicals) or observable natural behavior or occurrences (e.g., counting how many people enter the medical treatment facility on a certain day) can be used. For the Army, stress- and health-related issues could be measured using health care data. Frequency of health care utilization and severity of stress- and health-related diagnoses, for example, are routinely collected and stored by the Army. These metrics could also augment statistics on soldiers' readiness for deployment.

Aggregating measures at the company-level and using non-reactive measures have several key strengths in this context. First, the concerns related to self-presentation bias and under-reporting of health issues would not have as great an influence on the measure as the data would be routinely collected for other purposes. Second, using these non-reactive measures can minimize the time and effort associated with collecting data directly from soldiers; this is true for both researchers and soldiers themselves. Finally, these kinds of aggregated, non-reactive measures are more easily available (e.g., in a military data repository) for military-sponsored projects than direct measures.

DIRECTIONS FOR FUTURE RESEARCH ON JOB PERFORMANCE, STRESS, AND HEALTH

While the research on stress, health, and job performance highlights opportunities for the Army to improve job performance metrics, this research also points to opportunities for the future research efforts to refine job performance measures when examining the connections between soldiers' stress and job performance. First and foremost, there is a wide field for rigorous investigation of the associations between stress, health, and job performance within the Army. In addition, existing data available from military sources, such as the Person-event Data Environment (PDE), can be a boon for researchers in this field. With these secondary data come several constraints, however, that researchers must consider and address. Along with this, Army leadership can receive better information about the performance of the force and the critical ways to continue to increase health, reduce stress, and improve performance.

The Person–Event Data Environment

One emerging research opportunity within the Department of Defense (DoD) is the use of extant population-level data housed within databases supporting the Army's and other services' operational missions; this may be especially useful because of military leaders' concern over service member survey fatigue and over exposure to research studies. The PDE is a cloud-based computing environment that houses data on millions of past and current DoD employees and their dependents (Vie, Griffith, Scheier, Lester, & Seligman, 2013; Vie et al., 2015). As of this writing, the system merges data from major military databases, which include over 700 major data files and over 19,000 individual variables. The PDE holds an array of human resources, medical, combat deployment, family, social services, and survey data. Since the PDE is a cloud-based computing environment, the data do not leave the PDE. Rather, researchers access the PDE cloud virtually from anywhere in the world, provided they are cleared to do so and have the proper equipment and permissions.

Published research is emerging from the use of the PDE. For example, researchers using data from the PDE recently published a study identifying vulnerable populations of those who are at significantly higher risk of developing PTSD, even before those individuals were exposed to combat operations (Shen, Arkes, & Lester, 2017). Another group of researchers used PDE data to validate a psychometric instrument given to all soldiers in the Army annually, known as the Global Assessment Tool (GAT; Vie, Scheier, Lester, & Seligman, 2016). Finally, data from the PDE were used to examine the link between attrition from the Army and soldiers' mental health, along with the associated economic impact to the Army (Cunha, Arkes, Lester, & Shen, 2015). In sum, the PDE and its data are being used to meet the needs of the Army while also advancing generalizable scientific knowledge.

Data Constraints

Using existing Army data can be extremely beneficial for researchers interested in Army job performance. These data, however, have several constraints that researchers should address. Researchers examining Army soldiers' job performance, for instance, often do not have the luxury of administering their preferred measure of job performance. Instead, they are limited to information that is already gathered on soldiers. These kinds of Army records are collected for administrative purposes, not research purposes, and often have data quality and methodological concerns. For example, administrative data could have data entry errors or incomplete records that researchers must identify and correct. In addition, existing data may not be as precise or specific as a researcher would prefer. In these cases, it can be helpful to utilize proxy measures that assess concepts related to job performance (e.g., promotions and awards). Researchers can also consider using multiple measures of job performance to help triangulate concepts of interest.

Using existing Army data can also present unique challenges for longitudinal studies. Unlike carefully constructed longitudinal research designs, which collect baseline measures at a single time point and administer follow-up measures at equally spaced intervals, the timing of Army records varies widely. Soldiers enter the Army at different times, deploy at different times, complete paperwork at different times, and experience outcomes of interest (e.g., receive an early promotion) at different times. Researchers examining longitudinal research questions for Army soldiers can apply gating criteria to impose a temporal structure in their data. This can involve specifying a baseline period, which can be arbitrary (e.g., fiscal year 2010) or meaningful (e.g., first 12 months of a soldier's service), and gating can involve specifying spacing requirements for follow-up records (e.g., measures must be 9–15 months apart). Researchers can choose to be more restrictive (which reduces unwanted variation in spacing between measures but decreases the sample size) or less restrictive (which yields a larger sample size with greater variation between time points) based on what is most important for the research question. In addition, conducting analyses that use variables originally assessed in different forms requires additional gating criteria (e.g., Forms X, Y, and Z must be completed during FY 2010). As the number of forms required during a specified time window increases, the number of soldiers who meet the gating criteria decreases. Additional forms can also add unintended variation in timing to a set of measures (e.g., baseline characteristics), depending on the gating criteria set (e.g., Form X could be completed on October 1, 2009, while Form Y could be completed on September 30, 2010). In these instances, researchers must weigh the value added by including each additional measure against the loss in sample size and the statistical power to capture an effect, if one exists.

CONCLUSION

Continued research on military job performance, stress, and health can have significant benefits for the fields of military psychology and industrial/organizational psychology. As we continue to better understand these factors and their associations, we can improve our theories, definitions, and the measures we use. Accurate, robust, and psychometrically sound measures of job performance can lead to improvements within both academic and military communities. As the quality of our indicators increases, so do the rigor and reliability of our research findings. These improvements also translate into increased efficiency and productivity within organizations such as the Army.

REFERENCES

Abramis, D. J. (1994). Work role ambiguity, job satisfaction, and job performance: Meta-analyses and review. *Psychological Reports*, *75*(3 suppl), 1411–1433. doi:10.2466/pr0.1994.75.3f.1411

AbuAlRub, R. F. (2004). Job stress, job performance, and social support among hospital nurses. *Journal of Nursing Scholarship*, *36*(1), 73–78. doi:10.1111/j.1547-5069.2004.04016.x

Adler, D. A., McLaughlin, T. J., Rogers, W. H., Chang, H., Lapitsky, L., & Lerner, D. (2006). Job performance deficits due to depression. *American Journal of Psychiatry*, *163*(9), 1569–1576. doi:10.1176/ajp.2006.163.9.1569

American Psychological Association. (2017). *Stress in America: Coping with change*. Stress in America™ Survey. Retrieved from https://www.apa.org

Anderson, C. R. (1976). Coping behaviors as intervening mechanisms in the inverted-U stress–performance relationship. *Journal of Applied Psychology*, *61*(1), 30–34. doi:10.1037/0021-9010.61.1.30

Arshadi, N., & Damiri, H. (2013). The relationship of job stress with turnover intention and job performance: Moderating role of OBSE. *Procedia-Social and Behavioral Sciences*, *84*, 706–710. doi:10.1016/j.sbspro.2013.06.631

Babin, B. J., & Boles, J. S. (1996). The effects of perceived co-worker involvement and supervisor support on service provider role stress, performance and job satisfaction. *Journal of Retailing*, *72*(1), 57–75. doi:10.1016/S0022-4359(96)90005-6

Bakker, A. B., Demerouti, E., & Verbeke, W. (2004). Using the job demands–resources model to predict burnout and performance. *Human Resource Management*, *43*(1), 83–104. doi:10.1002/hrm.20004

Barrick, M. R., & Mount, M. K. (1991). The big five personality dimensions and job performance: A meta-analysis. *Personnel Psychology*, *44*(1), 1–26. doi:10.1111/j.1744-6570.1991.tb00688.x

Borman, W. C., & Motowidlo, S. J. (1997). Task performance and contextual performance: The meaning for personnel selection research. *Human Performance*, *10*(2), 99–109. doi:10.1207/s15327043hup1002_3

Brief, A. P., & Motowidlo, S. J. (1986). Prosocial organizational behaviors. *Academy of Management Review*, *11*(4), 710–725. doi:10.5465/AMR.1986.4283909

Burton, W. N., Conti, D. J., Chen, C. Y., Schultz, A. B., & Edington, D. W. (1999). The role of health risk factors and disease on worker productivity. *Journal of Occupational and Environmental Medicine*, *41*(10), 863–877. Retrieved from http://journals.lww.com

Burton, W. N., Pransky, G., Conti, D. J., Chen, C. Y., & Edington, D. W. (2004). The association of medical conditions and presenteeism. *Journal of Occupational and Environmental Medicine*, *46*(6), S38–S45. Retrieved from http://journals.lww.com

Cohen, S. (1980). Aftereffects of stress on human performance and social behavior: A review of research and theory. *Psychological Bulletin*, *88*(1), 82. doi:10.1037/0033-2909.88.1.82

Collins, S. M., Karasek, R. A., & Costas, K. (2005). Job strain and autonomic indices of cardiovascular disease risk. *American Journal of Industrial Medicine*, *48*(3), 182–193. doi:10.1002/ajim.20204

Conn, V. S., Hafdahl, A. R., Cooper, P. S., Brown, L. M., & Lusk, S. L. (2009). Meta-analysis of workplace physical activity interventions. *American Journal of Preventive Medicine*, *37*(4), 330–339. doi:10.1016/j.amepre.2009.06.008

Cunha, J. M., Arkes, J., Lester, P. B., & Shen, Y. C. (2015). Employee retention and psychological heath: Evidence from military recruits. *Applied Economic Letters*, *22*(18), 1505–1510. doi:10.1080/13504851.2015.1042136

Frey, J. J., Osteen, P. J., Berglund, P. A., Jinnett, K., & Ko, J. (2015). Predicting the impact of chronic health conditions on workplace productivity and accidents: Results from two US Department of Energy national laboratories. *Journal of Occupational and Environmental Medicine*, *57*(4), 436–444. doi:10.1097/JOM.0000000000000383

Fritz, C., & Sonnentag, S. (2005). Recovery, health, and job performance: Effects of weekend experiences. *Journal of Occupational Health Psychology*, *10*(3), 187–199. doi:10.1037/1076-8998.10.3.187

Gandy, W. M., Coberley, C., Pope, J. E., & Rula, E. Y. (2014). Well-being and employee health – How employees' well-being scores interact with demographic factors to influence risk of hospitalization or an emergency room visit. *Population Health Management*, *17*(1), 13–20. doi:10.1089/pop.2012.0120

Gandy, W. M., Coberley, C., Pope, J. E., & Rula, E. Y. (2016). Comparison of the utility of two assessments for explaining and predicting productivity change: Well-being versus an HRA. *Journal of Occupational and Environmental Medicine*, *58*(1), 69–75. doi:10.1097/JOM.0000000000000598

George, J. M., & Brief, A. P. (1992). Feeling good-doing good: A conceptual analysis of the mood at work-organizational spontaneity relationship. *Psychological Bulletin*, *112*(2), 310–329. doi:10.1037/0033-2909.112.2.310

Gilboa, S., Shirom, A., Fried, Y., & Cooper, C. (2008). A meta-analysis of work demand stressors and job performance: Examining main and moderating effects. *Personnel Psychology*, *61*(2), 227–271. doi:10.1111/j.1744-6570.2008.00113.x

Glass, D. C., & Singer, J. E. (1972). *Urban stress: Experiments on noise and social stressors*. New York, NY: New York Academic Press.

Grossmeier, J., Mangen, D. J., Terry, P. E., & Haglund-Howieson, L. (2015). Health risk change as a predictor of productivity change. *Journal of Occupational and Environmental Medicine*, *57*(4), 347–354. doi:10.1097/JOM.0000000000000408

Hilton, M. F., Scuffham, P. A., Sheridan, J., Cleary, C. M., & Whiteford, H. A. (2008). Mental ill-health and the differential effect of employee type on absenteeism and presenteeism. *Journal of Occupational and Environmental Medicine*, *50*(11), 1228–1243. doi:10.1097/JOM.0b013e31818c30a8

Hoge, C. W., Auchterlonie, J. L., & Milliken, C. S. (2006). Mental health problems, use of mental health services, and attrition from military service after returning from deployment to Iraq or Afghanistan. *JAMA*, *295*(9), 1023–1032. doi:10.1001/jama.295.9.1023

Hourani, L. L., Williams, T. V., & Kress, A. M. (2006). Stress, mental health, and job performance among active duty military personnel: Findings from the 2002 Department of Defense Health-Related Behaviors Survey. *Military Medicine*, *171*(9), 849–856. Retrieved from https://search.proquest.com

Jain, G., Roy, A., Harikrishnan, V., Yu, S., Dabbous, O., & Lawrence, C. (2013). Patient-reported depression severity measured by the PHQ-9 and impact on work productivity: Results from a survey of full-time employees in the United States. *Journal of Occupational and Environmental Medicine*, *55*(3), 252–258. doi:10.1097/JOM.0b013e31828349c9

Jamal, M. (2011). Job stress, job performance and organizational commitment in a multinational company: An empirical study in two countries. *International Journal of Business and Social Science*, *2*(20), 20–29. Retrieved from www.ijbssnet.com

Janis, I. L., & Mann, L. (1977). *Decision-making: A psychological analysis of conflict, choice, and commitment*. New York, NY: Free Press.

Kaufman, K. R., Brodine, S., & Shaffer, R. (2000). Military training-related injuries: Surveillance, research, and prevention. *American Journal of Preventive Medicine*, *18*(3), 54–63. doi:10.1016/S0749-3797(00)00114-8

Kazmi, R., Amjad, S., & Khan, D. (2008). Occupational stress and its effect on job performance. A case study of medical house officers of district Abbottabad. *Journal of Ayub Medical College Abbottabad*, *20*(3), 135–139. Retrieved from http://www.ayubmed.edu

Lang, J., Thomas, J. L., Bliese, P. D., & Adler, A. B. (2007). Job demands and job performance: The mediating effect of psychological and physical strain and the moderating effect of role clarity. *Journal of Occupational Health Psychology*, *12*(2), 116–124. doi:10.1037/1076-8998.12.2.116

Lauder, T. D., Baker, S. P., Smith, G. S., & Lincoln, A. E. (2000). Sports and physical training injury hospitalizations in the army. *American Journal of Preventive Medicine*, *18*(3), 118–128. doi:10.1016/S0749-3797(99)00174-9

LeCheminant, J. D., Merrill, R. M., & Masterson, T. (2015). Health behaviors and work-related outcomes among school employees. *American Journal of Health Behavior*, *39*(3), 345–351. doi:10.5993/AJHB.39.3.7

Lerner, D., Adler, D. A., Chang, H., Berndt, E. R., Irish, J. T., Lapitsky, L., … Rogers, W. H. (2004). The clinical and occupational correlates of work productivity loss among employed patients with depression. *Journal of Occupational and Environmental Medicine/American College of Occupational and Environmental Medicine*, *46*(60), S46–S55. Retrieved from https://www.ncbi.nlm.nih.gov

Lerner, D., & Henke, R. M. (2008). What does research tell us about depression, job performance, and work productivity? *Journal of Occupational and Environmental Medicine, 50*(4), 401–410. doi:10.1097/JOM.0b013e31816bae50

Lin, Y. W., & Lin, Y. Y. (2014). A multilevel model of organizational health culture and the effectiveness of health promotion. *American Journal of Health Promotion, 29*(1), e53–e63. doi:10.4278/ajhp.121116-QUAN-562

McEwen, B. S. (2005). Glucocorticoids, depression, and mood disorders: Structural remodeling in the brain. *Metabolism, 54*(5), 20–23. doi:doi:10.1016/j.metabol.2005.01.008

Merchant, J. A., Kelly, K. M., Burmeister, L. F., Lozier, M. J., Amendola, A., Lind, D. P., … & Buikema, B. S. (2014). Employment status matters: A statewide survey of quality-of-life, prevention behaviors, and absenteeism and presenteeism. *Journal of Occupational and Environmental Medicine, 56*(7), 686–698. doi:10.1097/JOM.0000000000000149

Merrill, R. M., Aldana, S. G., Pope, J. E., Anderson, D. R., Coberley, C. R., Grossmeier, J. J., & Whitmer, R. W. (2013). Self-rated job performance and absenteeism according to employee engagement, health behaviors, and physical health. *Journal of Occupational and Environmental Medicine, 55*(1), 10–18. doi:10.1097/JOM.0b013e31827b73af

Merrill, R. M., Aldana, S. G., Pope, J. E., Anderson, D. R., Coberley, C. R., Whitmer, R. W, & the HERO Research Study Subcommittee. (2012). Presenteeism according to healthy behaviors, physical health, and work environment. *Population Health Management, 15*(5), 293–301. doi:10.1089/pop.2012.0003

Motowidlo, S. J., Packard, J. S., & Manning, M. R. (1986). Occupational stress: Its causes and consequences for job performance. *Journal of Applied Psychology, 71*(4), 618–629. doi:10.1037/0021-9010.71.4.618

Motowidlo, S. J., & Van Scotter, J. R. (1994). Evidence that task performance should be distinguished from contextual performance. *Journal of Applied Psychology, 79*(4), 475–480. doi:10.1037/0021-9010.79.4.475

Muse, L. A., Harris, S. G., & Feild, H. S. (2003). Has the inverted-U theory of stress and job performance had a fair test? *Human Performance, 16*(4), 349–364. doi:10.1207/S15327043HUP1604_2

Nerurkar, A., Bitton, A., Davis, R. B., Phillips, R. S., & Yeh, G. (2013). When physicians counsel about stress: Results of a national study. *JAMA Internal Medicine, 173*(1), 76–77. doi:10.1001/2013.jamainternmed.480

Organ, D. W. (1988). A restatement of the satisfaction-performance hypothesis. *Journal of Management, 14*(4), 547–557. doi:10.1177/014920638801400405

Park, J. (2007). *Work stress and job performance*. Ottawa, Canada: Statistics Canada.

Sears, L. E., Shi, Y., Coberley, C. R., & Pope, J. E. (2013). Overall well-being as a predictor of health care, productivity, and retention outcomes in a large employer. *Population Health Management, 16*(6), 397–405. doi:10.1089/pop.2012.0114

Selye, H. (1956). *The stress of life*. New York, NY: McGraw-Hill.

Shen, Y. C., Arkes, J., Lester, P. B. (2017). Resourcing psychological health in demanding workplaces: An empirical examination. *BMC Psychology*. Retrieved from https://bmcpsychology.biomedcentral.com

Spence, J. T., & Spence, K. W. (1966). The motivational components of manifest anxiety: Drive and drive stimuli. In C. D. Spielberger (Ed.), *Anxiety and behavior* (pp. 291–326). New York, NY: Academic Press.

Stanley, G., & Burrows, G. D. (1987). *Stress: Theory and practice*. Sydney, Australia: Grune & Stratton.

Stewart, W. F., Ricci, J. A., Chee, E., Hahn, S. R., & Morganstein, D. (2003). Cost of lost productive work time among US workers with depression. *JAMA, 289*(23), 3135–3144. doi:10.1001/jama.289.23.3135

Tanielian, T., Jaycox, L. H., Schell, T. L., Marshall, G. N., Burnam, M. A., Eibner, C., … Vaiana, M. E. (2008). *Invisible wounds of war. Summary and recommendations for addressing psychological and cognitive injuries*. Santa Monica, CA: RAND. Retrieved from http://www.dtic.mil/get-tr-doc/pdf?AD=ADA480992

Tubre, T. C., & Collins, J. M. (2000). Jackson and Schuler (1985) revisited: A meta-analysis of the relationships between role ambiguity, role conflict, and job performance. *Journal of Management, 26*(1), 155–169. doi:10.1177/014920630002600104

Van den Heuvel, S. G., Geuskens, G. A., Hooftman, W. E., Koppes, L. L., & Van den Bossche, S. N. (2010). Productivity loss at work; health-related and work-related factors. *Journal of Occupational Rehabilitation*, *20*(3), 331–339. doi:10.1007/s10926-009-9219-7

Vie, L. L., Griffith, K. N., Scheier, L. M., Lester, P. B., & Seligman, M. E. P. (2013). The person-event data environment: Leveraging big data for studies of psychological strengths in soldiers. *Frontiers in Psychology*, *4*(934), 1–7. doi:10.3389/fpsyg.2013.00934

Vie, L. L., Scheier, L. M., Lester, P. B., Ho, T. E., Labarthe, D. R., Seligman, M. E. P. (2015). The U.S. army person-event data environment: A military-civilian big data enterprise. *Big Data*, *3*(2), 67–79. doi:10.1089/big.2014.0055

Vie, L. L., Scheier, L. M., Lester, P. B., & Seligman, M. E. (2016). Initial validation of the US army global assessment tool. *Military Psychology*, *28*(6), 468–487. doi:10.1037/mil0000141

Webb, E. J., Campbell, D. T., Schwartz, R. D., & Sechrest, L. (1999). *Unobtrusive measures* (Vol. 2). Thousand Oaks, CA: SAGE.

Westman, M., & Eden, D. (1996). The inverted-U relationship between stress and performance: A field study. *Work & Stress*, *10*(2), 165–173. doi:10.1080/02678379608256795

Yerkes, R. M., & Dodson, J. D. (1908). The relation of strength of stimulus to rapidity of habit formation. *Journal of Comparative Neurology and Psychology*, *18*(5), 459–482. doi:10.1002/cne.920180503

WORK, STRESS, AND HEALTH OF MILITARY COUPLES ACROSS TRANSITIONS

Wylie H. Wan, Sarah N. Haverly and Leslie B. Hammer

ABSTRACT

This chapter focuses on military couples and factors that affect their experiences of work, stress, and health using a life course perspective. An introduction to the definition of military couples is provided followed by a brief review of previous research on marital quality and divorce among military couples. The core of the chapter describes the advantages of using a life course perspective to examine the military life course for couples, and two critical transitions of military life are more fully examined. Specifically, periodic relocation and deployment and their impacts on military couples are reviewed in detail. Future directions for research on military couples are provided, and the use of the Convoy Model of Social Relations as an integrative approach to examine military personnel and family members' stress and health across the military life course is introduced.

Keywords: Military; couples; work and family; stress; health; life course; transitions

WHY STUDY MILITARY COUPLES?

It is widely known that close relationships and health are intricately tied, and there is now an emphasis on placing social connections as a public health priority (Dunkel Schetter, 2017; Holt-Lunstad, Robles, & Sbarra, 2017). While there

Occupational Stress and Well-being in Military Contexts
Research in Occupational Stress and Well-being, Volume 16, 69–90
Copyright © 2018 by Emerald Publishing Limited
All rights of reproduction in any form reserved
ISSN: 1479-3555/doi:10.1108/S1479-355520180000016005

are many important close relationships in a service member's life, this chapter focuses on military couples because spouses and partners are often the primary source of support for a service member, thus impacting stress, health, and well-being of the service member and the family (Norwood, Fullerton, & Hagen, 1996).

Whereas couples in the civilian workforce can experience day-to-day stress from work and family demands (e.g., work–family conflict or living in different locations), military couples have to manage these stresses within the context of military settings. There are many defining characteristics and contexts that shape the military way of life; for example, the distinct military language and culture, risk of injury and death, and the priorities of placing service before self (Segal, 1986). The military occupation inherently involves difficult and strenuous tasks that are physically and psychological demanding, and at times dangerous. When a person joins the military, their family and friends become an integral part of the military experience, as they share the lifestyle, joys, and hardships of being part of the larger military community.

Studying the contexts in which military couples live and work is important because military couples with a service member(s) in active duty, in the National Guard and Reserves (NG/R), or separated from the military can have significantly different lifestyles and challenges. During active duty, service members could be separated from friends and family periodically for prolonged periods. Daily anxiety can occur in the face of potential injury or death. Spouses and partners often have to adapt to being separated from their military partner, uproot their family and jobs to relocate, and cope with the ambiguity and stressors during military missions (Drummet, Coleman, & Cable, 2003). The task of caregiving to elderly relatives and children also fall on the spouse/partner while the service member is in training or on missions. Thus, the need to adjust to the absence and return of the service member can take a toll on the family, especially because service members are sometimes deployed for multiple times.

Service members who are transitioning out of the military have different needs and challenges than active duty service members. These veterans need to reintegrate into civilian life and adjust to being at home permanently, which may include maintaining feelings of worthiness and seeking new identities at work and at home. If they were deployed for long periods, the family also has to readjust to how the service member fits in their daily routine. The spouse/partner can play a significant role during this time, and the need for support is exemplified for veterans with severe injuries or post-traumatic stress disorder (PTSD). As a result, the marital or dating relationship can be strained during the long-term transition and recovery process. Feelings of guilt, stress, and shame may arise as spouses and partners are expected to provide support but do not receive enough support themselves, which can impact their own health and well-being. These couples may be faced with different stressors than couples with a service member in the NG/R.

For those in the NG/R, many couples have to navigate the life of the "weekend warrior" where service members are gone from home life for at least one weekend a month, also known as drill. These spouses and partners may need to adjust to their military partner's multiple work needs on a daily or weekly basis; for example, scheduling home activities may have to accommodate the civilian job on weekdays and drills on weekends. Part-time soldiers in the NG/R have also been called upon duty more frequently than ever for domestic deployments such as hurricanes, floods, and fires. Finally, these couples also face complexities during different stages of home life. For example, birth of a newborn, increasing demands of an aging parent, and teenagers testing the limits are all cases of challenging periods in a family life and are compounded by service members' relocation and deployment cycles.

Thus, military couples can have vastly different experiences depending on their military and home life stages, and researchers need to take into account these diverse circumstances when studying military couples. In addition, although there may be differences in the working environment of the military and civilian workforces, studying military couples can generalize to mainstream occupational stress and health research in terms of understanding communication, relationship maintenance, and work and home resources and stressors. Having greater understanding of military couples can, therefore, help service members manage military and civilian work roles, reintegrate into society after their military service, provide support for their families, and be a statement of acknowledgement and appreciation for those who have served the country.

The purpose of this chapter is to understand the stress, health, and well-being of military couples within the work–family context based on available research. First, the definition of the term "military couples" is discussed, followed by a brief overview of previous research on military couples that has focused on marital quality and divorce. Next, because the military lifestyle is filled with transitions, such as team changes, base relocation, deployment, and reintegration, the core of the chapter is on a review of studies on work–family transitions using the life course perspective as a guiding theoretical framework. Mainstream occupational stress and health research on couples has been examined predominately using the demands–resources model (Bakker & Demerouti, 2013), conservation of resources theory (Grandey & Cropanzano, 1999; Hobfoll, 1989), border and boundary theories (Ashforth, Kreiner, & Fugate, 2000; Clark, 2000), spillover–crossover theory (Westman, 2001), role conflict and enhancement theories (Barnett & Hyde, 2001; Greenhaus & Beutell, 1985; Greenhaus & Powell, 2006), as well as other general stress/strain models (e.g., Frone, Yardley, & Markel, 1997). These theories and perspectives tend to focus on current contexts and health with less attention paid to changes and transitions over time. The life course perspective is unique and insightful because it focuses on changes in couples' work and personal lives over time, allowing for an examination of major work–family transitions. In particular, two work–family transitions that are important and often experienced by military couples as part of the military lifestyle, namely periodic relocation and deployment, are examined. Lastly, future directions are suggested with the aim to enhance the health and well-being of military couples by striving for a more comprehensive understanding of their work and family experiences.

WHO ARE MILITARY COUPLES?

The term "military couples" used in this chapter broadly includes couples who are married or in a committed relationship in which one or both partners is/are currently active in the military or have separated from the military. This inclusive definition was selected because military couples are an extremely diverse population with varied racial, ethnic, gender, socioeconomic, and geographical backgrounds (Blaisure, Saathoff-Wells, Pereira, MacDermid Wadsworth, & Dombro, 2015; Clever & Segal, 2013). Thus, studying military couples can be challenging because they can be difficult to identify and differentiate. For example, there are differences between military branches on how relationship status is measured. The Navy asks soldiers to select "married" or "never married" on demographic forms, whereas other branches offer "divorced" and "other" options. As a result, much of the research available on military couples has focused on married spouses due to the ease of differentiating between service members who are married and those who are not, yet committed partners who are not married but who may still be pillars of support are often left out of consideration. Therefore, the term "spouse" is used in this chapter to refer to individuals who are married and the term "partner" refers to partners in a couple in general, including couples who are married, cohabitating, and dating, to be inclusive of and recognize these partners who may be strong supports for service members and play important roles in their military and personal lives.

Another reason for research to focus on married military couples is that the Department of Defense (DoD) recognizes marital relationships for the purpose of receiving benefits. Based on the reports of 2013, 2.2 million service members reported 3 million family members, of which 1.1 million were spouses (Office of the Deputy Assistant Secretary of Defense, 2014). Approximately 57% of active duty service members and 55% of reserve personnel reported family obligations (Office of the Deputy Assistant Secretary of Defense, 2014). Thirty-seven percent of reported family members were spouses and 63% were children. Across both active and reserve components, enlisted members and junior officers are less likely to be married than are senior enlisted members and senior officers. This may be, in large part, due to age differences, as junior service members are traditionally younger. Fifty-six percent of active duty personnel and 46% of reservists were married (Office of the Deputy Assistant Secretary of Defense, 2014). Furthermore, approximately 2.2% of the military personnel are lesbian, gay, and bisexuals (Gates, 2010). It is unclear as to how many of them are in committed relationships or married, but they are important to be taken into account, particularly in light of recent changes in both military policies and federal laws that allow same-sex spouses and families to receive benefits.

Based on the current research, one shortcoming of the literature on military couples is that it often focuses exclusively on married military couples, specifically military husbands and civilian wives (due to a majority of military couples identifying as such), with limited attention given to female service members with partners, same-sex couples, and marriages where both partners are service members (officially called dual-military couples). As a result, despite the fact that the majority of research covered in this chapter examined the male/female partnership, future research should examine military marriages and partnerships outside of traditional heterosexual relationships.

UNDERSTANDING RESEARCH ON MILITARY COUPLES

Previous Research on Married Military Couples

Much of the research on military couples in the past two decades has focused on examining influences within the marital relationship, such as marital satisfaction and divorce (Karney & Crown, 2007; Renshaw, Rodrigues, & Jones, 2008), communication skills (Blanchard, Hawkins, Baldwin, & Fawcett, 2009), and aggression and conflict (Heyman & Neidig, 1999; Marshall, Panuzio, & Taft, 2005). There are a considerable amount of studies on the effects of PTSD and the effects of alcohol use on couples' relationship quality (e.g., Allen, Rhoades, Stanley, & Markman, 2010; Cunradi, Caetano, & Schafer, 2002; Monson, Taft, & Fredman, 2009), as well as developments of couples therapy and programs to improve couples' communication (e.g., Gottman, Gottman, & Atkins, 2011). These studies have provided important knowledge to understand the trends of marriage and divorce of military couples, as well as risk factors that contribute to the likelihood of divorce.

Karney and Crown (2007) offers the thoughtful idea that there is a selection issue within military marriages. It is possible that some divorce cases among service members may stem from potentially premature marriages. Service men and women consistently marry at younger rates than the general US population, a fact, which Karney and Crown argue, is incentivized by the military due in part to the increased richness of benefits available to married service members. For example, married service members are compensated at a higher rate during deployments than are their single counterparts to account for "separation." Fortunately, recent research suggests that divorce rates are not as high as previously believed (Karney & Crown, 2007). Some researchers (e.g., Lundquist & Smith, 2005) have pointed out that since the institution of an all-volunteer force, military policies have been increasingly friendly to families and marriages, which may help marriages remain intact. While research is needed to examine the efficacy of these family-friendly military policies on family relationships and well-being, their existence has provided military families with access to potentially advantageous support systems (e.g., doctors and employment assistance) not available to civilian families.

However, in addition to research on military couples' marriages, researchers have repeatedly called for an expansion of the range of relevant predictors and outcomes of military couples beyond predictors of divorce (Karney & Crown, 2007; MacLean & Elder, 2007). The rest of this chapter answers this call by closely examining major work transitions that can impact military couples' stress, health, and well-being beginning with an examination of the military life course.

Military Service and the Life Course

Military life for both the service member and the partner begins when the service member decides to join the military, but it does not end when they end their service as the effects of being in the military continue throughout life. The life course perspective posits that earlier experiences in life, such as deployment and combat exposure, can shape the trajectories of our lives and the outcomes that occur later in life (e.g., stress, health, and well-being; MacLean & Elder, 2007). These trajectories can further be changed during major life transitions, for example, getting married or having children can have significant impact on later life outcomes. It is well-known that a defining characteristic of military life is that service members have to go through many transitions, from training and rotations to pre- and post-deployment to reintegration to civilian life. Personal lives also go through multiple transitions, such as parenthood, caregiving, re-employment, and relocation, which lead to the need for military couples to adapt quickly and frequently. As such, military service is a prime example that illustrates the principles of the life course perspective.

The idea of examining military service in the life course is not new (Clever & Segal, 2013; Elder, Gimbel, & Ivie, 1991; Gade, 1991; Modell & Haggerty, 1991; MacLean & Elder, 2007). Adopting a life course perspective was even hailed as a turning point for military personnel research in the early 1990s (Gade, 1991). One reason for this push to view military service through a life course lens was to change from an outcome-based approach in research, which links outcomes to antecedent events, to an event-based model, which links events to subsequent outcomes (Gade, 1991). Rather than focusing on a particular outcome, this approach is particularly useful in determining whether a transition, event, or intervention leads to positive or negative short-term and long-term consequences for service members and their families. Another major reason for adopting the life course perspective is that it emphasizes that the service member and partner are embedded within larger family, community, societal, and historical contexts, thus connecting the couple's life story to that of their changing relationships and environments throughout their military career, civilian career, and personal lives (MacLean & Elder, 2007).

The life course perspective has been increasingly considered as a vigorous and holistic framework for understanding military life (e.g., Drummet et al., 2003; Lundquist & Xu, 2014). In 2010, a report by the DoD published the Composite Life Cycle Model, which was based on Transitional Psychology and the Life Stage Theory (Chiarelli, 2010). The report focused on the idea of examining the effects of transitions, major life events, and stressors in the military. The model proposes that, in order to enhance service member well-being and reduce stress, the military needs "to focus on the whole person through a composite view of three separate strands: the Unit Life Cycle, the Soldier Life Cycle, and the Family Life Cycle" (Chiarelli, 2010, pp. 90–91). The Unit Life Cycle mainly comprises transitions that occur for the military unit, including pre-deployment, deployment, post-deployment, and reintegration or reset. The Soldier Life Cycle comprises transitions and events related to the military career, such as recruitment, reassignment, promotion, death of a squad member, and retirement. Finally, the Family Life Cycle recognizes major life events of a personal nature, such as marriage, childbirth, and geographic separation. The Composite Life Cycle Model portrays the complexities of military and family lives by showing that transitions in one strand do not necessarily synchronize with transitions in another strand, which can amplify the amount of stress felt by service members and their partners. It also suggests that if stress is not properly managed or reduced before the next transition (e.g., redeployment and financial difficulties after childbirth), it can accumulate over time with adverse impacts (Chiarelli, 2010).

In a follow-up report, one of the Army's major goals was to "set conditions to incorporate the Composite Life Cycle Model" and "to include identification of stress clusters in the Life Cycle strands of Unit, Soldier, and Family" (Chiarelli, 2010, p. 14). Since then, much of the attention to these reports has been on suicide prevention and couples' relationship education. Recommendations from researchers and the Army report indicate that more research is needed to identify stressors that relate to all three strands of the model to understand their effects on the service member and families (Chiarelli, 2010; Karney & Crown, 2007).

Although relatively little research on the military has explicitly drawn from the Composite Life Cycle Model (George, 2003; MacLean & Elder, 2007), researchers have examined military service using the broader life course perspective or with an event-based approach. A few studies on military families, including the Millennium Cohort Family Study (Crum-Cianflone, Fairbank, Marmar, & Schlenger, 2014), the Deployment Life Study (Meadows et al., 2016), and the Study on Employment Retention of Veterans (SERVe; Hammer, Wan, Brockwood, Mohr, & Carlson, 2017) have included spouses in their longitudinal studies and are discussed later in the section.

Transitions in the Military Life Course

The life course perspective emphasizes the ways in which transitions can have significant positive and negative impact on the trajectories of our lives. There are many important and common transitional events that can occur during a military life course, including the timing of recruitment and separation, the timing of when two individuals become a couple (e.g., before recruitment, during active service, or post-service), transitions within the military service (e.g., reassignment, relocation, and base closure), marriage and caregiving for children and relatives, and reintegration and reset. Resilience and adjustment to transitions can be key to creating positive experiences and outcomes for military couples. In this section, two specific transitional events – periodic relocation and deployment – are discussed because they are often experienced by military couples due to the military lifestyle and have been studied relatively more extensively in the literature.

Relocation

Periodic relocation is one of the hallmark transitions of military life. The active duty lifestyle, in particular, is inherently mobile and moves are frequent. For example, the Army relocates service members and their families, on average, every two to three years (Blaisure et al., 2015; Burrell, 2006). In the United States, a permanent change of station occurs when the military assigns a service member to a new duty station, leading to a relocation of military and personal lives. Military families move two to four times more than civilian families, and at times with little notice (Clever & Segal, 2013; Drummet et al., 2003). Compared to moves among civilian families, military relocation is more likely to be international or involve longer distances domestically (Booth et al., 2007; Griffith, Stewart, & Cato, 1988; Pittman & Bowen, 1994). Spouses, partners, and dependents are likely to move with the service member if the new station is at a significant distance from the former station. Each move can be considered as a new transition (i.e., a new turning point in the life course) that requires adjusting for both partners.

Although service members can indicate a preference as to where they would like to be stationed, the assignment ultimately depends on the needs of the military (Blaisure et al., 2015). As a result, while deployment was cited most often by spouses as the most stressful situation in the past five years, relocation was the next most cited stressful adjustment associated with military life for the couple (Dimiceli, Steinhardt, & Smith, 2010; Henry & Robichaux, 1999). Surveys of Army soldiers revealed that problems with the move, little notice for the move, finding and waiting for permanent housing, setting up the new household, and financial costs and delays in reimbursements all contribute to the stress associated with relocating (Booth et al., 2007; Bowen, Orthner, Zimmerman, & Meechan, 1992).

Relocation Effects on Couples. "Trailing spouses" is a term used to describe spouses (and partners) who frequently relocate due to their partner's employment (Keenan, 2011). Some partners adjust well to relocation and find exciting the opportunity to move to different places. One study found that the number of relocations was positively associated with well-being (Burrell, Adams, Durand, & Castro, 2006), whereas another found no relationship between relocation and well-being (Brett, 1982). For couples with children, research has found that children can have positive experiences (particularly academically) and not be significantly affected by relocations (Burland & Lundquist, 2013), whereas parents may be emotionally and physically spent due to the move (Drummet et al., 2003; Puskar, Wilson, & Moonis, 1990; Segal, 1986). Although relocation is a well-known part of military life and can be considered normative, some partners may have difficulties adapting to such frequent changes and unfamiliar surroundings and routines. Cumulative risk can also build up if partners have to relocate again before they have fully adjusted to the current living situation (Black, 1993). In cases where the couple has to relocate overseas, research has found negative influences of relocating on psychological and emotional health, although the effects varied depending on individual circumstances (Blakely, Hennessy, Chung, & Skirton, 2012; Burrell et al., 2006). Thus, over time, although there can be cumulative positive impact of relocating, such as exposure to different cultures, cumulative negative impact of relocating can be detrimental not only to the couple's relationship due to increased conflict, but also to their individual physical and psychological well-being later in life due to prolonged stress and maladjustment.

One reason for increased stress associated with moving is the loss of social support networks. This loss can occur within the military, for example, soldiers can return from deployment to find that they need to relocate because of a base closure and realignment, resulting in a fractured network support and loss of familiar access to military services. Loss can also occur outside the military as the service member and partner have to leave behind friends and family (Dimiceli et al., 2010), which can result in decreased social support and increased social isolation during an already stressful transition (Jervis, 2009; McNulty, 2003). Some couples may also experience cultural shock at their new location, which may add to the difficulty of establishing new close relationships, or they may think that the temporary nature of the move makes the emotional investment needed to form new friendships less worthwhile. Over time, lack of an adequate support network may take a toll on the couple's psychological health. Fortunately, research has found that social support from the community (e.g., military support personnel and participation in recreational programs) and from friends has a positive impact on military spouses' adjustment to relocation, with an even greater impact than the family's internal resources (e.g., supportive communication and family cohesion; Blakely et al., 2012; Lavee, McCubbin, & Patterson, 1985). Therefore, in addition to considering relocation as an opportunity for a positive bonding experience for the couple (Copeland & Norell, 2002), having greater external social support is essential to reducing stress and facilitating adjustment to frequent relocations. However, the use of military support services is affected by stigma and the military culture of sacrifice and putting duty first (Drummet et al., 2003). Given that the retention of service members can depend on spouses' satisfaction with the military (Bowen, 1987; Lakhani et al., 1985; Lundquist & Xu, 2014), reducing stigma and providing opportunities to maintain social support with existing support systems may be crucial for military couples as they adjust to their new location and build new supports. Having a supportive network during relocation may then promote a more positive trajectory for the couple's military life course, as well as enhance the quality of and extend the service member's active service.

Apart from a loss of external support due to relocation, military partners are also at risk of a loss of self-identity, including loss of individuality (i.e., being known as the "partner of" the service member) and loss of career identity. While some partners are content with either finding temporary jobs or not working, others experience feelings of worthlessness and stress associated with not being able to develop a career of their own (Jervis, 2009). Among civilian partners of service members, relocating is associated with difficulties in finding employment, a significant decline in employment, as well as a decline in work hours among those who remained employed (Cooke & Speirs, 2005; Southwell & MacDermid Wadsworth, 2016). Research has repeatedly shown that spouses believed that relocating has affected their employment opportunities, earning potential, career goals, difficulties in obtaining childcare, and employer bias and unwillingness to invest in an employee who may leave soon (Booth & Lederer, 2012; Castaneda & Harrell, 2008; Trougakos, Bull, Green, MacDermid, & Weiss, 2007). Compared to their civilian counterparts, wives of service members earn significantly less even if they are working for similar hours (Meadows, Griffin, Karney, & Pollak, 2016). Over the life course, military partners may be at a cumulative disadvantage in terms of employment and educational opportunities due to relocation. Since military partners' well-being and their satisfaction with the military depends on the quality of their employment (in addition to the quality of family life), employment assistant programs are effective and are needed to help partners obtain employment and boost their self-efficacy in order to lessen any long-term disadvantage accrued due to multiple relocations (Trougakos et al., 2007).

Based on the studies reviewed on relocation, most were conducted cross-sectionally or retrospectively, which makes it difficult to determine whether relocation, or which part of a relocation, has significant impact on couples. Examining the life course of military couples by taking into account pre-, during, and post-relocation (over multiple relocations) can greatly improve our understanding of their experiences, which is important, especially because relocation is a common, normative part of military life for couples. In addition, the majority of these studies examined only married spousal outcomes. Most of the studies did not include both partners of the same couple, making it difficult to understand how these partners help each other or cause strain for each other during a relocation transition. Lastly, the current literature focused mainly on active duty military couples in which a service member is married to a civilian partner. Dual military couples and NG/R have significantly different sets of challenges when there is a need to relocate. For example, NG/R who would like to relocate for personal or professional reasons in their civilian career may be unable to do so due to their military service. By expanding the study of relocation to identify the needs and challenges that occur over time for military couples among different branches and components, researchers may be able to help service members and their families establish a positive trajectory with better performance and quality of life.

Deployment

Apart from periodic relocation, deployment is another major transitional event that is commonly experienced by military couples. In the United States, there was a surge in deployment post-9/11 with peak deployments occurring in the mid-to-late 2000s (Meadows et al., 2016). Since then, deployments have been declining for both active duty and NG/R, but the nature of a volunteer military and the increased dependence on reserve components mean a greater likelihood of being deployed multiple times (Werber, Harrell, Varda, Hall, & Beckett, 2009). Deployments are assigned in all military branches and components, and can range from one week to 12 or 18 months or longer (Blaisure et al., 2015). Missions can be for combat, peacekeeping, or humanitarian purposes, which mean that deployments can be planned ahead of time with lengthy notice to make preparations, or with little notice, such as a response to a natural disaster.

Deployments can affect military couples in many ways. For the service member, especially for those with post-deployment PTSD symptoms and higher levels of stress, deployment has been associated with more marital conflict, increased risk of divorce, less satisfaction with the military, greater need for support, and greater economic strain (Allen et al., 2010; Allen, Rhoades, Stanley, & Markman, 2011; Karney & Crown, 2007; Negrusa, Negrusa, & Hosek, 2014). As for the spouse, deployment has consistently been linked to a wide range of mental health diagnoses (Mansfield et al., 2010). Longer deployment periods, deployment extensions, and combat exposure have been associated with more psychological problems for the spouse (Allen et al., 2011; De Burgh, White, Fear, & Iversen, 2011). Moreover, although deployment status was not associated with weight status, decreased social support was associated with the risk of being overweight or obese for spouses, which highlights the importance of perceived social support for spouses regardless of whether or not their military partner is deployed (Fish, Harrington, Bellin, & Shaw, 2014).

Deployment is also a unique transition to study because there may be gender differences in deployment effects for couples. Female service members are less likely to relocate and deploy less frequently than male service members (Southwell & MacDermid Wadsworth, 2016). At the same time, husbands of female service members work for more hours than wives of male service members, and are more likely to report lower marital satisfaction, less community support, and less satisfaction with the military lifestyle (Southwell & MacDermid Wadsworth, 2016). Given the importance of social support, support programs may be critical for both spousal satisfaction and service member retention. One study using data from the Military Family Life Project, a longitudinal study on active duty military spouses that started in 2010 (2010 Military Family Life Project, 2011; 2011 Military Family Life Project, 2012), found that although few spouses utilized support programs requiring active engagement (e.g., family readiness and spousal support groups, in-person or web-based counseling, and reunion planning class), the programs were effective when utilized (Clark, Jordan, & Clark, 2013). This finding suggests that more work is needed to engage spouses to participate in these programs to overcome challenges that accompany deployment.

Deployment as a Cycle. Deployment is a transition in a military life course with several adjustment stages as exemplified by the Emotional Cycle of Deployment Model (DeVoe & Ross, 2012; Logan, 1987; Pincus, House, Christenson, & Adler, 2001). The stages include pre-deployment, during deployment/sustainment, and post-deployment (after deployment) (Blaisure et al., 2015; Pincus et al., 2001). Although the studies reviewed so far have examined the impact of deployment on the service member, the spouse, or the couple as a whole, one limitation is that most of these studies were cross-sectional or longitudinal but within one deployment stage (e.g., two-wave study post-deployment), which limits the investigation of deployment as multiple stages that occur over time.

The cycle of deployment is normative in the military life course and couples may react to each deployment stage with normative responses (e.g., stress, uncertainty, anxiety, and stabilization). However, there can be different sets of issues that couples face at each stage (Laser & Stephens, 2011). During the pre-deployment stage, couples may experience stress and an anticipation of loss while having to prepare the family financially, legally, and emotionally for the deployment. During deployment, an adaptation period is needed as partners settle into a new communication pattern in terms of both form (e.g., phone and online) and frequency. Spouses may experience isolation or lack of social support, increased stress from household responsibilities, and emotional or psychological health issues while the service member is away (Lufkin, 2017; Southwell & MacDermid Wadsworth, 2016). It is clear from research that social support is imperative to build and maintain resiliency among spouses during this time (Skomorovsky, 2014). Finally, during the post-deployment stage, service members and partners who are able to adapt to new roles during each transition, including the absence and return of the service member to home life, are typically able to adjust well (MacDermid Wadsworth, 2010).

In order to better understand how military couples experience and cope with the challenges of deployment, the following studies examined health and well-being outcomes of married individuals or couples across two or more deployment stages. For marital functioning, one study examined changes in marital satisfaction from pre-deployment to post-deployment (Parcell & Maguire, 2014). While some couples experience a decrease in marital satisfaction post-deployment, the majority are able to rebound to the level of marital satisfaction pre-deployment or perceive even higher marital satisfaction post-deployment. These distinct martial trajectories reflect the diversity of military couples and the varied experiences they have in military and personal lives, suggesting that most couples are able to adjust well in spite of going through multiple stages of major transition over a short period.

As for psychological functioning, Erbes, Kramer, Arbisi, DeGarmo, and Polusny (2017) found distinct trajectories of depressive symptoms and alcohol misuse across the deployment stages among partners of deployed NG personnel. The majority of the partners were considered as part of the "resilience" group, meaning they showed low distress and alcohol misuse over time, whereas other groups of partners showed varying levels of distress and alcohol misuse at different points of different stages (e.g., increase during pre-deployment vs increase at beginning of deployment or decrease during deployment vs decrease post-deployment). The significance of examining trajectories as part of the military life course lies in the identification of predictors of trajectories, such as neuroticism, family readiness, and low social support. This allows for more targeted interventions to prevent at-risk couples from continuing on a high-risk trajectory prior to the development of distress and alcohol problems.

Due to the motivation to understand the impact of deployment on military families, identify predictors of trajectories, and inform policy, one recent landmark study, "The Deployment Life Study," investigated family readiness across the cycle of deployment (Meadows et al. 2016). It is currently the only study specifically designed to measure a wide array of relational, health, and well-being outcomes across the deployment cycle of multiple family members. The study involved the service member, spouses, and one child aged between of 11 and 17 years (if available). Notably, service members (and their families) were eligible only if the service member was not deployed at baseline. This design allows for a clear examination of changes in individual, couple, and family functioning from pre-, mid- to post-deployment. Based on analysis of the deployment cycle over three years, Meadows et al. (2016) reported that couples, on average, became less satisfied with their marriage over time, and that this decrease did not significantly differ between couples with a deployed and non-deployed service member. The systematic comparison between deployed and non-deployed couples allowed researchers to determine that the decrease in marital satisfaction is normative for those who had a deployment. Examining pre-, mid-, and post-deployment changes also revealed that more frequent communication with the service member during deployment predicted greater marital satisfaction for spouses at post-deployment, thus providing a clear, attainable point of intervention specifically to increase communication during deployment for better post-deployment outcomes. Similarly, the findings for health and well-being indicated separation from the military is another potential intervention point because those who separated or retired were at increased risk of psychological symptoms.

It can be seen that these studies examining longitudinal changes from pre-deployment to post-deployment and include both partners of the same couple can provide valuable information on the health and well-being of military couples over time. The Millennium Cohort Family Study, an expansion of the Millenium Cohort Study, which has been ongoing for 20+ years, is another example of a longitudinal study that started in 2011 to include spouses in addition to service members (Crum-Cianflone et al., 2014). Since these studies are expensive, time-consuming, and require significant resources and effort, secondary data analysis is encouraged to make use of this wealth of data if it is made available publically. One possible future direction is to examine the effects of multiple deployments when more waves of data become available, and determine whether stress across multiple deployments is additive or cumulative and whether it is similar for each family member. It is exciting that longitudinal couple data are increasingly valued and recognized as important to our understanding of the military life course for couples. Using the life course perspective as a way of studying the military transitions of relocation and deployments among military couples can be an important and useful framework for understanding their health and well-being. Next, we provide some potential avenues for future research.

FUTURE DIRECTIONS

In the previous section, we focused on examining married military individuals, military spouses and partners, and military couples embedded within the larger military life course. We discussed and provided critical assessment of studies on two major transitions that have significant impact on military couples. Based on this review, we suggest several priorities for future research on military couples and on the military life course in general.

Expand Research on Military Couples

Studies to Include Both Partners of a Couple and Expand Range of Outcomes

The most noteworthy observation of the studies included in this chapter is that many studies examined married individuals and comparatively fewer studies included both partners from the same couple. Whereas there is an abundance of dyadic research on civilian couples, we have less knowledge of how military couples interact and influence each other within their larger family and military contexts. Several studies, for example, have examined the effects of work–family conflict, burnout, and job stress among military couples (Westman, 2005; Westman & Etzion, 1995; Westman & Vinokur, 1998; Westman, Vinokur, Hamilton, & Roziner, 2004). However, these studies did not examine the effects of work–family conflict and burnout during major transitions, which may be more stressful and have greater impact on the couple. In addition, reviews of the literature on military marriages (Karney & Crown, 2011; MacLean & Elder, 2007) have pointed out that we need to examine relevant predictors and outcomes of military couples beyond their communication styles, marital quality, and divorce risk. For example, the timing of romantic formation (before recruitment, during service, or after service) may play an important role on the development of the relationship and the couple's resilience to stressors during and after military service.

Another future direction is to expand military couples' research on reintegration into the civilian workforce. Studies on reintegration have mainly focused on service members' employment and financial well-being (Elbogen, Johnson, Wagner, Newton, & Beckham, 2012; Hall, Harrell, Bicksler, Stewart, & Fisher, 2014; Kleykamp, 2013) and NG/R who have periodic drills and have to transition frequently between military and civilian work roles (Nagl & Sharp, 2010). Less is understood about the impact of military service on spouse's/partner's employment and earning potential after the military service has ended. For example, military partners earn less than their civilian counterparts even if they work for a similar number of hours (Meadows et al., 2016). Thus, remain the following major questions: Does the employment and wage gap between military partners and civilian counterparts dissipate over time? Moreover, are there differences between couples in which the service member separated from the military recently versus 5, 10, or 20 years ago? Longitudinal panel studies, such as the Deployment Cycle Study (Meadows et al., 2016), the Millennium Cohort Family Study (Crum-Cianflone et al., 2014), and the Military Family Life Project (2011 Military Family Life Project, 2012), may be able to provide these answers in time.

While understanding that funding resources are becoming scarcer and that longitudinal studies can be costly in terms of time and effort, we echo the call from previous researchers to involve both partners in longitudinal studies to better understand the dynamics and processes in which military couples function and adapt, particularly on a day-to-day basis (Meadows et al., 2016). At least two studies to our knowledge have answered this call. The Study for Employment Retention of Veterans (SERVe) focuses on improving employment retention, health, and well-being of (current and former) military service members who hold civilian jobs (for more information, see Hammer et al., 2017). In addition to longitudinal evaluation of the service members, SERVe also recruited and surveyed spouses and partners to examine matched dyads of military couples. In addition, an upcoming study on Military Employees Sleep and Health (Hammer et al., 2017) also evaluates the experiences of full-time NG/R and their partners.

Studies such as these provide in-depth understanding of the day-to-day life of military couples during and after their service.

Studies that Allow for Systematic Comparison

Another priority is to develop ways to conduct research that allows for systematic comparison of couples within and outside the military. The current state of the literature on military couples is scattered with regards to membership in different service branches and components, single versus repeated deployments and relocations, gender of the service member(s), and single versus dual military career couples. Past studies have often excluded NG/R because they were not expected to be deployed and separated from their families as frequently as they are now, which contribute to our lack of understanding of the differences between active duty and NG/R (Clever & Segal, 2013). In addition, the majority of studies examined in this chapter were on US military couples. It is important to note that different country and military policies can add another layer of complexity when examining the health and well-being of military families. The difficulty for systematic comparison lies in the feasibility of finding comparable samples of couples within the military to examine differences between branches and components, as well as comparable samples of military and civilian couples (e.g., of similar age, gender, relationship status, and background) to examine the effects of military service. For example, caregivers affiliated with a deployed NG member and with the Navy (regardless of component) reported poorer well-being compared to other branches and components (Lara-Cinisomo et al., 2012). Given that there are likely significant differences in stress, health, and well-being based on service branch, component, and life experiences, we need to tease apart variability within each of these dimensions (e.g., within a branch) and across dimensions (e.g., across branches; between military and civilian populations). Close collaboration between the military and academic researchers could be a first step in finding appropriate dimensions for systematic comparisons.

Expand the Composite Life Cycle Model

The Composite Life Cycle Model provides a holistic view of understanding service members and their families by encompassing three strands of life (unit, soldier, and family; Chiarelli, 2010). However, many service members in the NG/R may have an additional life cycle strand that influences their relationships, performance, and well-being. Since many NG/R hold a civilian job while serving in the military, we suggest that a civilian workplace strand is needed in addition to the current three strands when assessing NG/R. Similar to the solider strand, the civilian workplace strand would include professional and personal transitions in the civilian workplace, such as starting a new career, promotions, unemployment, and change in leadership. While the original Composite Life Cycle Model was intended to be viewed from a military standpoint, adding a workplace strand can highlight the importance of civilian employers' roles to learn and understand the challenges that their military employees face in their (multiple lines of) work and family lives. This could help to increase appreciation of their efforts and skills, and to build an organizational culture that supports our military. The workplace strand is also likely to continue longer throughout life after the service member separates from the military. In this case, be it for active duty personnel or NG/R, the process of reintegration can be highlighted as part of the model (e.g., from obtaining a new job to retirement).

Move Toward an Integrative Understanding of Soldier, Family, and Military Lives

Finally, researchers have indicated the importance of conducting longitudinal and integrated research (Blaisure et al., 2015; Chiarelli, 2010; Gade, 1991; Karney & Crown, 2011; MacLean & Elder, 2007). Specifically, researchers have suggested that future work should "explore ways in which the data can be collected from multiple family members at the same time" (Meadows et al., 2016, p. xxvii), and the military has recommended that research should "identify and track support and stressors related to *all* strands of the life cycle model" (Chiarelli, 2010, p. 109). We propose that examining social support systems is an area prime for integrated research. Social support and strain occurs across all strands, from supervisor and co-worker support in the unit and workplace strands to partner, family, and friend support in the family (or more broadly, personal life) strand.

One method that could be used to determine and assess the various support systems is based on the Convoy Model of Social Relations (Antonucci, 2001; Kahn & Antonucci, 1980; Sherman, Wan, & Antonucci, 2016). Intended as a multidisciplinary model based on sociological and psychological theories and traditionally used to examine civilian populations, the convoy model can easily be applied to study the military. A convoy is defined as a group of vehicles or ships that travel together and offer protection. In this model, a "convoy" refers to a group of people, or social network, which surrounds and protects an individual as they travel through life. The model takes into account personal characteristics (e.g., age, gender, socioeconomic status, and race) and situational characteristics (e.g., work and family roles and living environment) that may influence the amount and type of social support received.

The main goal of the Convoy Model of Social Relations is to examine the nature of these dynamic close relationships and their influence on health and well-being over the life course. An individual can be close to different people at different points in life. For example, parents and teachers may play more important roles in childhood, friends in adolescence, and partners, children, colleagues, and comrades in adulthood. First, researchers need to measure the convoy, which can be assessed with the hierarchical mapping technique (Fig. 1). Using this technique, researchers can ask individuals (e.g., service members and partners) to look at a diagram with three concentric circles imagining that the individual is at the center. Each of the three circles represents different levels of closeness or importance to the individual. The individual nominates the person(s) to whom they feel closest (or people who are so important that it is hard to imagine work/personal life without them) to the smallest circle, then nominates person(s) who are not as close but still very important to their life in the outer circles.

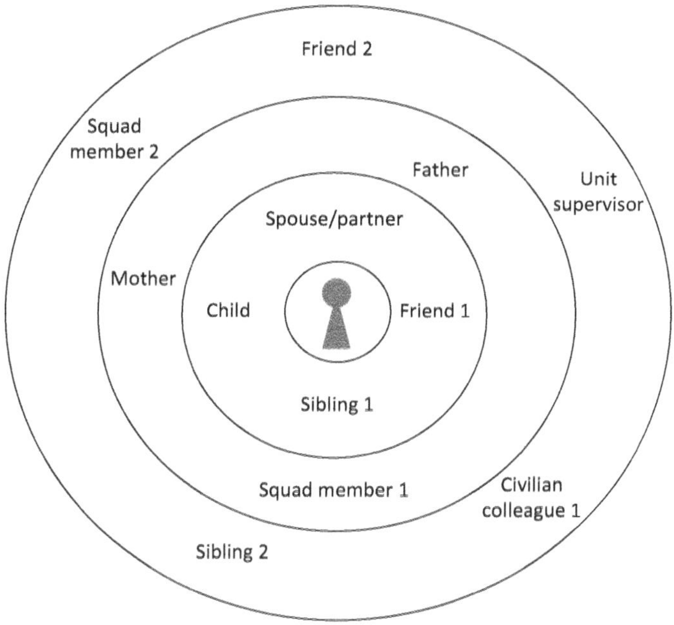

Fig. 1. Hierarchical Mapping Technique as an Integrative Method to Identify and Track Support Networks across Unit, Family/Personal Life, and Workplace Strands. *Source:* Adapted from Antonucci (1986).

The resulting diagram graphically depicts the individual's convoy and allows the individual to nominate as many people from as many strands. Studies have typically allowed up to 20 total nominations to capture the complexity and breadth of the convoy. Not only does this method allow researchers to collect data about social networks across strands, it also avoids any bias or misconceptions about close network membership as opposed to having researchers define the relationships that should be considered as important. As a result, this method provides a person-centered view of their support system. With this information, researchers can assess social convoy structure (e.g., how many people are in the social network and how far away do they live), function (e.g., aid and affect), and quality (e.g., positive support, negative strain, and reliability). Note that service members and partners can have no or few nominations in a particular strand, and they can feel more support or strain from one relationship or one strand. In addition, both structure and quality of a social convoy can change over time. By assessing the social convoy of service members and their partners across branches and components at regular intervals, we can have greater understanding of the various support systems that may be beneficial to military families. This understanding could lead to the identification of target points of intervention, particularly in strands where more support is needed that may impact performance and well-being in other strands of life.

CONCLUSION

Military service is life defining for service members and their close friends and family. Throughout a service member's life, the spouse or partner is often the primary support with the most consistent presence, and therefore the understanding of military couples is of utmost importance. In this chapter, we focused on the various definitions, experiences, and challenges of the armed services and specifically of military couples. Using a life course perspective, this chapter explored factors related to the transitions of periodic relocation and deployment that have significant impact on military couples. We hope that this chapter will help to expand research on military couples and direct research toward a more integrative understanding of the life cycle of service members and their support systems from different strands of life.

ACKNOWLEDGMENTS

Portions of this chapter were supported by the Office of the Assistant Secretary of Defense for Health Affairs through the USAMRMC Broad Agency Announcement Award No. W81XWH-13-2-0020. The U.S. Army Medical Research Acquisition Activity, 820 Chandler Street, Fort Detrick MD 21702-5014 is the awarding and administering acquisition office. Portions of this chapter were also funded by grant #T03OH008435 awarded to Portland State University—funded by the Centers for Disease Control and Prevention, National Institute for Occupational Safety and Health. Opinions, interpretations, conclusions, and recommendations are those of the authors and are not necessarily endorsed by the Department of Defense or by NIOSH. Leslie B. Hammer is Principal Investigator on both awards.

REFERENCES

Allen, E. S., Rhoades, G. K., Stanley, S. M., & Markman, H. J. (2010). Hitting home: Relationships between recent deployment, posttraumatic stress symptoms, and marital functioning for Army couples. *Journal of Family Psychology*, *24*(3), 280.

Allen, E. S., Rhoades, G. K., Stanley, S. M., & Markman, H. J. (2011). On the home front: Stress for recently deployed army couples. *Family Process*, *50*(2), 235–247.

Antonucci, T. C. (2001). Social relations: An examination of social networks, social support, and sense of control. In J. E. Birren & K. W. Schaie (Eds.), *Handbook of the psychology of aging* (pp. 427-453). San Diego, CA, US: Academic Press.

Antonucci, T. C. (1986). Hierarchical mapping technique. Generations, *Journal of the American Society on Aging*, *10*(4), 10–12.

Ashforth, B. E., Kreiner, G. E., & Fugate, M. (2000). All in a day's work: Boundaries and micro role transitions. *Academy of Management Review*, *25*(3), 472–491.

Bakker, A. B., & Demerouti, E. (2013). The spillover–crossover model. In J. Grzywacz, & E. Demerouti (Eds.), *New frontiers in work and family research* (pp. 53–69), Hove: Psychology Press.

Barnett, R. C., & Hyde, J. S. (2001). Women, men, work, and family: An expansionist theory. *American psychologist*, *56*(10), 781.

Blanchard, V. L., Hawkins, A. J., Baldwin, S. A., & Fawcett, E. B. (2009). Investigating the effects of marriage and relationship education on couples' communication skills: A meta-analytic study. *Journal of Family Psychology*, *23*(2), 203–214. http://dx.doi.org/10.1037/a0015211

Black, W. G., Jr. (1993). Military-induced family separation: A stress reduction intervention. *Social Work, 38*(3), 273–280.

Blaisure, K. R., Saathoff-Wells, T., Pereira, A., Wadsworth, S. M., & Dombro, A. L. (2015). *Serving military families: Theories, research, and application*. New York, NY: Routledge.

Blakely, G., Hennessy, C., Chung, M. C., & Skirton, H. (2012). A systematic review of the impact of foreign postings on accompanying spouses of military personnel. *Nursing & Health Sciences, 14*(1), 121–132.

Booth, B., & Lederer, S. (2012). Military families in an era of persistent conflict. In J. H. Laurence & M. D. Matthews (Eds.), *The Oxford handbook of military psychology* (pp. 365–380). New York, NY: Oxford University Press.

Booth, B., Segal, M. W., Bell, D. B., Martin, J. A., Ender, M. G., Rohall, D. E., & Nelson, J. (2007). *What we know about army families: 2007 update*. Arlington, VA: Family and Morale, Welfare and Recreation Command.

Bowen, G. L. (1987). Wives' employment status and marital adjustment in military families. *Psychological Reports, 61*(2), 467–474.

Bowen, G. L., Orthner, D. K., Zimmerman, L. I., & Meehan, T. (1992). *Family patterns and adaptation in the US army*. Research Triangle Park, NC: Research Triangle Institute.

Brett, J. M. (1982). Job transfer and well-being. *Journal of Applied Psychology, 67*(4), 450.

Burland, D., Lundquist, J. H. (2013). The best years of our lives: Military service and family relationships --A life-course perspective. In Wilmoth, J. M., London, A. S. (Eds.), *Life-course perspectives on military service* (pp. 165–184). New York, NY: Routledge.

Burrell, L. M. (2006). Moving military families: The impact of relocation on family well-being, employment, and commitment to the military. In C. A. Castro, A. B. Adler, & T. W. Britt (Eds.), *Military life: The psychology of serving in peace and combat: The military family* (Vol. 3, pp. 39–63). Westport, CT: Praeger Security International.

Burrell, L. M., Adams, G. A., Durand, D. B., & Castro, C. A. (2006). The impact of military lifestyle demands on well-being, army, and family outcomes. *Armed Forces & Society, 33*(1), 43–58.

Castaneda, L. W., & Harell, M. C. (2008). Military spouse employment: A grounded theory approach to experiences and perceptions. *Armed Forces & Society, 34*(3), 389–412.

Chiarelli, P. W. (2010). *Army health promotion, risk reduction, suicide prevention report 2010*. Washington, DC: Department of Defense.

Clark, S. C. (2000). Work/family border theory: A new theory of work/family balance. *Human Relations, 53*(6), 747–770.

Clark, M. G., Jordan, J. D., & Clark, K. L. (2013). Motivating military families to thrive. *Family and Consumer Sciences Research Journal, 42*(2), 110–123.

Clever, M., & Segal, D. R. (2013). The demographics of military children and families. *The Future of Children, 23*(2), 13–39.

Cooke, T. J., & Speirs, K. (2005). Migration and employment among the civilian spouses of military personnel. *Social Science Quarterly, 86*(2), 343–355.

Copeland, A. P., & Norell, S. K. (2002). Spousal adjustment on international assignments: The role of social support. *International Journal of Intercultural Relations, 26*(3), 255–272.

Crum-Cianflone, N. F., Fairbank, J. A., Marmar, C. R., & Schlenger, W. (2014). The millennium cohort family study: A prospective evaluation of the health and well-being of military service members and their families. *International Journal of Methods in Psychiatric Research, 23*(3), 320–330.

Cunradi, C. B., Caetano, R., & Schafer, J. (2002). Alcohol-related problems, drug use, and male intimate partner violence severity among US couples. *Alcoholism: Clinical and Experimental Research, 26*(4), 493–500.

De Burgh, H. T., White, C. J., Fear, N. T., & Iversen, A. C. (2011). The impact of deployment to Iraq or Afghanistan on partners and wives of military personnel. *International Review of Psychiatry, 23*(2), 192–200.

DeVoe, E. R., & Ross, A. (2012). The parenting cycle of deployment. *Military Medicine, 177*(2), 184–190.

Dimiceli, E. E., Steinhardt, M. A., & Smith, S. E. (2010). Stressful experiences, coping strategies, and predictors of health-related outcomes among wives of deployed military servicemen. *Armed Forces & Society, 36*(2), 351–373.

Drummet, A. R., Coleman, M., & Cable, S. (2003). Military families under stress: Implications for family life education. *Family Relations*, *52*(3), 279–287.

Dunkel Schetter, C. (2017). Moving research on health and close relationships forward – A challenge and an obligation: Introduction to the special issue. *American Psychologist*, *72*(6), 511–516.

Elbogen, E. B., Johnson, C. S. C., Wagner, H. R., Newton, V. M., & Beckham, J. C. (2012). Financial well-being and post-deployment adjustment among Iraq and Afghanistan war veterans. *Military Medicine*, *177*(6), 669.

Elder, G. H., Jr, Gimbel, C., & Ivie, R. (1991). Turning points in life: The case of military service and war. *Military Psychology*, *3*(4), 215.

Erbes, C. R., Kramer, M., Arbisi, P. A., DeGarmo, D., & Polusny, M. A. (2017). Characterizing spouse/partner depression and alcohol problems over the course of military deployment. *Journal of Consulting and Clinical Psychology*, *85*(4), 297.

Fish, T. L., Harrington, D., Bellin, M. H., & Shaw, T. V. (2014). The effect of deployment, distress, and perceived social support on army spouses' weight status. *US Army Medical Department Journal* (October–December), 87–95.

Frone, M. R., Yardley, J. K., & Markel, K. S. (1997). Developing and testing an integrative model of the work–family interface. *Journal of vocational behavior, 50*(2), 145–167.

Gade, P. A. (1991). Military service and the life-course perspective: A turning point for military personnel research. *Military Psychology*, *3*(4), 187.

Gates, G. J. (2010). *Lesbian, gay, and bisexual men and women in the US military: Updated estimates*. Retrieved from the Williams Institute website http://www3.law.ucla.edu/williamsinstitute/pdf/GLBmilitary Update.pdf

George, L. K. (2003). Life course research: Achievements and potential. In J. T. Mortimer & M. J. Shanahan (Eds.), *Handbook of the life course* (pp. 671–680). New York: Kluwer Academic/Plenum Publishers.

Gottman, J. M., Gottman, J. S., & Atkins, C. L. (2011). The comprehensive soldier fitness program: Family skills component. *American Psychologist*, *66*(1), 52.

Grandey, A. A., & Cropanzano, R. (1999). The conservation of resources model applied to work–family conflict and strain. *Journal of vocational behavior, 54*(2), 350–370.

Greenhaus, J. H., & Beutell, N. J. (1985). Sources of conflict between work and family roles. *Academy of management review, 10*(1), 76–88.

Greenhaus, J. H., & Powell, G. N. (2006). When work and family are allies: A theory of work-family enrichment. *Academy of management review, 31*(1), 72–92.

Griffith, J. D., Stewart, L. S., & Cato, E. D. (1988). *Annual survey of army families: A report on army spouses and families in 1987*. Alexandria, VA: US Army Community and Family Support Center.

Hall, K. C., Harrell, M. C., Bicksler, B. A., Stewart, R., & Fisher, M. P. (2014). *Veteran employment*. Santa Monica, CA: Rand Corporation.

Hammer, L. B., Wan, W. H., Brockwood, K. J., Mohr, C. D., & Carlson, K. F. (2017). Military, work, and health characteristics of separated and active service members from the study for employment retention of veterans (SERVe). *Military Psychology*, *29*(6), 491–512. Retrieved from http://dx.doi.org/10.1037/mil0000196

Henry, R., & Robichaux, R. J. (1999). Understanding life in the army: Military life from a service member and family member perspective. In J. G. Daley (Ed.). *Social work practice in the military* (pp. 217–233). New York, NY: The Haworth Press.

Heyman, R. E., & Neidig, P. H. (1999). A comparison of spousal aggression prevalence rates in US Army and civilian representative samples. *Journal of Consulting and Clinical Psychology*, *67*(2), 239.

Hobfoll, S. E. (1989). Conservation of resources: A new attempt at conceptualizing stress. *American psychologist, 44*(3), 513.

Holt-Lunstad, J., Robles, T. F., & Sbarra, D. A. (2017). Advancing social connection as a public health priority in the United States. *American Psychologist*, *72*(6), 517.

Jervis, S. (2009). *Military wives and relocation: A psycho-social perspective*. Doctoral Dissertation, University of West of England, Bristol, UK.

Kahn, R.L., & Antonucci, T.C. (1980). Convoys over the life course: Attachment, roles, and social support. In P.B. Baltes, & O. Brim (Eds.), *Life-span development and behavior* (Vol. 3).

New York: Academic Press. Reprinted 1989 in Joep Munnichs & Gwenyth Uildris (Eds.), Psychogerontologie (pp. 81–102). Van Loghum Slaterus.

Karney, B. R., & Crown, J. S. (2007). *Families under stress: An assessment of data, theory, and research on marriage and divorce in the military* (Vol. 599). Santa Monica, CA: Rand Corporation.

Karney, B. R., & Crown, J. S. (2011). Does deployment keep military marriages together or break them apart? Evidence from Afghanistan and Iraq. In MacDermid Wadsworth, S., Riggs, D. (Eds.),*Risk and resilience in US military families* (pp. 23–45). New York, NY: Springer.

Keenan, B. (2011). *Diplomatic baggage: The adventures of a trailing spouse*. London: Hachette.

Kleykamp, M. (2013). Unemployment, earnings and enrollment among post 9/11 veterans. *Social Science Research*, *42*(3), 836–851.

Lakhani, H., Thomas, S., & Gilroy, C. (1985). Army european tour extension: a multivariate approach. *Journal of Behavioral Economics, 14*(2), 15–41.

Lara-Cinisomo, S., Chandra, A., Burns, R. M., Jaycox, L. H., Tanielian, T., Ruder, T., & Han, B. (2012). A mixed-method approach to understanding the experiences of non-deployed military caregivers. *Maternal and Child Health Journal, 16*(2), 374–384.

Laser, J. A., & Stephens, P. M. (2011). Working with military families through deployment and beyond. *Clinical Social Work Journal, 39*(1), 28–38.

Lavee, Y., McCubbin, H. I., & Patterson, J. M. (1985). The double ABCX model of family stress and adaptation: An empirical test by analysis of structural equations with latent variables. *Journal of Marriage and the Family*, *47*(4), 811–825.

Logan, K. V. (1987, February). The emotional cycle of deployment. *US Naval Institute Proceedings 113*(1), 43–47.

Lufkin, K. P. (2017). An exploratory study of marital and quality of life ratings among male spouses of military members. *Contemporary Family Therapy*, *39*(3), 162–171.

Lundquist, J., & Smith, H. L. (2005). Family formation among women in the US military: Evidence from the NLSY. *Journal of Marriage and Family*, *67*(1), 1–13.

Lundquist, J., & Xu, Z. (2014). Re-institutionalizing families: Life course policy and marriage in the military. *Journal of Marriage and Family*, *76*(5), 1063–1081.

MacDermid Wadsworth, S. M. (2010). Family risk and resilience in the context of war and terrorism. *Journal of Marriage and Family*, *72*(3), 537–556.

MacLean, A., & Elder Jr, G. H. (2007). Military service in the life course. *Annual Review of Sociology*, *33,* 175–196.

Mansfield, A. J., Kaufman, J. S., Marshall, S. W., Gaynes, B. N., Morrissey, J. P., & Engel, C. C. (2010). Deployment and the use of mental health services among US Army wives. *New England Journal of Medicine*, *362*(2), 101–109.

Marshall, A. D., Panuzio, J., & Taft, C. T. (2005). Intimate partner violence among military veterans and active duty servicemen. *Clinical Psychology Review*, *25*(7), 862–876.

McNulty, A. F. (2003). Does deployment impact the health care use of military families stationed in Okinawa, Japan? *Military Medicine*, *168*(6), 465.

Meadows, S. O., Griffin, B. A., Karney, B. R., & Pollak, J. (2016). Employment gaps between military spouses and matched civilians. *Armed Forces & Society*, *42*(3), 542–561.

Meadows, S. O., Tanielian, T., Karney, B. R., Ayer, L., Chandra, A., Friedman, E. M., ... & Troxel, W. M. (2016). The deployment life study: Longitudinal analysis of military families across the deployment cycle (No. RR1388). RAND Arroyo Center Santa Monica United States.

2010 Military Family Life Project. (2011). *Tabulations of responses*. DMDC Report No. 2010-029. Defense Manpower Data Center, Washington, DC.

2011 Military Family Life Project. (2012). *Tabulations of responses*. DMDC Report No. 2012-027. Defense Manpower Data Center, Washington, DC.

Modell, J., & Haggerty, T. (1991). The social impact of war. *Annual Review of Sociology*, *17*(1), 205–224.

Monson, C. M., Taft, C. T., & Fredman, S. J. (2009). Military-related PTSD and intimate relationships: From description to theory-driven research and intervention development. *Clinical Psychology review*, *29*(8), 707–714.

Nagl, J., & Sharp, T. (2010). *An indispensable force: Investing in America's National Guard and Reserves*. Washington, DC: Center for a New American Security.

Negrusa, S., Negrusa, B., & Hosek, J. (2014). Gone to war: Have deployments increased divorces? *Journal of Population Economics*, *27*(2), 473–496.
Norwood, A. E., Fullerton, C. S., & Hagen, K. P. (1996). Those left behind: Military families. In R. J. Ursano & A. E. Norwood (Eds.), *Emotional aftermath of the Persian Gulf War: Veterans, families, communities, and nations* (pp. 163–196). Arlington, VA, US: American Psychiatric Association.
Office of the Deputy Assistant Secretary of Defense [DASD]. (2014). 2014 demographics: Profile of the military community. Retrieved from http://download.militaryonesource.mil/12038/MOS/Reports/2014-Demographics-Report.pdf.
Parcell, E. S., & Maguire, K. C. (2014). Turning points and trajectories in military deployment. *Journal of Family Communication*, *14*(2), 129–148.
Pincus, S. H., House, R., Christenson, J., & Adler, L. E. (2001). The emotional cycle of deployment: A military family perspective. *US Army Medical Department Journal*, *4*(5), 6.
Pittman, J. F., & Bowen, G. L. (1994). Adolescents on the move: Adjustment to family relocation. *Youth & Society*, *26*(1), 69–91.
Puskar, K. R., Wilson, G., & Moonis, L. J. (1990). The effect of group support on relocated corporate and military wives: A secondary analysis. *Minerva*, *8*(2), 36.
Renshaw, K. D., Rodrigues, C. S., & Jones, D. H. (2008). Psychological symptoms and marital satisfaction in spouses of Operation Iraqi Freedom veterans: Relationships with spouses' perceptions of veterans' experiences and symptoms. *Journal of Family Psychology*, *22*(4), 586.
Segal, M. W. (1986). The military and the family as greedy institutions. *Armed Forces & Society*, *13*(1), 9–38.
Sherman, C. W., Wan, W. H., & Antonucci, T. C. (2016). Social convoy model. In S.K. Whitbourne (Ed.), *The Encyclopedia of Adulthood and Aging*. Hoboken, New Jersey: Wiley-Blackwell.
Skomorovsky, A. (2014). Deployment stress and well-being among military spouses: The role of social support. *Military Psychology*, *26*, 44–54.
Southwell, K. H., & MacDermid Wadsworth, S. M. (2016). The many faces of military families: Unique features of the lives of female service members. *Military Medicine*, *181*(1S), 70–79.
Trougakos, J. P., Bull, R. A., Green, S. G., MacDermid, S. M., & Weiss, H. M. (2007). Influences on job search self-efficacy of spouses of enlisted military personnel. *Human Performance*, *20*(4), 391–413.
Werber, L., Harrell, M. C., Varda, D. M., Hall, K. C., & Beckett, M. K. (2009). *Deployment experiences of guard and reserve families: Implications for support and retention*. Santa Monica, CA: Rand Corporation.
Westman, M. (2001). Stress and strain crossover. *Human Relations*, *54*(6), 717–751.
Westman, M. (2005). The crossover of work–family conflict from one spouse to the other. *Journal of Applied Social Psychology*, *35*(9), 1936–1957.
Westman, M., & Etzion, D. (1995). Crossover of stress, strain and resources from one spouse to another. *Journal of Organizational Behavior*, *16*(2), 169–181.
Westman, M., & Vinokur, A. D. (1998). Unraveling the relationship of distress levels within couples: Common stressors, empathic reactions, or crossover via social interaction? *Human Relations*, *51*(2), 137–156.
Westman, M., Vinokur, A. D., Hamilton, V. L., & Roziner, I. (2004). Crossover of marital dissatisfaction during military downsizing among Russian army officers and their spouses. *Journal of Applied Psychology*, *89*(5), 769.

FIGHTING FOR FAMILY: CONSIDERATIONS OF WORK–FAMILY CONFLICT IN MILITARY SERVICE MEMBER PARENTS

Maura J. Mills and Leanne M. Tortez

ABSTRACT

We review the state of the literature concerning work–family conflict in the military, focusing on service members' parenting roles and overall family and child well-being. This includes recognition that for many women service members, parenting considerations often arise long before a child is born, thereby further complicating work–family conflict considerations in regard to gender-specific conflict factors such as pregnancy, childbirth, postpartum, and breastfeeding. Subsequently, we consider more gender-invariant conflict factors, such as the nature of the work itself as causing conflict for the service member as parent (e.g., nontraditional hours, long separations, and child care challenges) as well as for the child (e.g., irregular contact with parent, fear for parent's safety, and frequent relocations), and the ramifications of such conflict on service member and child well-being. Finally, we review formalized support resources that are in place to mitigate negative effects of such conflict, and make recommendations to facilitate progress in research and practice moving forward.

Keywords: Military; service members; work–family conflict; work–life conflict; parenting; breastfeeding; pregnancy; postpartum; gendered occupations; support

Occupational Stress and Well-being in Military Contexts
Research in Occupational Stress and Well-being, Volume 16, 91–116
Copyright © 2018 by Emerald Publishing Limited
All rights of reproduction in any form reserved
ISSN: 1479-3555/doi:10.1108/S1479-355520180000016008

Serving in the military is hard. Parenting is hard. The combination – serving in the military while simultaneously trying to sustain a healthy and happy family life – can be doubly difficult. Such domain conflict is grounded in theories such as work–family conflict theory (see Greenhaus & Beutell, 1985), which suggests that one domain (e.g., work) interferes with one's optimal functioning in an alternate domain (e.g., home), and can do so via time-, strain-, and/or behavior-based conflict(s). However, while such conflict is well-recognized regardless of profession, the military context provides a particularly unique landscape for such conflict to manifest itself. Bell and Schumm (2013) acknowledged this, describing the struggle of the military service member as being trapped between "two very greedy institutions: the military and the family" (p. 83; see also Segal, 1988). Indeed, both are high-demanding domains that often warrant near-full commitment from an individual. Some (e.g., Huffman, Culbertson, & Barbour, 2015, p. 280) have even conceptualized the military as being "more of a lifestyle than an occupation," contributing to its "unforgiving" nature wherein the "mission comes first" and is expected to supersede all competing obligations – including family (à la time-based conflict). One must wonder, then, whether that makes them mutually exclusive. However, with over half of all service members reporting dependents (a number higher than in the past; Blaisure, Saathoff-Wells, Pereira, MacDermid Wadsworth, & Dombro, 2012; Flake, Davis, Johnson, & Middleton, 2009), there exists a need to align these two domains, as well as to align current and future service members' perceptions that the supports are in place to facilitate effective management of these oft-competing roles.

Even from a strategic perspective, one must consider that a military incompatible with family life does not a strong military make. Specifically, from a recruitment and retention perspective, poor work–family considerations may lead to high-potential would-be service members failing to enlist or re-enlist (Kelley et al., 2001), or, when they do enlist, subsequently leaving the service prematurely (Heilmann, Bell, & McDonald, 2009) due to the strains of incompatibility. From a recruitment perspective, this translates into many of the best individuals for the job, objectively, self-selecting out of military careers at the recruitment stage. From a retention perspective, this risks substantial sunk cost when service members on whom considerable training dollars have been invested ultimately leave the service (à la behavior-based conflict). Previous estimates indicate that the Navy alone loses $126 million in recruiting and training investments on recruits who leave the service within six months (Government Accountability Office, 1997). The solution, then, lies in a critical examination of the extent to which (and how) military membership impacts the stress and well-being of service members and their families (à la strain-based conflict), and recommendations for remedial strategies for aligning the demands of the two domains. To serve this purpose, we address these issues through consideration of the demands of military service roles, both at home and abroad (deployments and overseas stations), the extent to which they are compatible with effective and meaningful parenting roles and parent–child relationships,[1] and the resultant stress and impact on service members' well-being.

THE EARLY DAYS: FOR SOME, IT BEGINS BEFORE IT BEGINS

For some service members, coming face-to-face with the duality of military life and parenting comes long before the child is even born. That is, women in particular are more likely to reflect on the future familial considerations in deciding whether to even enter the military (Silva, 2008), as is the case in many professions that pose uniquely challenging career hurdles for those ultimately desiring to have children (to name just a few, police officers, lawyers, doctors, academics, chemists, and anthropologists; Culbertson, Huffman, Mills, & Imhof, 2017; Lucas-Thompson & Goldberg, 2015; Stanfors, 2014; Tremblay, 2016). There is good reason for this, as in most circumstances of biological family creation, women are faced with negotiating the physiological, physical, and logistical considerations of pregnancy alongside their occupation in a way that men are not. Likewise, post-birth, many women are also faced with negotiating the demands (again, physiological, physical, and logistical) of breastfeeding maintenance subsequent to their return to work.[2] In both of these cases, the extent to which these circumstances are possible (and successful) is often largely dependent upon individuals' job responsibilities and demands, as well as the extent to which her employer can be supportive of relevant logistical needs.

The Gendered Occupation: Leaky Military Pipelines

Prior to discussion of mother-specific childrearing considerations, it is first warranted to address the military as a highly gendered occupation, as individuals in such divergent-gendered occupations (e.g., women serving in the male-dominated military) are often faced with unique work–family pressures (Huffman et al., 2015). Although the proportion of women service members is growing,[3] it is doing so slowly (Mackenzie, 2012), and the preponderance of literature suggests that in gendered occupations, the minority gender (here, women) typically experiences greater work–family conflict than does the majority gender (Cook & Minnotte, 2008). This may result from the degree to which male-dominant occupations (such as the military) accommodate (or fail to) family life, thereby creating room for subsequent domain conflict (Haas & Hwang, 2007; Mills, Pervez, & Mandeville, 2018). Indeed, Evans and Rosen (1997) found that half of women in the military felt as though there was no ideal time to have children while serving in the armed forces. Likewise, Pierce (1998) found that approximately 25% of women who voluntarily left military service identified work–family conflict as a contributing factor in that decision – a finding more recently substantiated qualitatively by Dichter and True (2014). Unfortunately, this is not surprising when we consider the many ways that military service may impact demands of parenting differentially for women service members as compared to men.

Pregnancy and Childbirth

Perhaps the most apparent considerations regarding women's differential work–family needs may be the obvious issues of pregnancy and childbirth. A large majority of active duty servicewomen is of childbearing age, with an estimated 10% of servicewomen becoming pregnant each year (Mulhall, 2009). Thus, these women often face issues around contraception access, pregnancy, pregnancy outcomes after environmental exposures, and other challenges (Krulewitch, 2016). However, research regarding these issues and women service members' reproductive and gynecological well-being has received little attention (Segal & Lane, 2016). Most of the existing research has focused on the extent to which pregnancy can impact organizational readiness, which has (in the past) resulted in the exclusion of women from certain military roles (Segal & Lane, 2016).

Some research has indicated that around 54% of pregnancies in active duty servicewomen may be unplanned (Enewold et al., 2010; Grindlay & Grossman, 2013), which may lead to a host of other unique challenges such as low birth weight and preterm birth (Shah et al., 2011). In general, active duty women are at greater risk for maternal and infant complications, including being five times more likely to have a preterm birth as compared to civilian women (McNeary & Lomenick, 2000). Nevertheless, mothers in the military have access to health care services at no cost, including breastfeeding classes, infant care, and counseling (Sylvia, McMullen, Levine, & Cruz, 2001). Further, they seem responsive to such services, as one study reported that almost 100% of mothers in the military attended check-ups during their pregnancies (Sylvia et al., 2001). Despite these benefits, however, mothers in the military face several unique challenges, often including increased pregnancy risks resulting from above-average stress levels, sleep disturbances, and fatigue. Stinson and Lee (2003) found that sleep disturbance and fatigue were predictive of preterm labor among active duty military births, further finding that service member rank also served as a risk factor, such that officers delivered prematurely at a significantly higher rate than did enlisted women. Compounding this is the consideration that compared to civilian women, military women tend to work longer into their pregnancies and experience less social support as a result of factors such as frequent relocations and spousal and coworker deployments (Drummet, Coleman, & Cable, 2003; Klaman & Turner, 2016; Messersmith-Heroman, Heroman, & Moore, 1994).

There is also the consideration of the extent to which pregnancy affects deployment and troop readiness. Today, a pregnant woman serving in the military is protected from deployment for six months (McGraw, Koehlmoos, & Ritchie, 2016). Unfortunately, although this deployment protection is undoubtedly legitimate, it has also resulted in claims that female service members may attempt to get pregnant to avoid a deployment (Manski, Grindlay, Burns, Holt, & Grossman, 2014; Ritchie, 2001). In addition to such an accusation stigmatizing the "condition" of pregnancy (and women service members more broadly), such an accusation also has not been supported in the literature (Custer, Waller, Vernon, & O'Rourke, 2008; Grindlay, Yanow, Jelinska, Gomperts, & Grossman, 2011; Uriell & Burress, 2009). Moreover, a study of primarily enlisted postpartum women service members across all branches of the military indicated that 64% of the women felt that their military plans were not changed as a result of pregnancy, although the majority (57–60%) also planned to leave the military upon completing their service obligations (Biggs, Douglas, O'Boyle, & Rieg, 2009). Indeed, compared to male service members, women have consistently lower re-enlistment rates, regardless of branch (Military Leadership Diversity Commission, 2010). Similar research has demonstrated lower retention rates across branches for servicewomen, even at senior officer levels (Asch, Miller, & Malchiodi, 2012). Such gender differences may be related to the consideration that pregnant service members (or those planning a pregnancy) may experience a "motherhood penalty" that negatively affects their rank, ability to be promoted, and advancement potential (Fitzgerald et al., 2013). Therefore, a woman may refrain from asking for advice within her chain of command in order to avoid others' misrepresentations of her reproductive intentions (Fitzgerald et al., 2013). Indeed, qualitative research has echoed servicewomen's concerns about being "kicked out" of the military, losing their rank, and being formally penalized as a direct or indirect result of their pregnancies (Grindlay et al., 2011).

However, such challenges of pregnancy are not limited to active duty service members. Even women who become pregnant having left the service are not likely to escape the military-related challenges of pregnancy. Likely due to the unique stressors of a military career (e.g., frequent uncertainty, limited autonomy, repeated relocations, compromised social support, threats to physical safety, and exposure to traumatic events), many women veterans face mental health-related issues (Haskell et al., 2009) that may exacerbate pregnancy complications such as preterm deliveries and lower birth weights (Copper et al., 1996). Mattocks and colleagues (2010) found that 32% of pregnant veterans had one or more mental health diagnoses – a significantly higher rate than the 21% of women veterans who were not pregnant. Specifically, veterans with a pregnancy were more likely to be diagnosed with major or mild depression, post-traumatic stress disorder (PTSD), anxiety, schizophrenia, bipolar disorder, and alcohol and drug abuse or dependency (Mattocks et al., 2010). Such heightened likelihood of mental health issues for pregnant veterans as compared to those not bearing children may come down to an increased need or desire for social support during emotionally challenging pregnancies, as well as, more holistically, the compounding of military-related stressors with hormonally induced pregnancy-related stressors, the combination of which may make mental health problems more probable.

Postpartum

Birth, however, is only the beginning. Recovery from childbirth can be a feat unto itself, depending on the circumstances surrounding the birth. Moreover, in a physically demanding occupation such as the military, the extent to which – and how quickly – a woman is able to return to her "pre-baby body" is spotlighted. Indeed, US Navy regulation (OPNAVINST 6110.1J) explicates the expectation that active duty women return to Navy body weight standards six months post-birth. Chauhan et al. (2013) examined the reality of this, noting that only 48% of women in their cohort study were in compliance with Naval body weight standards six months postpartum. With a cesarean delivery as one of only two factors predictive of this outcome in their study, Chauhan et al. (2013) further boldly concluded that "avoiding" a cesarean delivery could improve the number of women meeting Naval body standards six months postpartum, although also admitted that "the evidence supporting [the] directive appears to be arbitrary" (p. 406). We further suggest that it could also be detrimental to women's emotional well-being by way of postpartum body image, in addition to increasing risk for eating disorders or compromising the nutrition necessary for successful breastfeeding.

Similarly, the US Air Force exempts pregnant women from completing the required physical fitness test; however, they must successfully pass it six months postpartum (Armitage, Severtsen, Vandermause, & Smart, 2014). Unsurprisingly, research has found that active duty women are more likely to fail a fitness test six months postpartum as compared to before pregnancy (Armitage & Smart, 2012; Weina, 2006). A number of factors may influence postpartum servicewomen's ability to prepare for their fitness tests, including physical, emotional, and social issues. In a qualitative study of active duty postpartum women serving in the Air Force, participants reported not being able to train because their health care provider advised them not to do so due to perinatal health concerns (e.g., incisional healing problems, infections, etc.) and issues around breastfeeding (e.g., decreased milk supply as a result of intense training, scheduling around training times, etc.; Armitage et al., 2014).

Related to this is a mother's likelihood of experiencing postpartum depression. Appolonio and Fingerhut (2008) determined that 20% of active duty mothers experience postpartum depression, as predicted by psychosocial factors such as poor social support, low marital satisfaction, and life and child care stressors – all of which may be heightened in a military career (Nguyen et al., 2013; Rychnovsky & Beck, 2006). The likelihood of experiencing postpartum depression is also considerably higher when servicewomen are exposed to combat. In a study of military servicewomen who were deployed after childbirth, those with combat-associated exposures had a significantly higher prevalence of maternal depression as compared to servicewomen who were never deployed and those without combat-associated exposures (Nguyen et al., 2013). This is in addition to some studies having found that the rate of postpartum depression among active duty servicewomen may be somewhat higher than the rate found in civilian populations (~20% vs. ~13% respectively; Appolonio & Fingerhut, 2008; Gavin et al., 2005; O'Boyle, Magaan, Ricks, Doyle, & Morrison, 2005; O'Hara & Swain, 1996). The Armed Forces Surveillance Study found that servicewomen diagnosed with postpartum depression were 42 times more likely to also be diagnosed with suicidality (Do, Hu, Otto, & Rohrbeck, 2013). This is further relevant when we consider that service members tend to underreport emotional and mental health concerns for fear of occupational retribution or stigma, so the percentage may in actuality be even more disparate (Kim, Britt, Klocko, Riviere, & Adler, 2011; Porter & Johnson, 1994). As such, the risk of military women experiencing compromised mental and emotional health postpartum – and their reluctance to seek remedial care to attend to those concerns – puts this population at a unique risk as compared to non-military mothers and even as compared to military fathers.

Breastfeeding

Although maintaining breastfeeding after returning to work is a challenge for all new mothers (Spitzmueller et al., 2016), active duty women face a number of additional challenges. Despite the fact that there are official breastfeeding policies associated with each branch of the military (Fitzgerald et al., 2013), service member perceptions of support for breastfeeding have been found to vary across branches. For instance, Martin, Drake, Yoder, Gibson, and Litke (2015) found that these perceptions varied by branch of service and rank. Specifically, women in the Air Force perceived the most breastfeeding support, followed by women in the Navy and Marines, while those in the Army had the lowest perceptions of support. Martin et al. further found that, across branches, officers had significantly higher perceptions of breastfeeding support as compared to enlisted women. Such support is crucial, as an unsupportive work environment can further hamper a servicewoman's breastfeeding success (Martin, 2015).

To the extent that they are linked with breastfeeding duration, these variable support perceptions are particularly notable in light of the aforementioned deployment protection for six months postpartum. That is, the duration of that protection starkly contrasts with widespread medical recommendations that infants be breastfed for at least one year (American Academy of Pediatrics, 2012), and more optimally two years (World Health Organization, 2002). Considering this, it is unsurprising that servicewomen in particular struggle to meet these recommendations. Notably, servicewomen and civilian women breastfeed at similar rates immediately after birth (i.e., at hospital discharge; Farwell, 2017; Rishel & Sweeney, 2005). However, differences arise in the duration of breastfeeding. In a study of women who were breastfeeding at hospital discharge, Rishel and Sweeney (2005) found that only one-third of servicewomen continued to breastfeed at the fourth month, compared to over half of civilian women. Similar results have been found in more recent studies (Uriell, Perry, Kee, & Burress, 2009; also at the four-month mark) and considering different durations (Bales, Washburn, & Bales, 2012; at the six-month mark).

Farwell (2017) identified a number of factors that affect breastfeeding duration in active duty servicewomen. Specifically, continuation of breastfeeding through at least 12 months (as recommended) was most strongly predicted in cases with annual income exceeding $50,000 and education level beyond high school (Mao, Narang, & Lopreiato, 2012). In addition to these more universal considerations, there are also a number of military-specific issues at play. Rank, for instance, played an important role, with enlisted servicewomen less likely to continue breastfeeding at 12 months as compared to officers (Mao et al., 2012). Also important are physical separations from the baby (in multiple forms, including long working hours compounded with inflexible schedules, temporary duty assignments, and deployments after six months), pressures related to meeting physical readiness standards, and negative responses from other service members (Bales et al., 2012). Concern about potential exposure to toxic elements (e.g., petroleum) in combat environments, which may be contraindicated during breastfeeding, was also given as a hindrance to continuation (Bales et al., 2012; McGraw et al., 2016).

In addition, common logistical issues that lactating civilian women often face in the workplace (e.g., difficulty scheduling pumping breaks, lack of appropriate "mothers' rooms", milk storage challenges, etc.; Bettinelli, 2012; Bruck-Lee, Albert, & Stone, 2016) are again magnified in the military population. Despite policies across all military branches calling for private and clean places for mothers to express milk (Farwell, 2017), even when in a non-combat environment such as the garrison, it may be difficult for women to pump milk in a hygienic manner (Bell & Ritchie, 2003). As such, it is also highly recommended that servicewomen discuss their pumping needs with their supervisor and/or commander to ensure that they are receiving adequate accommodations and time allotments (Fitzgerald et al., 2103). However, the predominantly masculine culture of the military environment can make such a conversation awkward and may overly reflect the servicewoman's femininity in a culture that is not always accepting of that. Nevertheless, progress is on the horizon. Today, although some branches (e.g., Navy and Air Force) are specific about time allotted for pumping (e.g., 15–30 minutes every 3–4 hours), other branches (e.g., Army) allow for more flexible arrangements to align with individual needs (Fitzgerald et al., 2103).

SERVICE MEMBER AS PARENT: MILITARY JOB CHARACTERISTICS

Nevertheless, while work–family conflict in this gendered occupation is indeed likely to differ between male and female service members, particularly such that women have more pre-birth conflict, it is also true that service members of both genders are at high risk of experiencing work–family conflict (Adams, Jex, & Cunningham, 2006) simply by virtue of the uniquely demanding (emotionally, physically, and temporally) nature of military occupations (Stansfeld & Candy, 2006). Indeed, research has indicated that job characteristics such as extended involuntary separations from family, frequent relocations, unpredictability, lack of flexibility, nontraditional working hours, physically and emotionally demanding work, and high-risk assignments – all of which are characteristic of the military (Adams et al., 2006; Blaisure et al., 2012) – have negative implications for service members' mental health, stress, and well-being (Odle-Dusseau et al., 2013; Tucker, Sinclair, & Thomas, 2005). The same has often been found to hold for the stress and well-being of service members' spouses (Seo, Lloyd, & Nam, 2014; Skomorovsky, Hujaleh, & Wolejszo, 2015), children (Foreman, Pike, DuPont, & Lughi, 2001; Lester & Flake, 2013), and overall family functioning (Kaczmarek & Sibbel, 2008).

Service Members' Work–Family Strain

Undoubtedly, the physical and emotionally demanding nature of military service can result in significant strain on service members. Although this can result for all service members, combat exposure in particular accounts for the most consistent and negative consequences of military service (MacLean & Elder, 2007). Service members exposed to combat are more likely to be diagnosed with PTSD (LeardMann,

Smith, Smith, Wells, & Ryan, 2009; Smith et al., 2008), and develop depression, anxiety, and other mental health problems (Hoge et al., 2004; Milliken, Auchterlonie, & Hoge, 2007). Unsurprisingly, deployment (and even the threat of it) serves as a primary stressor for service members and their families (Galovski & Lyons, 2004). Further, each stage of deployment impacts the family in different ways (DeVoe & Ross, 2012). The pre-deployment period raises stress related to concerns about parenting, saying goodbye, and worries about managing family needs with increasing military demands such as training and preparation (both logistical and emotional). During the deployment, the home-based parent reacts to child stress, and finds new routines and new ways to cope with daily challenges. Importantly, these challenges often continue well into the post-deployment phase (Thomas et al., 2010), thereby directly impacting service members' home lives and work–family conflict (Adams et al., 2006; Huffman et al., 2015). During this reintegration phase, parents may disagree and clash over new roles, children may be resistant to change, and the returning service member may be insensitive to changes that have occurred in the family during their deployment (DeVoe & Ross, 2012). Indeed, a substantial proportion (23–36%) of service members' spouses identified the restoration of co-parenting as one of the most difficult aspects of restoring family life post-deployment (US Army Community and Family Support Center, 2005). Moreover, recurrent deployments have been associated with poorer family adjustments – specifically greater dysfunction in affective involvement, family communication, problem solving, marital instability, and general family functioning (Lester et al., 2016). With 43% of deployed service members experiencing multiple deployments (IOM, 2013), the effects of deployment on the family unit warrant considerable attention.

However, while deployment is perhaps the most extreme strain faced by service members, it is far from the only one. Other challenges include the potential for frequent relocations, long and inflexible working hours, and long periods of separation during training exercises (MacDermid Wadsworth, 2010; Milliken et al., 2007). Relocations in particular can disrupt established social networks, moving service members, their spouses, and their children away from friends, family, and other forms of support (Le, Tissington, & Budhwar, 2010). Further, military work often represents nonstandard shift work at its most extreme, which can negatively affect the individual's experience at work, their physical and mental health, as well as family dynamics (Rosiello & Mills, 2015). Half of military spouses report that the amount of time that the service member spends away from home is problematic (US Army Community and Family Support Center, 2005). Other research has illustrated the disruptive nature of an individual service member's work strain on the family system as a whole. For instance, Huffman, Matthews, and Irving (2017) found that both the service member's self-reported work–family conflict and the spouse's perception of their work–family conflict relate to fairness perceptions in the division of household labor: When either partner perceived the service member to be experiencing conflict, they were more likely to believe that the division of household labor was unfair. Such perceived inequities can be detrimental to marital satisfaction and stability, as well as to family cohesion more broadly (Huffman, Craddock, Culbertson, & Klinefelter, 2017).

Children's Strain

Not to be neglected is the impact on service members' children. Although some research (Jeffreys & Leitzel, 2000; Jensen, Xenakis, Wolf, & Bain, 1991) has found limited support for negative effects of parents' military occupations on their children, the preponderance of research has identified some additional challenges in this regard. For instance, an Army data collection effort identified that approximately one-fifth of soldiers' children cope poorly with a parent's deployment, as characterized by fears about the parent being in harm's way, negative affect, inability to concentrate, and aggressive behavior (US Army Community and Family Support Center, 2005). In a more recent study of Army families, 42% of parents with a deployed spouse reported high levels of parenting stress, with about one-third also reporting psychological symptoms in their children (Flake et al., 2009).

In line with this, the preponderance of research generally indicates deployment's negative impact on the mental and behavioral health of service members' children (Chandra et al., 2010; Gorman, Eide, & Hisle-Gorman, 2010; Lincoln, Swift, & Shorteno-Fraser, 2008; Mansfield, Kaufman, Engel, & Gaynes, 2011). Gorman et al. (2010) found that children showed a 19% increase in behavioral disorders and an 18% increase in stress disorders when a parent was deployed. Similarly, Hisle-Gorman et al. (2015) found that, compared to children of non-deployed parents, children of deployed parents experienced an 11% increase in doctor visits for reasons of both mental and physical health. However, the effects of parental deployment on children, and the ability for children to cope with a parent's deployment, can vary depending on the age of the child (Bello-Utu & DeSocio, 2015). Research has suggested that younger children are especially affected by a parent's deployment, as they have fewer resources compared to older children (Paris, DeVoe, Ross, & Acker, 2010). Parental deployment during a child's early and middle childhood may pose significant emotional and social adjustment problems (Lester et al., 2016; Mustillo, MacDermid Wadsworth, & Lester, 2016). In older children, however, distress about the deployment is more likely to manifest as increased social anxiety (in the case of repeated deployments; Lester et al., 2016) or substance use (Acion, Ramirez, Jorge, & Arndt, 2013).

Of course, the well-being of military children can be strongly influenced by their parents. Lester et al. (2016) found that depression of the home-based parent – not uncommon in military spouses (IOM, 2013) – predicted separation anxiety in younger children (e.g., infants, toddlers, and preschool age). It also predicted emotional and behavioral problems, including challenges interacting with peers, in children aged 6–10 years, and general and social anxiety in older children. Notably, Lester et al. (2010) found that depression levels of the at-home parent were even more predictive of child outcomes than other factors such as duration of deployment. Ultimately, functional coping by the home–based parent is an important protective factor for children of all ages when faced with a parental deployment (Bello-Utu & DeSocio, 2015).

Regardless of the at-home parent's coping, however, a parental deployment has the potential to negatively impact the quality of children's parental attachments. This results from both directly limiting the relationship between the child and deployed parent for prolonged periods (Paris et al., 2010) and indirectly influencing the quality of the relationship between the child and the at-home parent due to stressful demands (Flake et al., 2009). This deployment-related stress may negatively influence parenting practices, such as through compromised problem solving, reduced involvement and encouragement, and more frequent aversive behavior (Gewirtz, Erbes, Polusny, Forgatch, & DeGarmo, 2011). Child neglect and other forms of maltreatment may also be heightened at times of deployment (Gibbs, Martin, Kupper, & Johnson, 2007; Rentz et al., 2007). In a study of at-home mothers married to military service members, Posada et al. (2015) found that child attachment behaviors were significantly related to the father's exposure to combat, father's involvement when not deployed, and mother's depression symptoms. Interestingly, however, Posada et al. (2015) found no relation between children's attachment behavior and the cumulative frequency of paternal deployments or the number of days deployed in the previous year.

Finally, challenges may also arise during the reintegration stage, when the deployed parent returns home, and may be just as stressful as periods of separation (Goff, Crow, Reisbig, & Hamilton, 2007). Research has found that greater challenges exist as children increase in age, possibly a result of older children having more responsibilities and therefore finding the shifting of roles upon reintegration difficult (Chandra et al., 2010). Further, the longer the parent is deployed, the more difficult is the experience of reintegration for the child (Chandra et al., 2010). Undoubtedly, successful family reintegration for children depends on the mental health and coping of both parents (Bello-Utu & DeSocio, 2015).

FORMALIZED SUPPORT RESOURCES

Without sufficient personal resources (Orthner, 2002a) and institutionalized support from the military (McFadyen, Kerpelman, & Adler-Baeder, 2005), the above combination of occupational characteristics can be a recipe for disaster on the home front, including the potential for increased familial instability (Karney & Crown, 2007; Southwell & MacDermid Wadsworth, 2016). Consequently, as emphasized by Harms, Krasikova, Vanhove, Herian, and Lester (2013), family supports are an important protective factor buffering the extent to which such risk factors ultimately affect both overall service member and familial well-being as well as job-relevant factors such as on-the-job performance. As such, we further consider relevant federal policies as applicable to military personnel and their families, as well as more targeted formal work–family management programs facilitated predominantly through the US Department of Defense (DoD) and individual military bases and units (installations).

Federal Policy and Leave Availability

Most widely available are the relevant federal policies applicable to military personnel and their families in order to facilitate military–family balance and quality of home life. For instance, service members and their employed immediate family members who qualify for the Family and Medical Leave Act (FMLA) are also eligible for military-specific leaves such as Military Caregiver Leave (MCL) and Qualifying Exigency Leave (QEL). The former allows for service members' immediate family or next of kin[4] to take up to 26 weeks of leave to care for an injured or ill service member, inclusive of active duty, reserve, and veteran. The latter (QEL) is targeted toward active duty service members and their families, allowing for temporary employment leave when an immediate family member (spouse, child, parent) is called to active duty either domestically or internationally (e.g., deployment). It also allows for familial leave for a variety of other commitments related to the service member's military duty, including for military events/ceremonies (broadly defined), counseling sessions, and during a deployed member's temporary return home for rest and recuperation (R&R) leave, among other such obligations.

These leaves can serve as crucial crutches to help military families manage their family lives during a variety of military commitments. However, their utility is limited by some important parameters. First, as aforementioned, they are only available to family members who otherwise qualify for FMLA, which is heavily reliant on the nature of the family member's own employment. For instance, individuals working at small companies, working part-time (defined as <1,250 hours/year), and newly hired employees (tenure <12 months) are not eligible for FMLA. The latter restriction in particular may be unduly problematic for military families, who often find themselves moving more frequently than the general population as a result of installation (base) reassignments. Another problematic consideration that limits the utility of these leave options is that FMLA (and likewise MCL and QEL) leaves are unpaid. Unpaid leave can force parents to resume work before they are able to recover from childbirth, establish breastfeeding, or develop a strong bond with the baby (Rowe-Finkbeiner, Martin, Abrams, Zuccaro, & Dardari, 2016). Beyond the expected financial issues that unpaid leave can cause, unpaid leave also has the potential to impact infant and maternal health, including a 20% increase in infant mortality (Tanaka, 2005). Such findings drive home the importance of accessible and realistic leave options for military families.

Whole-family Functioning and Parenting Supports

In addition to the aforementioned leave options, facilitating familial coping is also critical to helping military parents and their children successfully manage the demands of military life. Indeed, the DoD boasts approximately 26 distinct policies related to family resilience, helping service members and their families "bounce back" from the stressors of military life (Meadows et al., 2015). Not only are such programs beneficial to service members' families, but they are also advantageous to the service member him or herself. That is, stress from a service member's family life has been known to spillover into their service role, potentially compromising their productivity, focus, and even safety on the job (Bray et al., 2010; Carter et al., 2015; Kennedy et al., 2009). Similarly, service members are more likely to meet the demands of their missions, especially when deployed, when they are confident that their family is receiving sufficient support on the home front (Burnam, Meredith, Sherbourne, Valdez, & Vernez, 1992; Haas, Pazdernik, & Olsen, 2005). With this in mind, various programs have been developed to assist with navigating the challenges of raising a family in the military. This includes resource-focused programs such as Military OneSource – a military-contracted community support program that connects military families to a variety of resources, including youth programs, parenting resources, and support for topics related to deployment, relocation, and reintegration, as well as access to nonmedical counseling services. There also exist assistance-based programs such as Operation Homefront, which provides more tangible assistance to military families in the form of relief, recovery, and recognition for military families during difficult times. This type of support ranges from financial assistance to baby showers and military child recognition programs.

A number of not-for-profit organizations have similar missions, including the National Military Family Association, Give an Hour, the United Service Organizations, and Families OverComing Under Stress (FOCUS), all dedicated to supporting and strengthening military families (Conforte et al., 2017; Johnson & Ling, 2013). The National Military Family Association provides resources related to navigating military life, educational scholarships for spouses, and camps for children. Specifically, the Operation Purple Camp project aims to build psychological strength and resilience, and has already served more than 45,000 children of wounded service members (Easterbrooks, Ginsburg, & Lerner, 2013). "Give an Hour" creates nationwide networks of health professionals who volunteer their services to meet the mental health needs of service members and their families. Such free services include help with substance abuse, counseling, PTSD, grief, anxiety, and sexual health and intimacy (Kudler & Porter, 2013). The United Service Organizations aim to provide morale, welfare, and recreation-type services to service members and their families. Their centers, located worldwide, offer free internet, library access, housing assistance, family crisis counseling, support groups, game rooms, and nursing facilities for service members and their families. Finally, FOCUS is a family-centered program aimed at helping military families and children cope with deployment by building resiliency and improving psychological health (Saltzman et al., 2011). Through eight modules and a web-based component, the program focuses on core elements such as psych-education, emotional regulation skills, goal setting, problem solving skills, traumatic stress management techniques, and family communication skills (Beardslee et al., 2011).

Such structured supports for families continue to be valuable at all stages of the military cycle, even into the post-deployment phase. Indeed, some research has suggested that service members returning from deployment may prefer family-based interventions over individual therapy (Khaylis, Polusny, Erbes, Gewirtz, & Rath, 2011). For example, at the time of this writing, one of the most widely used resilience-building family-based programs in the military is the Comprehensive Soldier and Family Fitness (CSF2), which aims at improving and sustaining the mental and emotional health and well-being of the service member and his/her family (spouse and children), recognizing that the latter are an important part of overall service member well-being (Gottman, Gottman, & Atkins,

2011; Park, 2011). Programs focused specifically on the challenges of parenting military children are also popular, and include Parent Management Training – Oregon (PMTO), and After Deployment: Adaptive Parenting Tools (ADAPT), which are social interaction learning frameworks for parenting (Gewirtz et al., 2011). Such programs are built on the premise that stressful life circumstances such as deployment impact parenting practices and child outcomes (Patterson, 2005). Using a curriculum and materials modified for a military population, the ADAPT program incorporates psych-education and emotion-regulation to target post-deployment adjustment reactions such as avoidance, hypervigilance, and irritability (Gewirtz et al., 2011).

The majority of supports still target such active duty families, however. In response, the Joint Family Support Assistance Program was developed to provide support and meet the ongoing needs of reservist families and others who are not geographically co-located with their installation (MacDermid Wadsworth & Southwell, 2011). The program utilizes Military Family Life Consultants assigned to each state and provides support, short-term counseling, information, and referrals (Deputy Under Secretary of Defense, Military Community and Family Policy, 2010). Similarly, the DoD Yellow Ribbon Reintegration Program assists reservists and their families throughout the deployment cycle. This includes protecting service members from being called back to duty for 90 days following their return, allowing them instead to focus on reintegrating with their families and civilian life (MacDermid Wadsworth & Southwell, 2011).

Child-focused Resources

While many of the above-mentioned supports include resources that parents can access on behalf of their children, none has a singular focus on the military child. However, the DoD offers various such resources that focus specifically on supporting the children of service members. Military-sponsored programs focusing on youth often incorporate extracurricular activities that facilitate a fun and social environment. Research has evidenced the importance of such programs for the well-being of military children, particularly early adolescents (aged 11–14 years; Richardson, Mallette, O'Neal, & Mancini, 2016). An extreme example of such a program is Education Activity Schools – DoD-sponsored public schools. These institutions are tailored toward educating service members' children in an environment that understands the stressors of military life and how they can impact children's educational success (Esqueda, Astor, & de Pedro, 2012). However, the vast majority of military children attend non-DoD schools that are often ill-equipped to handle – or do not fully understand – the unique needs of military children (Brendel, Maynard, Albright, & Bellomo, 2014; Harrison & Vannest, 2008) and therefore lack military-specific support systems (Esqueda et al., 2012). Indeed, in a study comparing perceptions of military-connected and nonmilitary parents with children in public school, military-connected parents consistently reported more negative assessments of school climate and were more dissatisfied with the level of understanding from the staff (Berkowitz, de Pedro, Couture, Benbenishty, & Astor, 2014). Given that military children change schools approximately every 2.9 years (Esqueda et al., 2012), support around the challenges of military life is crucial. While school-based interventions for military children in these settings do exist, they – and the research surrounding them – are largely lacking. In a systematic review of the effects of school-based interventions for US military children, Brendel et al. (2014) found only one study to meet the inclusion criteria for review, highlighting the need for increased awareness around the stressors faced by military children and the need for school-based research.

However, a more widely available resource for military children is DoD's online program Military Kids Connect, which provides an integrated peer support community for children aged 6–17 years (Blasko, 2015). Focusing on children's experiences of military life (i.e., deployment, relocation, and reintegration of the parent upon returning from deployment), the program is designed to provide education about military life, teach coping strategies, and provide peer support. For younger children, the DoD collaborated with Sesame Street and Electric Company to introduce Military Families Near and Far, a bilingual website for service members' children. The website aims to develop social support networks with children from other military families to counter feelings of loneliness and distance (Russo & Fallon, 2015).

Localized Military Support Programs

In addition to the nationwide offerings described above, the military has also been proactive in organizing more localized efforts to provide necessary supports to military families and equip them to thrive not just in spite of, but sometimes because of, their military affiliation (Adams et al., 2006). These installation-specific formal work–family management programs are facilitated through individual military bases and units. For example, the Army provides Army Family Team Building (AFTB) and Family Readiness Groups (FRGs) (Schumm, Bell, Milan, & Segal, 2000). Developed by Army family members, the AFTB program aims to provide education around military life to improve work–family fit and satisfaction with the military (McFadyen et al., 2005). Orthner (2002b) found that the program facilitates development of coping skills and improves families' adaptation to Army life as compared to those family members who did not use the program. FRGs focus on providing social support to Army families, and have been hailed as important to overall familial well-being, in addition to valuing the foci on social support, facilitated communication with deployed service members, sponsored family activities, and education about available community resources (Goodman et al., 2013).

However, while the AFTB and FRGs do well to provide more general support resources, there is also a daily need for parents to manage more logistical constraints of parenting, such as child care considerations. While such logistics can be challenging for any parent, they are often more so in the military context given the unique job characteristics such as nontraditional work schedules and relocations. As such, recognizing that reliable and affordable child care is a priority for military families, the DoD developed programs to provide and subsidize child care for military families. Such programs may be on- or off-installation, and include Child Development Centers, Family Child Care, School-Age Care, Operation Military Child Care, and Military Child Care in Your Neighborhood (Government Accountability Office, 2012). Within each program exist additional child care options. For instance, the Marine Corps has an Enhanced Extended Child Care program that offers child care to family members who cannot use regularly scheduled care due to extended duty, family illness, or family emergency. Similarly, the Air Force's Extended Duty Care and the Navy's Child Development Group Homes offer child care during nontraditional hours (Floyd & Phillips, 2013).

RECOMMENDATIONS FOR MOVING FORWARD

As demonstrated by the wide variety of aforementioned resources, in recent years the military has made great strides in recognizing that in order to recruit and retain service members, they must also recognize service members' parenting responsibilities, in addition to supporting service members' families (Adams et al., 2006). This type of support has increasingly come to manifest in a number of ways, not only via the more tangible child care offerings, specialized schooling options, and reliable family housing, but also the equally as important mental and emotional healthcare and support resources (Kleykamp, Kelty, & Segal, 2017). Nevertheless, despite such developments, there remains room for improvement, as many organizations – the military included – continue to navigate and increasingly appreciate this necessary attention to service members' familial and, specifically, parental roles. Below we outline a number of recommendations and considerations that, we believe, would facilitate such continual improvement moving forward.

Interestingly enough, notable among these is that, despite the range of support services available to today's military families, so many such support services exist that service and family members searching for resources may experience a sort of information overload. As Conforte et al. (2017) suggests, this may result in the perception of resource redundancy, thereby leading to confusion as to which resource is most appropriate under which circumstances, and possibly even overwhelming the service or family member to the point of delaying or suspending resource-seeking. However, a complementary problem has also been identified – specifically, lack of knowledge about available resources. For instance, while a majority of spouses who reported an active FRG in their partner's unit participated in the FRG (US Army Community and Family Support Center, 2005), a concerning number remained entirely unaware of any FRG support (Orthner, 2002c). This evidences an important gap in awareness that, if remedied, could contribute toward improving perceived and actual support with comparatively minimal additional effort or expense. Such challenges may be easily overcome with overarching logistical considerations that formalize and clarify resource networks from a high-level (e.g., national) perspective, as well as from a more localized viewpoint.

Another factor that may serve to mitigate the above concern is the opportunity for individualized, often informal support from one's immediate leader. Research increasingly indicates that – formalized support programs (or lack thereof) notwithstanding – informal support by one's superiors (e.g., "family supportive supervisor behaviors"; Hammer, Kossek, Zimmerman, & Daniels, 2007) can go a long way in improving the extent to which employees (here, service members) feel supported in their efforts to effectively manage both their work role and parenting role, thereby bridging this oft-felt divide (Hammer, Kossek, Yragui, Bonder, & Hanson, 2009; Matthews, Mills, Trout, & English, 2014; Mills, Matthews, Henning, & Woo, 2014). This includes the arrangement of idiosyncratic deals, or i-deals, that target individuals' needs on a case-by-case basis (Rousseau, Ho, & Greenberg, 2006). While the usage of i-deals in the military may be somewhat bounded by unique occupational characteristics and job demands, as well as governmental regulations, it remains that frontline supervisors often hold the key to approving or denying leave, flexibility, or other such requests for family-friendly accommodations (Castro, Thomas, & Adler, 2006; MacDermid Wadsworth, 2010). As such, educating commanding officers on the importance of family-friendly accommodations, in addition to providing service members with a supportive organizational culture in which to make such requests, is a critical first step in maximizing supervisors' impact.

This is particularly important when we consider the often differential family-related needs of women service members as they navigate the male-dominated military environment. For instance, some branches of the military (e.g., Air Force, Navy) are more progressive than others when it comes to policies for breastfeeding. In these and other branches, research recommends that women service members who need additional time for breastfeeding – or serve in branches that do not have specific policies – discuss their needs with their supervisors in hopes of arriving at an i-deal (Fitzgerald et al., 2013). However, the likelihood that a woman will approach her supervisor with such a request depends largely on external factors such as the culture of her unit and the extent to which she perceives her commanding officer as approachable and family-friendly. This speaks of the importance of an overall work–family supportive culture in driving important outcomes for service members, as previous research has also suggested (Huffman, Culbertson, & Castro, 2008). It also speaks to the need for greater research consideration given toward women service members, as while the number of women in the military is increasing (Mackenzie, 2012; Patten & Parker, 2011), most of what we know about the military has been derived predominantly from male service members (Southwell & MacDermid Wadsworth, 2016). This makes for a notable opportunity to increase the representativeness of our research – and, ultimately, practice – to the current military composition, thereby increasing the likelihood of representative practices and optimal outcomes.

Similarly, there is a need for increased research on and more inclusive practices regarding LGBTQ (lesbian, gay, bisexual, transgender, queer) military families. This includes targeted support services and resources for service members who identify as LGBTQ, as well as for their coming-of-age children who identify as such. Fortunately, repeal of the policy commonly known as "don't ask, don't tell," meant that these service members and their families are now no longer required to conceal their identities from their fellow service members or commanding officer, and can receive some benefits such as military identification cards and access to support programs such as FRGs. However, the recent controversy regarding the Defense of Marriage Act (DOMA) has meant that until very recently LGBTQ military families were unable to receive certain benefits associated with military affiliation, such as health benefits and housing considerations. For example, under DOMA, children with LGBTQ parents in the military were unable to live in an on-base residence with both parents. However, despite the 2013 repeal of DOMA, many service members may remain reluctant to come out (or to reveal their sexuality by enrolling spouse or dependents in military-provided services) in light of the military's stereotypically masculine, hetero-dominated culture. In this way, LGBTQ military families are still not afforded the same cultural, social, or logistic support as are heterosexual and cisgendered service members, even when formal policies allow for their inclusion. With an estimated 16,000+ LGBTQ military families currently serving (Oswald & Sternberg, 2014), the zeitgeist is ripe for this to be given greater consideration from a research front as well as in practice so as to maximize inclusion.

Finally, beyond the topical research needs identified above, more broadly there is also a notable need for more accessible, systematic, and methodologically rigorous research in military populations when it comes to work–family considerations. This includes more experimental and intervention-type designs that will allow for identification of actionable programs to ameliorate some of the challenges identified herein, as well as research critically evaluating the resulting programs. Unfortunately, as yet there has been considerably little work done to comprehensively evaluate the efficacy of such programs. This is perhaps due to limitations in accessing representative samples of military families for inclusion – particularly considering the relocations and deployments characteristic of military life – or to potential hurdles that researchers may encounter when attempting to publicly disseminate findings regarding these governmental populations. Rectifying this means improving non-governmental-affiliated researcher access to these populations and programs, and, relatedly, sustaining funding support for such research at a time when federally funded research is largely compromised across the board. Relatedly, there is also a need for more longitudinal research tracking work–family outcomes over time as well as the ever-changing dynamics of military family life. Again, the nature of military life, including relocations and deployments, not only presents some unique challenges to such rigorous, ongoing research, but also highlights why such research is so critical for this population in particular as family dynamics ebb and flow and children inevitably age in this unique environment.

CONCLUSION

Herein, we have aimed to give comprehensive consideration to the various parenting- and family-related stressors that interact with military service commitments to impact service members' parenting experiences and overall well-being, as well as that of their children. In so doing, we reviewed the state of the research in this regard, including both gender-differential and gender-invariant conflict considerations. We subsequently highlighted institutionalized and individualized supports that can mitigate the potential for negative effects, and finally put forth recommendations regarding additional considerations and supports that could further buffer the impact of such conflict moving forward.

NOTES

1. We recognize that another primary work–family consideration for military members is the extent to which their military involvement impacts their spouses/marriages and romantic partnerships as independent from their relationships with their children. We focus on the latter, and refer readers to Wan, Haverly and Hammer on page 69 of this special issue for a focus on the former.
2. This assumes, of course, that a woman took some leave from work post-birth; arguably a presumptive assumption considering that at the writing of this chapter, the United States is the only industrialized nation without any form of federally mandated paid leave post-birth.
3. The number of active duty women enlisted in the US military has increased from 42,000 (1973) to 167,000 (2010) (Patten & Parker, 2011).
4. This provision represented the first time that next of kin (i.e., grandparents, siblings, first cousins, etc.) were granted some form of federal job-protected leave (Karin, 2009).

REFERENCES

Acion, L., Ramirez, M. R., Jorge, R. E., & Arndt, S. (2013). Increased risk of alcohol and drug use among children from deployed military families. *Addiction, 108*, 1418–1425.

Adams, G. A., Jex, S. M., & Cunningham, C. J. L. (2006). Work–family conflict among military personnel. In C. A. Castro, A. B. Adler, & T. W. Britt (Eds.), *Military life: The psychology of serving in peace and combat* (pp. 169–192). Westport, CT: Praeger.

American Academy of Pediatrics. (2012). Breastfeeding and the use of human milk. *Pediatrics, 129*, 1035–1039.

Appolonio, K. K., & Fingerhut, R. (2008). Postpartum depression in the military sample. *Military Medicine, 173*, 1085–1091.

Armitage, N. H., Severtsen, B. M., Vandermause, R., & Smart, D. A. (2014). Training for the Air Force fitness assessment: The experience of postpartum women. *Military Medicine, 179*, 766–772.

Armitage, N. H., & Smart, D. A. (2012). Changes in Air Force fitness measurements pre- and post-childbirth. *Military Medicine, 177*, 1519–1523.

Asch, B. J., Miller, T., & Malchiodi, A. (2012). *A new look at gender and minority differences in officer career progression in the military*. Santa Monica, CA: RAND.

Bales, K., Washburn, J., & Bales, J. (2012). Breastfeeding rates and factors related to cessation in a military population. *Breastfeeding Medicine, 7*, 436–441.

Beardslee, W., Lester, P., Klosinski, L., Saltzman, W., Woodward, K., Nash, W., … Leskin, G. (2011). Family-centered preventive intervention for military families: Implications for implementation science. *Prevention Science, 12*, 339–348.

Bell, M. R., & Ritchie, E. C. (2003). Breastfeeding in the military: Part I. Information and resources provided to service women. *Military Medicine, 168*, 807–812.

Bell, D. B., & Schumm, W. R. (2013). Balancing work and family demands in the military: What happens when your employer tells you to go to war? In D. F. Halpern & S. E. Murphy (Eds.), *From work–family balance to work–family interaction* (pp. 83–98). New York, NY: Routledge.

Bello-Utu, C. F., & DeSocio, J. E. (2015). Military deployment and reintegration: A systematic review of child coping. *Journal of Child and Adolescent Psychiatric Nursing, 28*, 23–34.

Berkowitz, R., de Pedro, K. M., Couture, J., Benbenishty, R., & Astor, R. A. (2014). Military parents' perceptions of public school supports for their children. *Children & Schools, 36*, 1–8.

Bettinelli, M. E. (2012). Breastfeeding policies and breastfeeding support programs in the mother's workplace. *The Journal of Maternal-Fetal & Neonatal Medicine*, *25*, 73–74.

Biggs, R. L., Douglas, B. H., O'Boyle, A. L., & Rieg, T. S. (2009). The impact of pregnancy on the individual and military organization: A postpartum active duty survey. *Military Medicine*, *174*, 61–75.

Blaisure, K. R., Saathoff-Wells, T., Pereira, A., MacDermid Wadsworth, S., & Dombro, A. L. (2012). *Serving military families in the 21st century*. New York, NY: Routledge.

Blasko, K. A. (2015). MilitaryKidsConnect: Web-based prevention services for military children. *Psychological Services*, *12*, 261–266.

Bray, R. M., Pemberton, M. R., Lane, M. E., Hourani, L. L., Mattiko, M. J., & Babeu, L. A. (2010). Substance use and mental health trends among US military active duty personnel: Key findings from the 2008 DoD Health Behavior Survey. *Military Medicine*, *175*, 390–399.

Brendel, K. E., Maynard, B. R., Albright, D. L., & Bellomo, M. (2014). Effects of school-based interventions with US military-connected children: A systematic review. *Research on Social Work Practice*, *24*, 649–658.

Bruck-Lee, V., Albert, D., & Stone, K. L. (2016). Lactation and the working woman: Understanding the role of organizational factors, lactation support, and legal policy in promoting breastfeeding success. In C. Spitzmueller & R. A. Matthews (Eds.) *Research perspectives on work and the transition to motherhood* (pp. 217–240). New York, NY: Springer.

Burnam, A. M., Meredith, L. S., Sherbourne, C. D., Valdez, R. B., & Vernez, G. (1992). *Army families and soldier readiness*. Santa Monica, CA: RAND.

Carter, S. P., Loew, B., Allen, E. S., Osborne, L., Stanley, S. M., & Markman, H. J. (2015). Distraction during deployment: Marital relationship associations with spillover for deployed army soldiers. *Military Psychology*, *27*, 108–114.

Castro, C. A., Thomas, J. L., & Adler, A. B. (2006). Toward a liberal theory of military leadership. In A. B. Adler, C. A. Castro, & T. W. Britt (Eds.), *Military life: The psychology of serving in peace and combat* (pp. 192–212). Westport, CT: Praeger.

Chandra, A., Lara-Cinisomo, S., Jaycox, L. H., Tanielian, T., Burns, R. M., Ruder, T., & Han, B. (2010). Children on the home front: The experience of children from military families. *Pediatrics*, *125*, 16–25.

Chauhan, S. P., Johnson, T. L., Magann, E. F., Woods, J. Y., Chen, H., Sheldon, I. V., & Morrison, J. C. (2013). Compliance with regulations on weight gain 6 months after delivery in active duty military women. *Military Medicine*, *178*, 406–411.

Conforte, A. M., DeLeon, P. H., Engel, C. C., Ling, C., Bakalar, J. L., & Tanofsky-Kraff, M. (2017). Identifying policy implications and future research directions regarding military community support and child psychosocial adjustment. *Military Medicine*, *182*, 1572–1580.

Cook, A., & Minnotte, K. (2008). Occupational and industry sex segregation and the work–family interface. *Sex Roles*, *59*, 800–813.

Copper, R. L., Goldenberg, R. L., Das, A., Elder, N., Swain, M., Norman, G., … Jones, P. (1996). The preterm prediction study: Maternal stress is associated with spontaneous preterm birth at less than thirty-five weeks' gestation. *American Journal of Obstetrics and Gynecology*, *175*, 1286–1292.

Culbertson, S. S., Huffman, A. H., Mills, M. J., & Imhof, C. (2017). Balancing the badge: Work–family challenges within policing and recommended supports and initiatives. In C. D'Agostino & C. Cooper (Eds.) *Stress in policing: Sources, consequences, and interventions* (pp. 66–80). London: Gower.

Custer, M., Waller, K., Vernon, S., & O'Rourke, K. (2008). Unintended pregnancy rates among US military population. *Paediatric and Perinatal Epidemiology*, *22*, 195–200.

DeVoe, E. R., & Ross, A. (2012). The parenting cycle of deployment. *Military Medicine*, *177*, 184–190.

Deputy Under Secretary of Defense, Military Community and Family Policy (DUSD). (2010). *Profile of the military community: DoD 2008 demographics*. Alexandria, VA: ICF International.

Dichter, M. E., & True, G. (2014). This is the story of why my military career ended before it should have: Premature separation from military service among US women veterans. *Journal of Women and Social Work*, *30*, 187–199.

Do, T., Hu, Z., Otto, J., & Rohrbeck, P. (2013). Depression and suicidality during the postpartum period after first time deliveries, active component service women and dependent spouses, US Armed Forces, 2007–2012. *Medical Surveillance Monthly Report*, *20*, 2–7.

Drummet, A. R., Coleman, M., & Cable, S. (2003). Military families under stress: Implications for family life education. *Family Relations*, *52*, 279–287.

Easterbrooks, M. A., Ginsburg, K., & Lerner, R. M. (2013). Resilience among military youth. *The Future of Children*, *23*, 99–120.

Enewold, L., Brinton, L. A., McGlynn, K. A., Zahm, S. H., Potter, J. F., & Zhu, K. (2010). Oral contraceptive use among women in the military and the general US population. *Journal of Women's Health*, *19*, 839–845.

Esqueda, M. C., Astor, R. A., & de Pedro, K. M. T. (2012). A call to duty: Educational policy and school reform addressing the needs of children from military families. *Educational Researcher*, *41*, 65–70.

Evans, M. A., & Rosen, L. (1997). Pregnancy planning and the impact of work climate, psychological well-being and work effort in the military. *Journal of Occupational Health Psychology*, *2*, 352–361.

Farwell, A. L. (2017). An integrative review of breastfeeding duration and influencing factors among women serving active duty in the US military. *Journal of Obstetric, Gynecologic & Neonatal Nursing*, *46*, 171–181.

Fitzgerald, A. S., Duboyce, R. L., Ritter, J. B., Omori, D. J., Cooper, B. A., & O'Malley, P. G. (2013). A primer on the unique challenges of female soldiers' reproductive issues in a war-ready culture. *Military Medicine*, *178*, 511–516.

Flake, E. M., Davis, B. E., Johnson, P. L., & Middleton, L. S. (2009). The psychosocial effects of deployment on military children. *Journal of Developmental & Behavioral Pediatrics*, *30*, 271–278.

Floyd, M. L., & Phillips, D. A. (2013). Child care and other support programs. *The Future of Children*, *23*, 79–97.

Foreman, E., Pike, L., DuPont, S., & Lunghi, B. (2001). Psychosocial wellbeing of children from mobile and military families. Paper presented at the Helping Families Change conference. Melbourne, Victoria, Australia.

Galovski, T., & Lyons, J. A. (2004). Psychological sequelae of combat violence: A review of the impact of PTSD on the veteran's family and possible interventions. *Aggression and Violent Behavior*, *9*, 477–501.

Gavin, N. I., Gaynes, B. N., Lohr, K. N., Meltzer-Brody, S., Gartlehner, G., & Swinson, T. (2005). Perinatal depression: A systematic review of prevalence and incidence. *Obstetrics & Gynecology*, *106*, 1071–1083.

Gewirtz, A. H., Erbes, C. R., Polusny, M. A., Forgatch, M. S., & DeGarmo, D. S. (2011). Helping military families through the deployment process: Strategies to support parenting. *Professional Psychology: Research and Practice*, *42*, 56–62.

Gibbs, D. A., Martin, S. L., Kupper, L. L., & Johnson, R. E. (2007). Child maltreatment in enlisted soldiers' families during combat-related deployments. *Journal of the American Medical Association*, *298*, 528–535.

Goff, B. S. N., Crow, J. R., Reisbig, A. M., & Hamilton, S. (2007). The impact of individual trauma symptoms of deployed soldiers on relationship satisfaction. *Journal of Family Psychology*, *21*, 344–353.

Goodman, P., Turner, A., Agazio, J., Throop, M., Padden, D., Greiner, S., & Hillier, S. L. (2013). Deployment of military mothers: Supportive and nonsupportive military programs, processes, and policies. *Military Medicine*, *178*, 729–734.

Gorman, G. H., Eide, M., & Hisle-Gorman, E. (2010). Wartime military deployment and increased pediatric mental and behavioral health complaints. *Pediatrics*, *126*, 1058–1066.

Gottman, J. M., Gottman, J. S., & Atkins, C. L. (2011). The comprehensive soldier fitness program: Family skills component. *American Psychologist*, *66*, 52–57.

Government Accountability Office. (1997). *Military personnel: DoD could save millions by better screening of enlisted personnel*. GAO Publication No. 97-39. US Government Printing Office, Washington, DC.

Government Accountability Office. (2012). *Military child care: DoD is taking actions to address awareness and availability barriers*. GAO Publication No. 12-21. Government Printing Office, Washington, DC.

Greenhaus, J. H., & Beutell, N. J. (1985). Sources of conflict between work and family roles. *Academy of Management Review*, *10*, 76–88.

Grindlay, K., & Grossman, D. (2013). Unintended pregnancy among active-duty women in the United States military, 2008. *Obstetrics & Gynecology*, *121*, 241–246.

Grindlay, K., Yanow, S., Jelinska, K., Gomperts, R., & Grossman, D. (2011). Abortion restrictions in the US military: Voices from women deployed overseas. *Women's Health Issues*, *21*, 259–264.

Haas, L., & Hwang, C. P. (2007). Gender and organizational culture. *Gender and Society*, *21*, 52–79.

Haas, D. M., Pazdernik, L. A., & Olsen, C. H. (2005). A cross-sectional survey of the relationship between partner deployment and stress in pregnancy during wartime. *Women's Health Issues*, *15*, 48–54.

Hammer, L. B., Kossek, E. E., Yragui, N. L., Bodner, T. E., & Hanson, G. C. (2009). Development and validation of a multidimensional measure of family supportive supervisor behaviors (FSSB). *Journal of Management*, *34*, 837–856.

Hammer, L. B., Kossek, E. E., Zimmerman, K., & Daniels, R. (2007). Clarifying the construct of family-supportive supervisory behaviors (FSSB): A multilevel perspective. *Research in Occupational Stress and Well-Being*, *6*, 171–211.

Harms, P. D., Krasikova, D. V., Vanhove, A. J., Herian, M. N., & Lester, P. B. (2013). Stress and emotional well-being in military organizations. *Research in Occupational Stress and Well-Being*, *11*, 103–132.

Harrison, J., & Vannest, K. J. (2008). Educators supporting families in times of crisis: Military reserve deployments. *Preventing School Failure: Alternative Education for Children and Youth*, *52*, 17–24.

Haskell, S. G., Brandt, C. A., Krebs, E. E., Skanderson, M., Kerns, R. D., & Goulet, J. L. (2009). Pain among veterans of operations enduring freedom and Iraqi freedom: Do women and men differ? *Pain Medicine*, *10*, 1167–1173.

Heilmann, S. G., Bell, J. E., & McDonald, G. K. (2009). Work–home conflict: A study of the effects of role conflict on military officer turnover intention. *Journal of Leadership and Organizational Studies*, *16*, 85–96.

Hisle-Gorman, E., Harrington, D., Nylund, C. M., Tercyak, K. P., Anthony, B. J., & Gorman, G. H. (2015). Impact of parents' wartime military deployment and injury on young children's safety and mental health. *Journal of the American Academy of Child & Adolescent Psychiatry*, *54*, 294–301.

Hoge, C. W., Castro, C. A., Messer, S. C., McGurk, D., Cotting, D. I., & Koffman, R. L. (2004). Combat duty in Iraq and Afghanistan, mental health problems, and barriers to care. *New England Journal of Medicine*, *351*, 13–22.

Huffman, A. H., Craddock, E. B., Culbertson, S. S., & Klinefelter, Z. (2017). Decision-making and exchange processes of dual-military couples: A review and suggested strategies for navigating multiple roles. *Military Psychology*, *29*, 11–26.

Huffman, A. H., Culbertson, S. S., & Barbour, J. (2015). Gender roles in a masculine occupation: Military men and women's differential negotiation of the work–family interface. In M. J. Mills (Ed.), *Gender and the work–family experience: An intersection of two domains* (pp. 271–289). New York, NY: Springer.

Huffman, A. H., Culbertson, S. S., & Castro, C. A. (2008). Family-friendly environments and US army soldier performance and work outcomes. *Military Psychology*, *20*, 253–270.

Huffman, A. H., Matthews, R. A., & Irving, L. (2017). Family fairness and cohesion in marital dyads: Mediating processes between work–family conflict and couple psychological distress. *Journal of Occupational and Organizational Psychology*, *90*, 95–116.

Institute of Medicine. (2013). *Returning home from Iraq and Afghanistan: Assessment of readjustment needs of veterans, service members, and their families.* Washington, DC: National Academies Press.

Jeffreys, D. J., & Leitzel, J. D. (2000). The strengths and vulnerabilities of adolescents in military families. In J. A. Martin, L. N. Rosen, & L. R. Sparacino (Eds.), *The military family: A practice guide for human service providers* (pp. 225–240). Westport, CT: Praeger.

Jensen, C. P. S., Xenakis, S. N., Wolf, L. P., & Bain, M. W. (1991). The "military family syndrome" revisited: By the numbers. *The Journal of Nervous and Mental Disease*, *179*, 102–107.

Johnson, H. L., & Ling, C. G. (2013). Caring for military children in the 21st century. *Journal of the American Association of Nurse Practitioners*, *25*, 195–202.

Kaczmarek, E. A., & Sibbel, A. M. (2008). The psychosocial well-being of children from Australian military and fly-in/fly-out (FIFO) mining families. *Community, Work & Family*, *11*, 297–312.

Karin, M. (2009). Time off for military families: An emerging case study of a time of war... And the tipping point for future laws supporting work–life balance? *Rutgers Law Record, 33*, 46–64.

Karney, B., & Crown, J. (2007). *Families under stress: An assessment of data, theory, and research, on marriage and divorce in the military*. Arlington, VA: National Defense Research Institute (RAND). Retrieved from http://www.rand.org/pubs/monographs/2007/RAND_MG599.sum.pdf

Kelley, M. L., Hock, E., Bonney, J. F., Jarvis, M. S., Smith, K. M., & Gaffney, M. A. (2001). Navy mothers experiencing and not experiencing deployment: Reasons for staying in or leaving the military. *Military Psychology, 13*, 55–71.

Kennedy, H. P., Farrell, T., Paden, R., Hill, S., Jolivet, R., Willetts, J., & Rising, S. S. (2009). "I wasn't alone" – A study of group prenatal care in the military. *Journal of Midwifery & Women's Health, 54*, 176–183.

Khaylis, A., Polusny, M. A., Erbes, C. R., Gewirtz, A., & Rath, M. (2011). Post-traumatic stress, family adjustment, and treatment preferences among National Guard soldiers deployed to OEF/OIF. *Military Medicine, 176*, 126–131.

Kim, P. Y., Britt, T. W., Klocko, R. P., Riviere, L. A., & Adler, A. B. (2011). Stigma, negative attitudes about treatment, and utilization of mental health care among soldiers. *Military Psychology, 23*, 65–81.

Klaman, S. L., & Turner, K. (2016). Prevalence of perinatal depression in the military: A systematic review of the literature. *Maternal and Child Health Journal, 20*, 52–65.

Kleykamp, M., Kelty, R., & Segal, D. R. (2017). Military service in midlife. In L. M. Padilla-Walker & L. J. Nelson (Eds.) *Flourishing in emerging adulthood: Positive development during the third decade of life* (pp. 307–325). New York, NY: Oxford University Press.

Krulewitch, C. J. (2016). Reproductive health of active duty women in medically austere environments. *Military Medicine, 181*, 63–69.

Kudler, H., & Porter, C. R. I. (2013). Building communities of care for military children and families. *The Future of Children, 23*, 163–185.

Le, J. K., Tissington, P. A., & Budhwar, P. (2010). To move or not to move – A question of family? *The International Journal of Human Resource Management, 21*, 17–45.

LeardMann, C. A., Smith, T. C., Smith, B., Wells, T. S., & Ryan, M. A. (2009). Baseline self-reported functional health and vulnerability to post-traumatic stress disorder after combat deployment: Prospective US military cohort study. *British Medical Journal, 338*, b1273.

Lester, P., Aralis, H., Sinclair, M., Kiff, C., Lee, K. H., Mustillo, S., & MacDermid Wadsworth, S. M. (2016). The impact of deployment on parental, family and child adjustment in military families. *Child Psychiatry & Human Development, 47*, 938–949.

Lester, P., & Flake, L. C. E. (2013). How wartime military service affects children and families. *The Future of Children, 23*, 121–141.

Lester, P., Peterson, K., Reeves, J., Knauss, L., Glover, D., Mogil, C., ... Beardslee, W. (2010). The long war and parental combat deployment: Effects on military children and at-home spouses. *Journal of the American Academy of Child & Adolescent Psychiatry, 49*, 310–320.

Lincoln, A., Swift, E., & Shorteno-Fraser, M. (2008). Psychological adjustment and treatment of children and families with parents deployed in military combat. *Journal of Clinical Psychology, 84*, 984–992.

Lucas-Thompson, R. G., & Goldberg, W. A. (2015). Gender ideology and work–family plans of the next generation. In M. Mills (Ed.), *Gender and the work–family experience: An intersection of two domains* (pp. 3–20). New York, NY: Springer.

MacDermid Wadsworth, S. M. (2010). Family risk and resilience in the context of war and terrorism. *Journal of Marriage and Family, 72*, 537–556.

MacDermid Wadsworth, S. M., & Southwell, K. (2011). Military families: Extreme work and extreme "work–family". *The Annals of the American Academy of Political and Social Science, 638*, 163–183.

MacLean, A., & Elder, G. H. (2007). Military service in the life course. *Annual Review of Sociology, 33*, 175–196.

Mackenzie, M. H. (2012). Let women fight. *Foreign Affairs, 91*, 32–42.

Mansfield, A. J., Kaufman, J. S., Engel, C. C., & Gaynes, B. N. (2011). Deployment and mental health diagnoses among children of US Army personnel. *Archives of Pediatrics & Adolescent Medicine, 165*, 999–1005.

Manski, R., Grindlay, K., Burns, B., Holt, K., & Grossman, D. (2014). Reproductive health access among deployed US servicewomen: A qualitative study. *Military Medicine*, *179*, 645–652.

Mao, C. Y., Narang, S., & Lopreiato, J. (2012). Breastfeeding practices in military families: A 12-month prospective population-based study in the national capital region. *Military Medicine*, *177*, 229–234.

Martin, S. E., Drake, E., Yoder, L., Gibson, M., & Litke, C. A. (2015). Active duty women's perceptions of breast-feeding support in the military setting. *Military Medicine*, *180*, 1154–1160.

Matthews, R. A., Mills, M. J., Trout, R., & English, L. (2014). Family-supportive supervisor behaviors, work engagement, and subjective well-being: A contextually dependent mediated process. *Journal of Occupational Health Psychology*, *19*, 168–181.

Mattocks, K. M., Skanderson, M., Goulet, J. L., Brandt, C., Womack, J., Krebs, E., … Haskell, S. (2010). Pregnancy and mental health among women veterans returning from Iraq and Afghanistan. *Journal of Women's Health*, *19*, 2159–2166.

McFadyen, J., Kerpelman, J., & Adler-Baeder, F. (2005). Examining the impact of workplace supports: Work–family fit and satisfaction in the US military. *Family Relations*, *54*, 131–144.

McGraw, K., Koehlmoos, T. P., & Ritchie, E. C. (2016). Women in combat: Framing the issues of health and health research for America's servicewomen. *Military Medicine*, *181*, 7–11.

McNeary, A. M., & Lomenick, T. S. (2000). Military duty: Risk factor for preterm labor? A review. *Military Medicine*, *165*, 612–615.

Meadows, S. O., Beckett, M. K., Bowling, K., Golinelli, D., Fisher, M. P., …, Osilla, K. C. (2015). *Family resilience in the military: Definitions, models, and policies*. Santa Monica, CA: RAND.

Messersmith-Heroman, K., Heroman, W. M., & Moore, T. R. (1994). Pregnancy outcome in military and civilian women. *Military Medicine*, *15*, 577–579.

Military Leadership Diversity Commission. (2010). *Re-enlistment rates across the services by gender and race/ethnicity*. Issue Paper #31. Retrieved from https://www.hsdl.org/?view&did=716162

Milliken, C. S., Auchterlonie, J. L., & Hoge, C. W. (2007). Longitudinal assessment of mental health problems among active and reserve component soldiers returning from the Iraq war. *Journal of the American Medical Association*, *298*, 2141–2148.

Mills, M. J., Matthews, R. A., Henning, J. B., & Woo, V. A. (2014). Family-supportive organizations and supervisors: How do they influence employee outcomes and for whom? *International Journal of Human Resource Management*, *25*, 1763–1785.

Mills, M. J., Pervez, A., & Mandeville, A. (2018). We're not there yet: Gender and the work–family interface in the modern workscape. In J. Nicklin (Ed.) *Work-life balance in the 21st century: Perspectives, practices, and challenges* (pp. 66–80). Hauppauge, NY: Nova Science Publishers.

Mulhall, E. (2009). Supporting she 'who has borne the battle'. In *Women warriors. Iraq and Afghanistan veterans of America*. Retrieved from http://media.iava.org/IAVA_WomensReport_2009.pdf

Mustillo, S., MacDermid Wadsworth, S. M., & Lester, P. (2016). Parental deployment and well-being in children: Results from a new study of military families. *Journal of Emotional and Behavioral Disorders*, *24*, 82–91.

Nguyen, S., LeardMann, C. A., Smith, B., Conlin, A. M. S., Slymen, D. J., Hooper, T. I., … Smith, T. C. (2013). Is military deployment a risk factor for maternal depression? *Journal of Women's Health*, *22*, 9–18.

O'Boyle, A. L., Magaan, E. F., Ricks, R. E., Doyle, M., & Morrison, J. C. (2005). Depression screening in the pregnant soldier wellness program. *Southern Medical Journal*, *98*, 416–418.

Odle-Dusseau, H. N., Herleman, H. A., Britt, T. W., Moore, D. D., Castro, C. A., & McGurk, D. (2013). Family-supportive work environments and psychological strain: A longitudinal test of two theories. *Journal of Occupational Health Psychology*, *18*, 27–36.

O'Hara, M. W., & Swain, A. M. (1996). Rates and risk of postpartum depression: A meta-analysis. *International Review of Psychiatry*, *8*, 37–54.

Orthner, D. K. (2002a). *Relocation adjustment among Army civilian spouses*. 2001 Survey of Army Families (SAF) IV, US Army Community and Family Support Center. Retrieved from http://armymwr.com/corporateoperations/planning/surveys.asp

Orthner, D. K. (2002b). *Family readiness support and adjustment among Army civilian spouses*. Survey of Army Families IV, Survey Report, Army Research Institute. Retrieved from http://www.armymwr.com/corporate/ operations/planning/surveys

Orthner, D. K. (2002c). *Deployment and separation adjustment among Army civilian spouses*. SAF IV Survey Report, University of North Carolina at Chapel Hill. Retrieved from http://www.armymwr.com

Oswald, R. F., & Sternberg, M. M. (2014). Lesbian, gay, and bisexual military families: Visible but legally marginalized. In S. MacDermid Wadsworth & D. S. Riggs (Eds.), *Military deployment and its consequences for families* (pp. 133–149). New York, NY: Springer.

Paris, R., DeVoe, E. R., Ross, A. M., & Acker, M. L. (2010). When a parent goes to war: Effects of parental deployment on very young children and implications for intervention. *American Journal of Orthopsychiatry*, *80*, 610–618.

Park, N. (2011). Military children and families: Strengths and challenges during peace and war. *American Psychologist*, *66*, 65–72.

Patten, E., & Parker, K. (2011). *Women in the US military: Growing share, distinctive profile*. Pew Research Center. Retrieved from http://www.pewsocialtrends.org/2011/12/22/women-in-the-u-s-military-growing-share-distinctive-profile/

Patterson, G. (2005). The next generation of PMTO models. *The Behavior Therapist*, *28*, 27–33.

Pierce, P. F. (1998). Retention of Air Force women serving during Desert Shield and Desert Storm. *Military Psychology*, *10*, 195–213.

Porter, T. L., & Johnson, W. B. (1994). Psychiatric stigma in the military. *Military Medicine*, *159*, 602–609.

Posada, G., Walker, D., Cardin, J. F., Nyaronga, D., Schwarz, R., & MacDermid Wadsworth, S. M. (2015). Maternal perspectives on deployment and child–mother relationships in military families. *Family Relations*, *64*, 651–664.

Rentz, E. D., Marshall, S. W., Loomis, D., Casteel, C., Martin, S. L., & Gibbs, D. A. (2007). Effect of deployment on the occurrence of child maltreatment in military and nonmilitary families. *American Journal of Epidemiology*, *165*, 1199–1206.

Richardson, E. W., Mallette, J. K., O'Neal, C. W., & Mancini, J. A. (2016). Do youth development programs matter? An examination of transitions and well-being among military youth. *Journal of Child and Family Studies*, *25*, 1765–1776.

Rishel, P. E., & Sweeney, P. (2005). Comparison of breastfeeding rates among women delivering in military treatment facilities with and without a lactation consultant. *Military Medicine*, *170*, 435–438.

Ritchie, E. C. (2001). Issues for military women in deployment: An overview. *Military Medicine*, *166*, 1033–1037.

Rosiello, R., & Mills, M. J. (2015). Shift work as gendered and its impact on work–family balance. In M. J. Mills (Ed.), *Gender and the work–family experience: An intersection of two domains* (pp. 251–270). New York, NY: Springer.

Rousseau, D. M., Ho, V. T., & Greenberg, J. (2006). I-deals: Idiosyncratic terms in employment relationships. *Academy of Management Review*, *31*, 977–994.

Rowe-Finkbeiner, K., Martin, R., Abrams, B., Zuccaro, A., & Dardari, Y. (2016). Why paid family and medical leave matters for the future of America's families, businesses and economy. *Maternal and Child Health Journal*, *20*, 8–12.

Russo, T. J., & Fallon, M. A. (2015). Coping with stress: Supporting the needs of military families and their children. *Early Childhood Education Journal*, *43*, 407–416.

Rychnovsky, J., & Beck, C. T. (2006). Screening for postpartum depression in military women with the postpartum depression screening scale. *Military Medicine*, *171*, 1100–1104.

Saltzman, W. R., Lester, P., Beardslee, W. R., Layne, C. M., Woodward, K., & Nash, W. P. (2011). Mechanisms of risk and resilience in military families: Theoretical and empirical basis of a family-focused resilience enhancement program. *Clinical Child and Family Psychology Review*, *14*, 213–230.

Schumm, W. R., Bell, D. B., Milan, L. M., & Segal, M. W. (2000). *The family support group (FSG) leaders' handbook*. Alexandria, VA: US Army Research Institute for the Behavioral and Social Sciences.

Segal, M. W. (1988). The military and families as greedy institutions. In C. C. Moskos & F. R. Wood (Eds.), *The military: More than just a job?* (pp. 79–98). Washington, DC: Pergaman-Brassey's International Defense Publishers, Inc.

Segal, M. W., & Lane, M. D. (2016). Conceptual model of military women's life events and well-being. *Military Medicine*, *181*, 12–19.

Seo, J. Y., Lloyd, D. A., & Nam, S. I. (2014). Work–family conflict and intimate partner violence in the South Korean military: Mediating role of aggression and buffering effect of a counseling resource. *Journal of Family Violence*, *29*, 839–847.

Shah, P. S., Balkhair, T., Ohlsson, A., Beyene, J., Scott, F., & Frick, C. (2011). Intention to become pregnant and low birth weight and preterm birth: A systematic review. *Maternal and Child Health Journal*, *15*, 205–216.

Silva, J. M. (2008). A new generation of women? How female ROTC cadets negotiate the tension between masculine military culture and traditional femininity. *Social Forces*, *87*, 937–960.

Skomorovsky, A., Hujaleh, F., & Wolejszo, S. (2015). Intimate partner violence in the Canadian armed forces: The role of family stress and its impact on well-being. *Military Medicine*, *180*, 809–816.

Smith, T. C., Ryan, M. A., Wingard, D. L., Slymen, D. J., Sallis, J. F., & Kritz-Silverstein, D. (2008). New onset and persistent symptoms of post-traumatic stress disorder self reported after deployment and combat exposures: Prospective population-based US military cohort study. *British Medical Journal*, *336*, 366–371.

Southwell, K. H., & MacDermid Wadsworth, S. M. (2016). The many faces of military families: Unique features of the lives of female service members. *Military Medicine*, *181*, 70–79.

Spitzmueller, C., Wang, Z., Zhang, J., Thomas, C. L., Fisher, G. G., Matthews, R. A., & Strathearn, L. (2016). Got milk? Workplace factors related to breastfeeding among working mothers. *Journal of Organizational Behavior*, *37*, 692–718.

Stanfors, M. (2014). Fertility and the fast-track: Continued childbearing among professionals in Sweden, 1991–2009. *Demographic Research*, *31*, 421–458.

Stansfeld, S., & Candy, B. (2006). Psychosocial work environment and mental health – A meta-analytic review. *Scandinavian Journal of Work and Environmental Health, 32,* 443–462.

Stinson, J. C., & Lee, K. A. (2003). Premature labor and birth: Influence of rank and perception of fatigue in active duty military women. *Military Medicine*, *168*, 385–390.

Sylvia, B. M., McMullen, P., Levine, E., & Cruz, F. B. (2001). Prenatal care needs, availability, accessibility, use, and satisfaction: A comparison of military women within and outside the continental United States. *Military Medicine*, *166*, 443–448.

Tanaka, S. (2005). Parental leave and child health across OECD countries. *The Economic Journal*, *115*, F7–F28.

Thomas, J. L., Wilk, J. E., Riviere, L. A., McGurk, D., Castro, C. A., & Hoge, C. W. (2010). Prevalence of mental health problems and functional impairment among active component and National Guard soldiers 3 and 12 months following combat in Iraq. *Archives of General Psychiatry*, *67*, 614–623.

Tremblay, D. G. (2016). Work–family balance for women lawyers today: A reality or still a dream? In M. L. Connerley & J. Wu (Eds.), *Handbook on well-being of working women* (pp. 345–359). Dordrecht, The Netherlands: Springer.

Tucker, J. S., Sinclair, R. R., & Thomas, J. L. (2005). The multilevel effects of occupational stressors and soldiers' well-being, organizational attachment, and readiness. *Journal of Occupational Health Psychology*, *10*, 276–299.

US Army Community and Family Support Center. (2005). *Highlights: Survey of army families V*. Retrieved from http://www.army.mil/cfsc/documents/research/safv/SAFSummary.doc

US Navy Regulation (OPNAVINST 6110.1J). (2011). Physical readiness program. Retrieved from http://www.navy-prt.com/files/6110.1J_-_Physical_Readiness_program.pdf

Uriell, Z. A., & Burress, L. (2009). *Pregnancy and parenthood in the Navy: Results of the 2008 survey* (NPRST-AB-09-3). Millington, TN: Navy Personnel Research, Studies, and Technology Division, Bureau of Naval Personnel (NPRST/PERS-1).

Uriell, Z., Perry, A., Kee, A., & Burress, L. (2009). Breastfeeding in the Navy: Estimates of rate, duration, and perceived support. *Military Medicine*, *174*, 290–296.

Weina, S. U. (2006). Effects of pregnancy on the Army physical fitness test. *Military Medicine*, *171*, 534–537.

World Health Organization. (2002). *Global strategy on infant and young child feeding*. Retrieved from http://apps.who.int/gb/archive/pdf_files/WHA55/ea5515.pdf?ua

EXAMINING VETERAN TRANSITION TO THE WORKPLACE THROUGH MILITARY TRANSITION THEORY

Sara Kintzle and Carl A. Castro

ABSTRACT

The transition from military service to civilian employment is one of the most important factors related to post-service well-being and success. It is also one of the biggest challenges. The majority of veterans describe finding a job as the greatest challenge in transitioning to civilian life. While research has demonstrated a number of contributory factors related to difficulty in finding employment, a conceptual framework for understanding such challenges has yet to be proposed. Military transition theory describes the progression through which service members' transition out of the military and illustrates how certain factors may create susceptibility to negative transition outcomes. The purpose of this chapter is to utilize the military transition theory to provide a foundation for understanding the factors related to successful transition to the civilian workplace after military separation.

Keywords: Veteran; employment; military transition theory; military separation; transition outcomes; civilian employment

Securing employment post-transition from the military is one of the most important factors related to post-service well-being and success. It is also one of the biggest challenges. To those who serve the military, employment is often considered much more than a job. It is a call to service, an identity, a community, and a way of life that produces profound meaning. Finding post-service employment

Occupational Stress and Well-being in Military Contexts
Research in Occupational Stress and Well-being, Volume 16, 117–127
Copyright © 2018 by Emerald Publishing Limited
All rights of reproduction in any form reserved
ISSN: 1479-3555/doi:10.1108/S1479-355520180000016009

with the same attributes can be difficult. However, civilian employment after military separation not only provides financial stability, but also can aid in the development of new professional networks and colleagues, provide a new sense of purpose and meaning, and help transitioning service members foster their new identity as a veteran and a civilian.

The majority of veterans describe finding a job as the greatest challenge in transitioning to civilian life (Prudential.com, 2012). Over half of separating post-9/11 veterans will experience a period of unemployment after discharge from the military (Department of Veterans Affairs, 2015). This is most often attributed to the initial job-search period (Loughran, 2014). However, many veterans indicate that they need a break after separation from the military as well as time to figure out what they want to do with their life (Castro & Kintzle, 2017; Castro, Kintzle, & Hassan, 2014, 2015; Kintzle, Rasheed-Wallace, & Castro, 2016).

Research has demonstrated a number of contributory factors related to difficulty in finding employment. These include translating military qualifications, skills, and experiences to civilian jobs (Hall, Harrell, Bicksler, Stewart, & Fischer, 2014; Harrell & Berglass, 2014), challenges to resume-writing, interviewing, and professional networking (Prudential.com, 2012), stigma associated with hiring veterans (Stone & Stone, 2015), and physical and psychological health symptoms ((Burnett-Zeigler et al., 2011; Faberman & Foster, 2013). Despite the aforementioned findings, research on employment after military separation is still limited, and tends to focus narrowly on the issues outlined above. Further, the field has yet to provide a theoretical framework for understanding how such employment challenges emerge as well as what factors may predict workplace success. Military transition theory is a new and emerging theory that provides a conceptual framework for understanding the factors related to successful transition from the military and the impact of transition outcomes. The purpose of this chapter is to utilize the military transition theory to provide an understanding of veteran's transition to the civilian workplace after military separation.

MILITARY TRANSITION THEORY

The military transition theory describes the progression through which service members' transition out of the military (Castro & Kintzle, 2014). Military transition entails moving from the military culture to the civilian culture, producing changes in relationships, assumptions, work context, and personal and social identity. The theory postulates three phases describing individual, interpersonal, community, and military organizational factors that impact the military transition process. The military transition theory illustrates how certain factors may create susceptibility to negative outcomes, including challenges to finding and keeping civilian employment.

The military transition theory is defined by three interacting and overlapping components. The first segment of theory, approaching the military transition, outlines personal, cultural, and transitional factors that create the base of transition trajectory. These include military cultural factors such as type of military discharge and combat history, personal characteristics such as health, expectations, and personal preparedness, and lastly, factors describing the nature of the transition, that is, predictable or unpredictable, positive or negative.

The second segment, managing the transition, refers to factors affecting the individual progression from service member to civilian. Individual adjustment factors, such as coping styles, attitudes, and beliefs, impact how transition is managed. Social support in varying forms such as family, friends, community, and society may also affect transition. The military transition management includes navigating the resources provided by the military, that is, veterans' affairs (VA) benefits, education benefits, and career planning. Finally, community and civilian transition support describes the factors the civilian population can utilize in supporting transitioning service members.

The final segment, assessing the transition, describes outcomes associated with transition. These outcomes are measured through the categories of work, family, health, general well-being, and community. More specifically, these include whether the transitioning service member secured adequate employment, re-acclimation to family life and adjustment to new family roles, physical and psychological health, adaption to new social networks, and engagement in the community. Outcomes are interconnected as they impact one another. For example, challenges to physical health may create challenges in finding employment. However, success or failure in one outcome does not indicate success or failure in overall transition.

MILITARY TRANSITION THEORY: MILITARY TO CIVILIAN TRANSITION FACTORS

The theoretical framework outlined in the military to civilian transition provides insight into the factors that can impact veteran's ability to secure employment. Many of these factors can be used to demonstrate why some individuals find success and others do not, the barriers to finding employment as a transitioning service member, and the risk/protective factors associated with post-service employment success. Outlined below are the phases of this transition along with the variables associated with each phase that may impact employment.

APPROACHING MILITARY TRANSITION

Military and Cultural Factors

Military Skill

Applying for civilian jobs may be challenging for veterans as they attempt to translate military qualifications, skills, and experiences to civilian jobs (Hall et al., 2014; Harrell & Berglass, 2014). Skills translation and transferability can cause difficulties for civilian employers and veteran employees regarding suitable positions and workplaces (Hall et al., 2014; Harrell & Berglass, 2014). Service members enter the military with a varying degree of skills. Some may come in with skills they developed pre-service, others may join with little or no skills at all.

However, every service member develops skills while they are in the military. Some of these skills are transferrable to the civilian world, others are not. One could imagine that an individual serving an infantry unit might have more difficulty translating skills to a civilian workplace than an individual who served in a medical unit. Either way, not all service members want to do the same work post-service that they did while in the military. This ability to translate military skills to the civilian world is a significant barrier for transitioning service members. The type of skills developed during military service may be a predictor of how significant this barrier might be for a separating service member.

Military Identity

Socialization to the military culture begins during initial entry as members of the military learn customs, habits, practices, norms, and policies that will dictate their time of service (Smith & True, 2014). This process is seen as vital as it leads to the development of a strong military culture and viewing other members of the military like a family. Through this socialization, many individuals who serve in the armed forces develop a strong sense of military identity. This develops as their life becomes immersed in military culture through their service and most often continues even after leaving the military. However, military identity can have a significant impact on the post-service transition as individuals often experience "warring identities" between their strong sense of self as a service member and their new identity as a veteran. These competing identities can become problematic if separating service members are unable to adapt to this new sense of civilian identity (Ecclestone, Biesta, & Hughes, 2010; Smith & True, 2014).

Navigating a military identity in a civilian workplace environment can be difficult. The military system is structured through the application of strong work ethics with standard and equal rules for salary and advancement. Many veterans report a clash of culture in civilian work environments, one that can cause frustration and lead to workplace difficulty. Finding success in employment post-service often requires learning new norms, accepting differences between the cultures, and modifying expectations of the work environment. Individuals who have difficulty with this conversion may also have difficulty finding and keeping employment.

Military Discharge Status

Potential employers may ask about military service as well as the condition of discharge. Like any negative mark on a record, receiving a non-honorable discharge can severely limit employment options following military transition. Kintzle et al. (2015) found discharge status to be a common theme in chronically unemployed veterans. A non-honorable discharge status could be viewed as evidence of negative and/or unlawful behavior and cause hesitation on the part of the employer. This type of discharge status also limits access to veteran's benefits that could assist in securing employment. Non-honorable discharge statuses have also been linked with negative physical and mental health outcomes, which may also impact employability (Castro & Kintzle, 2017). The service members with a non-honorable discharge status are considered at risk for employment challenges.

Personal Characteristics

Preparation

Keeling, Ozuna, Kintzle, and Castro (in press) found preparation to be an essential factor for securing post-separation employment. Despite this, most veterans report that they were not at all prepared for finding employment post-service; 80% leave the military without having lined up for employment and most have not taken steps that would help them find employment after transition (Castro & Kintzle, 2017; Castro et al., 2014, 2015; Kintzle et al., 2016). There are many factors behind this lack of preparation (Keeling, Kintzle, & Castro, in press). Veterans indicate that they were not given the time or opportunities to look for work, prepare resumes, or go for interviews while they are still serving. This is exacerbated by the fact that many will be moving to a new community, which can make these tasks more difficult. Providing leave for service members to secure civilian employment while still on active duty is most often not a priority of the military.

An additional cause for this lack of preparation is that many service members leaving active duty are focused solely on getting out of the military, and haven't put much thought into the future. Transitioning service members also report needing a break before they move on to their next job, and some need time to figure out what they are going to do next in life (Castro & Kintzle, 2017; Castro et al., 2014, 2015; Kintzle et al., 2016). Regardless of the reason, lack of preparation is a significant barrier to post-service employment.

Expectations

Many service members leave the military with expectations that finding satisfactory employment will be easy (Keeling, Kintzle et al., in press). Some assume, as they have often been told, that their military status will provide them priority for certain positions. However, as we have displayed here, finding post-service employment can be quite challenging. Many report feeling as though after giving their life to military service, after separation they are suddenly forced to start over, often in entry level low paying jobs (Keeling, Ozuna et al., in press). Therefore, when separating service members experience these unexpected difficulties it can cause resentment, frustration, and anger.

Further complicating the issue are expectations of the income they will receive as civilians. The expectations of many separating service members are that they will earn more money as a civilian than as a service member; certainly no separating service member expects to earn less once they leave the military. Given that the military compensation of a sergeant/petty officer second class/staff sergeant (E-5), who is 26 years old, married with one child, has been on active duty for six years, and has some college experience, depending on duty location, can range from approximately $68,000–87,000, expecting similar civilian employment compensation is not realistic; especially given that the US national median income is around $53,000 for all workers. Many transitioning service members will be competing with civilians with college degrees and several years' of experience in a particular field. Therefore, unmet expectations for employment after military separation can create barriers to this work transition.

Health

Many service members leave the military with unmet physical and psychological health needs. It is reported that veterans facing health challenges as a result of their military service report greater employment concerns, especially in finding and maintaining work (Faberman & Foster, 2013). Veterans with physical and/or psychological health complaints have been found more likely to be unemployed (Prudential.com, 2012). Mental health difficulties have consistently been shown in various veteran and non-veteran studies to be associated with unemployment. Resnick and Rosenheck (2008) found veterans with post-traumatic stress disorder (PTSD) are 19% less likely to be employed. Studies on veteran populations have also found depression and anxiety to be associated with unemployment (Hamilton, Williams, & Washington, 2015; Horton et al., 2013; Zivin et al., 2016). Use of substances such as alcohol, prescription medicines, and other drugs to self-medicate for these uncared issues can also cause substance-use problems that interfere with employment (Kintzle et al., 2015). Kleylamp (2013) reports that a further challenge for those with mental health problems, especially PTSD, is employers' concerns that veterans have high rates of PTSD and are wary of incurring the costs of dealing with PTSD at the workplace. It is important to note that leaving the military with unmet physical and psychological health needs may impact veteran's ability to find and keep successful employment.

Nature of the Transition

Voluntary

Service members who leave the military voluntarily will more likely to have planned for their transition to civilian employment, allowing the opportunity for preparation. Those who are involuntarily discharged from the military may not have time to prepare adequately for employment post-service. These individuals may feel anger for their forced transition to civilian life, which may impact their view of this transition and their motivation to find new employment.

Predictability

Whether or not a service member had notice that he or she would be transitioning out of the military may impact their ability to be prepared to find employment. Unpredictable discharges can come from reduction in forces, injuries, or other than honorable discharges. Since the transition was not expected, service members never expected a need to find civilian employment.

Gradual / sudden
How much time individuals have before their transition will impact preparation time for thinking about their future career and finding employment. Sudden transitions can occur due to injury or involuntary exit. Service members who make a voluntary decision to leave the military know about their transition. Those who are injured or discharged unexpectedly with little notice will have had no opportunity for forethought regarding civilian employment.

MANAGING THE TRANSITION

Individual Adjustment Factors

Coping style
The difficulties veterans may have in transitioning to the civilian workplace in terms of things such as norms and work ethics have been described above. Veterans' ability to manage such friction may impact their ability to maintain employment. Some veterans describe that these challenges at the workplace lead to outbursts or unprofessional behavior (Kintzle et al., 2015). Individuals who demonstrate low frustration tolerance, anger management issues, and difficulties in self-regulation may have a more difficult time managing the emotions that come with this employment transition.

Attitude
Many of the factors that we have discussed above could impact the attitude in which veterans enter the civilian work force. These include expectations, preparations, and the nature of the transition. Veterans' attitude regarding learning new skills, finding meaning in new work, starting over, and feelings to adapt to a new environment may impact their employment success.

Military Transition Management

Supervisor Support
It is not in the interest of the military to make leaving service easy. The military has invested a tremendous amount of resources in recruiting and training its members, and thus does not want to lose them. Yet, without true supervisor support to the service member during the transition process, being prepared for a successful transition is improbable. Supervisors must allow separating service members the necessary time to adequately plan for their transition even if providing such time is not in the short-term interest of the military. In the long term, such behavior is seen as positive since all service members eventually leave the military.

Transition Assistance Program (TAP)
All military branches are required to provide transitional preparation and assistance to individuals transitioning from the military service to civilian life (Veterans

Education and Benefits Expansion Act, 2001). Unfortunately, data on the outcomes or effectiveness of such programs are limited. Many veterans report not attending TAPs, and the reviews of its usefulness are mixed. In a study by Keeling, et al., Ozuna et al. (in press), post-9/11 veterans described the TAP process as a "box checking exercise." While TAP addresses items such as job searching, resume-building, and translating skills, it most often does not include items such as military identity, expectations, and addressing unmet needs. In addition, in its current status, attendance at TAP occurs shortly before transition from the military. Therefore, for many service members, there is not much time to apply for what they have learned. The kind of support provided by the military through transition management is an essential element for preparing service members in securing post-service employment.

Career Planning

As described above, there are many reasons as to why transitioning service members may not have engaged in career planning. Service members who start planning early for a post-military career and then implement that planning during the military transition phase will be more likely to find employment that fits their long-term career plan. However, very little career planning occurs as part of the military transition management provided by the military. A more effective strategy would be to encourage service members the day they join the military to plan for their post-service period. Occurring early, this career planning could assist service members to think about their other passions, skills they have or are needed, and their goals for post-service employment. Career planning could also focus on the more psychological aspects of employment, including the following: What has serving in the military meant to me? What type of jobs could provide me the sense of purpose that I found in the military? What difficulties will I face moving to civilian employment, and how will I deal with them? Military transition theory argues that this level of career planning during military transition management can have a significant impact on employment success.

Job Search

Searching for employment is a job in itself. Along with the lack of career planning comes the lack of knowledge regarding the job search. Many veterans entering the civilian work force would have never looked for, applied for, or were interviewed for a civilian job. This means that new skills are to be developed, including conducting jobs searches, recognizing appropriate jobs, resume-writing, interview skills, and translating military abilities and duties to civilian terms. Regardless of when a service member intends to leave the military, they should always have a well-developed post-military employment strategy because eventually every person has to leave the military, with very few never having the need to work again.

Financial Management

A critical and often overlooked aspect of military-to-civilian life transition is financial management. Many service members had never fully appreciated the relatively generous salary and benefits they had received in the military. Indeed many service members dismiss or minimize the numerous benefits they had received, such as health and dental care, tax-free housing allowance, subsidized exchanges and commissaries to shop as well as significantly reduced life insurance and housing costs. All these benefits, which could easily approach $50,000–100,000 per year, are lost and must be replaced when service members leave the military, depending on where the service members choose to relocate and whether or not they have a family. In particular, service members who have a sizeable debt will most likely struggle financially during the transition. Conversely, service members with adequate savings will be placed in a better position to address significant financial stress that often occurs during the transition phase.

Community/Civilian Transition Support

Community Employment Support

The community the transitioning service member will enter and the supportive services available to that new veteran will also impact employment success. Those entering communities who are ready to welcome, support, train, and employ transitioning veterans will be more likely to find post-service employment. Programs that provide training in resume-writing, interview skills, and translating skill as well as programs that connect veterans with real opportunities of employment that result in securing suitable employment are essential. Less common, but just as important is the training to adjust to the civilian workforce. Community employment support can assist transitioning service members in finding civilian jobs, particularly for those hard to employ veterans. Considering the limited support provided by the military transition programs, community support is essential.

CONCLUSIONS

The effort to secure employment post-separation from the military is essential to transition success. Understanding how veterans find success and how they experience challenges is critical to building programs or interventions that can assist in workplace transition. The military transition theory provides a conceptual framework for understanding the complexities of the military to civilian employment shift. The theory also provides opportunities for developing strategies for addressing employment challenges. While many current veteran employment programs focus on translating skills, resume-building, and conducting interviews, little attention is provided to many of the important factors outlined in the military transition theory. These include preparation and expectations, military identity, and leader support. Professionals working with veterans in transition employment support should utilize this conceptual framework to ensure that their programs work to address the array of issues described in the theory.

Along with expanding current employment programs, the military transition theory also allows for identifying factors that may create susceptibility to negative outcomes, including challenges to finding and retaining civilian employment. By recognizing such factors, risks for employment challenges can be identified and addressed early before chronic challenges occur. Future research should examine the impact of these factors and how they manifest throughout the transition process.

The focus on employment after transition is an important issue. Inability to secure long-term employment after transition may lead to more chronic issues, such as long-term unemployment, financial and housing instability, family problems, and legal issues. The theoretical framework outlined in the military transition theory provides valuable insight into the factors that can impact veteran's ability to secure employment.

REFERENCES

Burnett-Zeigler, I., Valenstein, M., Ilgen, M., Blow, A. J., Gorman, L. A., & Zivin, K. (2011). Civilian employment among recently returning afghanistan and iraq national guard veterans. *Military Medicine, 176*(6), 639–646.

Castro, C. A., & Kintzle, S. (2014). Suicides in the military: The post-modern combat veteran and the Hemingway effect. *Current Psychiatry Reports, 16*(8), 460.

Castro, C. A., & Kintzle, S. (2017). *The state of the American veteran: The San Francisco veterans study.* Los Angeles, CA: USC CIR.

Castro, C. A., Kintzle, S., & Hassan, A. (2014). *The state of the American veteran: The Los Angeles county veterans study.* Los Angeles, CA: USC CIR.

Castro, C. A., Kintzle, S., & Hassan, A. (2015). *The state of the American veteran: The Los Angeles county veterans study.* Los Angeles, CA: USC CIR.

Department of Veterans Affairs. (2015). *2015 Veteran economic opportunity report.* Washington, DC: US Department of Veterans Affairs.

Ecclestone, K., Biesta, G., & Hughes, M. (2010). Transitions in the life course. The role of identity, agency, and structure. In K. Ecclestone, G. Biesta, & M. Hughes (Eds.), *Transitions and learning through the lifecourse* (pp. 1–15). New York, NY: Routledge.

Faberman, R. J., & Foster, T. (2013). Unemployment among recent veterans during the great recession. *Economic Perspectives, 37*(1), 1–13.

Hall, K. C., Harrell, M. C., Bicksler, B., A., Stewart, R., & Fisher, M. P. (2014). *Veteran employment: Lessons from the 100,000 jobs mission.* RAND. Retrieved from https://www.rand.org/pubs/research_reports/RR836.readonline.html

Hamilton, A. B., Williams, L., & Washington, D. L. (2015). Military and mental health correlates of unemployment in a national sample of women veterans. *Med Care, 53*(4, Suppl 1), S32–S38. doi:10.1097/mlr.0000000000000297

Harrell, M. C., & Berglass, N. (2014). *Employing America's veterans: Perspectives from businesses.* Washington, DC: CNAS. Retrieved from http://www.cnas.org/files/documents/publications/CNAS_EmployingAmericasVeterans_HarrellBerglass.pdf

Horton, J. L., Jacobson, I. G., Wong, C. A., Wells, T. S., Boyko, E. J., Smith, B., … Millennium Cohort Study, T. (2013). The impact of prior deployment experience on civilian employment after military service. *Occupational and Environmental Medicine, 70*(6), 408–417. doi:10.1136/oemed-2012-101073

Keeling, M., Kintzle, S., & Castro, C. A. (in press). Exploring the experiences of US veterans' post-service employment challenges. *Military Psychology.*

Keeling, M., Ozuna, S., Kintzle, S., & Casto, C. A. (in press). Veterans' civilian employment experiences: Lessons learnt from focus groups. *Journal of Career Development.*

Kintzle, S., Keeling, M., Xintarious, E., Taylor-Diggs, K., Munch, C., Hassan, A. M., & Castro, C. A. (2015). *Exploring the economic and employment challenges facing US veterans: A qualitative study of Volunteers of America service providers and veteran clients.* Los Angeles, CA: USC CIR.

Kintzle, S., Rasheed-Wallace, J., & Castro, C. A. (2016). *The state of the American veteran: The Chicagoland veterans study.* Los Angeles, CA: USC CIR.

Kleylamp, M. (2013). Unemployment, earnings and enrollment among post-9/11 veterans. *Social Science Research*, *42*(3), 836–851. doi:10.1016/j.ssresearch.2012.12.017

Loughran, D. S. (2014). *Why is veteran unemployment so high?* Santa Monica, CA: Rand Corporation.

Prudential.com. (2012). *Veterans' employment challenges: Perceptions and experiences of transitioning from military to civilian life*. Retrieved from http://www.prudential.com/documents/public/VeteransEmploymentChallenges.pdf

Veterans Education and Benefits Expansion Act of 2001. (2001). United States Code Title 38. Retrieved November 1st 2017 from https://www.congress.gov/107/plaws/publ103/PLAW-107publ103.pdf

Resnick, S. G., & Rosenheck, R. A. (2008). Posttraumatic stress disorder and employment in veterans participating in veterans health administration compensated work therapy. *Journal of Rehabilitation Research and Development*, *45*(3), 427.

Smith, R. T., & True, G. (2014). Warring identities identity conflict and the mental distress of American veterans of the wars in Iraq and Afghanistan. *Society and Mental Health*, *4*, 147–161.

Stone, C., & Stone, D. L. (2015). Factors affecting hiring decisions about veterans. *Human Resource Management Review*, *25*(1), 68–79. doi:http://dx.doi.org.libproxy2.usc.edu/10.1016/j.hrmr.2014.06.003

Zivin, K., Yosef, M., Levine, D. S., Abraham, K. M., Miller, E. M., Henry, J.,... Valenstein, M. (2016). Employment status, employment functioning, and barriers to employment among VA primary care patients. *Journal of Affective Disorders*, *193*, 194–202. doi:10.1016/j.jad.2015.12.054

PSYCHOSOCIAL HEALTH PREVENTION PROGRAMS IN MILITARY ORGANIZATIONS: A QUANTITATIVE REVIEW OF THE EVALUATIVE RIGOR EVIDENCE

Adam J. Vanhove, Tiffany Brutus and Kristin A. Sowden

ABSTRACT

In recent years, a wide range of psychosocial health interventions have been implemented among military service members and their families. However, there are questions over the evaluative rigor of these interventions. We conducted a systematic review of this literature, rating each relevant study (k = 111) on five evaluative rigor scales (type of control group, approach to participant assignment, outcome quality, number of measurement time points, and follow-up distality). The most frequently coded values on three of the five scales (control group type, participant assignment, and follow-up distality) were those indicating the lowest level of operationally defined rigor. Logistic regression results indicate that the evaluative rigor of intervention studies has largely remained consistent over time, with exceptions indicating that rigor has decreased. Analyses among seven military sub-populations indicate that interventions conducted among soldiers completing basic training, soldiers returning from combat deployment, and combat veterans have had, on average, the greatest evaluative rigor. However, variability in mean scores across evaluative rigor scales within sub-populations highlights the unique methodological

Occupational Stress and Well-being in Military Contexts
Research in Occupational Stress and Well-being, Volume 16, 129–156
Copyright © 2018 by Emerald Publishing Limited
All rights of reproduction in any form reserved
ISSN: 1479-3555/doi:10.1108/S1479-355520180000016010

hurdles common to different military settings. Recommendations for better standardizing the intervention evaluation process are discussed.

Keywords: health intervention; military intervention; preventive health; resilience; soldier health; stress management

INTRODUCTION

Over the course of less than two decades, attention to the stress associated with combat duty and its potential consequences for soldier mental health has drastically increased. Recent estimates suggest that a significant portion of combat veterans experience clinical-level post-traumatic stress, affective disorder symptoms, and/or substance abuse (Bagalman, 2013; Hoge & Castro, 2005; National Institutes of Health, 2009). This has placed considerable strain on the health care system, as mental health disorders represent the most prominent cause of hospitalization among active duty US service members (Armed Forces Health Surveillance Center, 2010).

In response, military organizations around the world have developed and implemented preventive interventions aimed at enhancing the psychosocial health and well-being of military personnel (see Bowles & Bates, 2010; Harms, Krasikova, Vanhove, Herian, & Lester, 2013; Meredith et al., 2011; Mulligan, Fear, Jones, Wessely, & Greenberg, 2011). Despite a proliferation of psychosocial health interventions being implemented among service members in various military settings, Slomski (2014) has argued that a lack of evidence exists, demonstrating these interventions' effectiveness. While Slomski acknowledges that some interventions have been shown to produce positive effects in non-military populations, unique characteristics associated with military populations (e.g., mental health stigma) have led to considerable concerns over the efficacy of such interventions in military settings (Lunasco, Goodwin, Ozanian, & Loflin, 2010; Sammons, 2005).

A cursory reading of the literature reveals that a plethora of empirical evidence does, in fact, exist evaluating the effectiveness of psychosocial health interventions among military populations. These interventions have varied greatly in terms of content and intended outcomes. Some have focused on developing mindfulness (Jha, Stanley, Kiyonaga, Wong, & Gelfand, 2010), resilience (Adler, Williams, McGurk, Moss, & Bliese, 2015), and self-esteem as a means of preventing the experience of stress; others have focused on developing skills associated with managing and coping with stress (Cigrang, Todd, & Carbone, 2000; Fornette et al., 2012; Williams et al., 2007); while still others have focused on alleviating trauma and stress-related symptoms (Boudewyns & Hyer, 1996; Gray et al., 2012; Murphy, Thompson, Murray, Rainey, & Uddo, 2009). Moreover, these interventions have been implemented among various military sub-populations, including those: completing basic training (Williams et al., 2004), preparing for deployment (Sharpley, Fear, Greenberg, Jones, & Wessely, 2008), returning from deployment

(Castro, Adler, McGurk, & Bliese, 2012), combat veterans (Polusny et al., 2015), and military families (Saltzman, Lester, Milburn, Woodward, & Stein, 2016).

What remains unclear despite the substantial evidence of intervention effects among military populations is the methodological rigor of this body of evidence. Meta-analysis of workplace resilience-building interventions shows stronger program effects among studies conducted with less evaluative rigor (see Vanhove, Herian, Perez, Harms, & Lester, 2016), suggesting that less rigorously evaluated interventions may be more likely to be implemented on a large scale. The consequences of diffusing psychosocial health interventions set to be effective based on weakly rigorous evidence are no less (and possibly more) severe than failing to evaluate intervention effectiveness at all. As such, research assessing aspects of methodological rigor across studies evaluating the effects of psychosocial health interventions conducted among military populations is a topic that warrants further investigation.

In this chapter, we provide a systematic quantitative analysis of the state of methodological rigor used to evaluate psychosocial health interventions implemented among current and former military service members and their families. We assess intervention studies according to five methodological design features indicative of evaluative rigor: type of control group, approach to participant assignment, outcome quality, number of measurement time points, and follow-up distality. We present summary analyses for each of these five features of evaluative rigor across studies, as well as separately, among seven different military sub-populations: service members completing basic training; active duty service members not deployed on combat duty; service members preparing for deployment, on-deployment, and returning from deployment; combat veterans; and military families. In addition, we present analyses assessing whether methodological rigor in evaluation studies has improved over time.

Findings provide a clear depiction of the current state of the quality of evidence pertaining to the effects of psychosocial health interventions implemented among military populations. Moreover, findings of sub-population analysis underscore relative methodological strengths and weaknesses associated with evaluation studies by sub-population in order to highlight the unique practical challenges inherent to different military contexts. Given the recent proliferation of psychosocial health interventions being implemented among military populations, we believe a review of the quality of evidence being produced is both timely and necessary to move forward research in this area in a manner that will best contribute to the psychosocial health of current and former service members and their families.

METHOD

Inclusion Criteria and Literature Search

We performed searches of PsycINFO and Google Scholar electronic databases using the search terms: "military" + "preventive"/"resilience"/"stress management"/"well-being" + "intervention"/"program". This resulted in a total of 9,824 articles returned. In addition, we examined studies included in reviews of various types of psychosocial health interventions, including: Martin, Sanderson, and Cocker (2009); Meredith et al. (2011); Meyers, van Woerkom, and Bakker (2013); Mulligan et al., (2011); Richardson and Rothstein (2008); Sherman (1998); Skeffington, Rees, and Kane (2013); Taylor and Schatz (2011); and Taylor, Schatz, Marino-Carper, Carrizales, and Vogel-Walcutt (2011).

Search techniques identified 136 psychosocial health intervention studies conducted among service members or their families. We found multiple cases where an intervention was evaluated in multiple studies, sometimes using the same sample. Since our focus is on reviewing the evaluative rigor of intervention studies, we treated each of these as independent studies as long as the evaluative design characteristics differed between the studies. For example, there were several interventions in which preliminary reports were published (e.g., report of treatment group-only reactions to intervention), followed by more complete reports (e.g., post-intervention comparison of treatment and control group on behavioral outcome measures). Further, we found multiple cases where more than one intervention was evaluated in a single study. In these cases, we coded each intervention as a separate study. Thus, we define "study" as an evaluation of an intervention using a unique evaluative design.

Each of the 136 studies was then evaluated against the following inclusion criteria. First, studies were required to include sufficient evaluative design and quantitative evaluative data. Case studies were not included, nor were studies that failed to provide adequate methodological information for study coding. Twenty-three studies (16.9%) failed to provide quantitative evaluative data and/or sufficient evaluative design information and were excluded from analyses. Second, studies were required to include psychological, social, or behavioral health outcomes. We did not include studies of physical or physiological outcomes. Two studies (1.5%) failed to meet this criterion and were excluded from analyses. This resulted in a total of 111 study samples (81.6%) being retained for analyses.

Study Coding: Evaluative Rigor

Five separate variables reflecting intervention evaluative design rigor were coded: type of control group, approach to participant assignment, outcome quality, number of measurement time points, and follow-up distality. *Control group type* was coded as "0" = no control group; "1" = non-intervention control group; or "2" = active comparison group. *Participant assignment* was coded as: "0" = completely non-random assignment; "1" = matched assignment between conditions; "2" = cluster randomized assignment between conditions (e.g., random assignment of platoons to intervention and control); and "3" = completely randomized assignment. *Outcome quality* was coded analogous to Kirkpatrick's (1994) taxonomy of training outcomes, which includes reaction, learning, behavior, and result outcomes. Most studies measured multiple outcomes, with some studies measuring outcomes representing different levels of the taxonomy. We coded studies based only on the highest level of outcome measured to capture the highest level of rigor achieved. Some adjustments were necessary for translating

Kirkpatrick's taxonomy to the population of outcomes used by studies included in our analyses. Reaction outcomes (e.g., satisfaction with intervention) were coded as "0". Learning outcomes (e.g., increased knowledge of concepts taught during interventions) were coded as "1." All studies, including learning outcomes, also included outcomes at higher levels on the taxonomy. Thus, no studies received a "1" score on outcome quality. The remaining outcomes assessed by the studies that we reviewed were psychosocial and behavioral in nature. Self-reported scores on these variables received a "2" score, and other-reports (e.g., Clinician-administered measures) and objective measures of behavior (e.g., completion of basic training) received a "3" score on quality of outcomes. *Number of measurement time points* was coded: "0" = no pre-test measurement, but at least one measurement time point following the beginning of the intervention; "1" = one pre-test measurement and one additional measurement time point following the beginning of the intervention; "2" = one pre-test measurement and two additional measurement time points following the beginning of the intervention; "3" = at least one pre-test measurement and three or more measurement time points following the beginning of the intervention. There were some cases where different measures were used at different time points. Among these, there were also situations in which some measures were employed more often than others. We relied on the number of time points at which the most frequently measured outcomes were measured to code the highest level of rigor achieved. In almost all cases, the first outcome measurement following the beginning of the intervention was taken immediately following the end of the intervention. However, there were a few exceptions (e.g., Williams et al., 2007) where outcome measurements were taken in correspondence with the delivery of separate intervention sessions (i.e., during intervention). Regarding post-intervention time-points assessed, the maximum was four. There were cases in which designs used diagnoses or other indicators of mental health symptoms/disorders as a means of determining study inclusion or condition assignment. In some of these cases, different, but comparable, outcome measures were used at subsequent time points. In these cases, we coded the comparable measures as sufficing the pre-test measurement requirement for being coded at a level greater than "0". *Follow-up distality* was coded: "0" = post-test only (no follow-up); "1" = follow-up measurement $\leq$3 months post-intervention; "2" = follow-up measurement $\leq$6 months post-intervention; and "3" = follow-up measurement >6 months post-intervention. Several studies included measurements at multiple follow-up time points. We coded studies based on the most distal post-intervention measurement time point to capture the highest level of evaluative rigor achieved.

Study Coding: Additional Variables

The total sample size was coded for each study, as were separate sample sizes for intervention and control groups. Sample size estimates reported are those from the final measurement time point – that is, the time point used to code each study on the follow-up distality scale. Year of publication was coded as a continuous variable. Finally, we coded the type of military sample. The following seven categories were included: "1" = soldiers going through basic training; "2" = active duty soldiers not deployed on combat duty; "3" = soldiers preparing for deployment; "4" = soldiers on deployment; "5" = soldiers returning from deployment; "6" = combat veterans; and "7" = samples including service members' family members.

Literature search techniques and study coding of all variables (evaluative rigor scales and additional variables) were completed by the second and third authors. Study coding was carried out independently for all studies by both study coders prior to establishing final coding consensus. Inter-rater agreement was more than 95%. All disagreements were handled by the first author.

RESULTS

Values for each included study on the five separate evaluative rigor scales and each additional variable described above are shown in Table 1. Table 2 depicts evaluative rigor scale trends through frequency estimates. As shown in Table 2, the greatest number of included studies were coded as using the lowest level of evaluative rigor on three of the five scales: control group type (M = 0.86, SD = 0.80, range = 0, 2) participant assignment (M = 1.17, SD = 1.36, range = 0, 3), and follow-up distality (M = 1.07, SD = 1.02, range = 0, 3) scales. Of these, Table 2 also shows a consistent decrease in the frequency of studies coded under each consecutive category of increased rigor on the control group type and follow-up distality scales, while a bi-modal trend exists among categories of the participant assignment scale. That is, completely non-random assignment (lowest rigor category) is the most common participant assignment technique used (55%), while completely random assignment (highest rigor category) is the second most common participant assignment technique used (30%). The number of measurement time points scale (M = 1.48, SD = 0.89, range = 0, 3) shows a relatively normal distribution, with the greatest frequency of studies using either pre-post (39%) or pre-post and follow-up (34%) designs. Relatively fewer studies used a post-test only or included multiple follow-up measurements. For the quality of outcome scale (M = 2.14, SD = 0.81, range = 0, 3), the majority of studies (60%) used self-reported psychosocial and behavioral measures (second highest rigor category), followed by other reports of those measures or objective outcomes (highest rigor category).

We conducted Chi-square independence tests to assess the extent to which coded values on each of the five evaluative criteria were related. Results are reported in Table 3 as a Chi-square matrix, which demonstrates statistically significant, positive associations between coded values on the majority of combinations of evaluative rigor scales. The exceptions include coded values on the control group type scale being independent of coded values on both number of measurement time points and follow-up distality scales. Coded values on the follow-up distality scale were also independent of coded values on the participant assignment and outcome quality scales, at the $p < 0.05$ threshold. However, across Chi-square independence tests, between two and nine cells contained $n < 5$, suggesting these analyses were underpowered.

Table 1. Evaluative Rigor Scores for Included Studies.

Study	Sub-Pop.	Treat *n*	Control *n*	Total *N*	Control Group Type	Part. Assign.	Outcome Quality	No. of Measurements	Follow-up
Adler et al. (2008) Debrief	4	75	79	154	1	2	2	2	3
Adler et al. (2008) SM	4	122	79	201	1	2	2	2	3
Adler et al. (2009) Debrief	5	271	243	514	2	2	2	2	2
Adler et al. (2009) Large group	5	274	243	517	2	2	2	2	2
Adler et al. (2009) Small group	5	272	243	515	2	2	2	2	2
Adler et al. (2015)	1	974	965	1,939	2	2	2	3	1
Baddeley and Pennebaker (2011) Expressive x^2	7	20	22	42	2	3	2	2	2
Baddeley and Pennebaker (2011) Soldier expressive	7	20	22	42	2	3	2	2	2
Baddeley and Pennebaker (2011) Spouse expressive	7	22	22	44	2	3	2	2	2
Beidel, Frueh, Uhde, Wong, and Mentrikoski (2011)	6	14	16	30	2	3	3	2	0
Bormann, Thorp, Wetherell, and Golshan (2008)	6	14	15	29	1	3	3	1	0
Bormann, Thorp, Wetherell, Golshan, and Lang (2013)	6	71	75	146	1	3	3	1	1
Boudewyns and Hyer (1990)/Boudewyns, Hyer, Woods, Harrison, and McCranie (1990)	6	19	19	38	2	3	2	1	1
Boudewyns and Hyer (1996) DTE	6	18	22	40	1	3	3	3	3
Boudewyns and Hyer (1996) EMDR	6	21	18	39	2	3	3	3	3
Brief et al. (2013)	6	183	120	303	1	3	2	2	1
Bryan and Morrow (2011)	4	192	–	192	0	0	2	0	0
Bush et al. (2017)	6	58	60	118	2	3	2	3	1
Cacioppo et al. (2015)	2	346	235	581	1	2	2	1	0
Carr et al. (2013)	4	160	–	160	0	0	2	1	0
Castro et al. (2012)	5	290	252	542	1	2	2	1	1
Chard, Schumm, Owens, and Cottingham (2010)	6	101	–	101	0	0	3	1	0
Chemtob, Tomas, Law, and Cremniter (1997)	6	14	–	14	0	0	2	2	3
Chongruksa, Prinyapol, Sawatsri, and Pansomboon (2015)	4	22	22	44	2	2	2	2	1
Cigrang et al. (2000)	1	94	84	178	2	3	3	0	1
Cigrang et al. (2011)	5	10	–	10	0	0	3	1	1
Cohn and Pakenham (2008)	1	101	73	174	1	2	2	2	1
Cooper and Clum (1989)	6	8	8	16	1	0	2	2	2

Table 1. *(Continued)*

Study	Sub-Pop.	Treat *n*	Control *n*	Total *N*	Control Group Type	Part. Assign.	Outcome Quality	No. of Measurements	Follow-up
Deahl, Gillham, Thomas, Searle, and Srinivasan (1994)	4	62	–	62	0	0	2	0	3
Deahl, Srinivasan, Jones, Neblett, and Jolly (2000)	5	54	52	106	1	3	3	3	3
Doss, Mitchell, Georgia, Biesen, and Rowe (2015)	7	161	–	161	0	0	3	1	0
Fischer, Sherman, Han, and Owen (2013)	7	96	–	96	0	0	2	3	0
Foran, Adler, McGurk, and Bliese (2012)	5	287	–	287	0	0	0	1	3
Forbes, Lewis, Parslow, Hawthorne, and Creamer (2008) Low-intensity program	6	197	–	197	0	0	2	2	2
Fornette et al. (2012)	1	10	11	21	1	1	2	1	1
Frappell-Cooke, Gulina, Green, Hacker Hughes, and Greenberg (2010) Coldstream Guards	3	86	–	86	0	0	2	2	2
Frappell-Cooke et al. (2010) Royal Marines	3	94	–	94	0	0	2	2	2
Frueh, Turner, Beidel, Mirabella, and Jones (1996)	6	11	–	11	0	0	3	1	0
Gewirtz, Pinna, Hanson, and Brockberg (2014)	7	33	–	33	0	0	0	0	0
Githens and Zalinski (1983) RJP + stress coping	1	1,767	3,316	5,083	2	0	3	0	1
Githins and Zalinski (1983) Stress coping	1	1,609	3,316	4,925	2	0	3	0	1
Glynn et al. (1999) Exposure	6	10	13	23	1	3	3	2	2
Glynn et al. (1999) Exposure + behavioral family therapy	7	10	13	23	1	3	3	2	2
Gould, Greenberg, and Hetherton (2007)	2	41	46	87	1	0	2	2	1
Gray et al. (2012)	2	44	–	44	0	0	2	1	0
Greenberg, Langston, Fear, Jones, and Wessely (2009)	2	845	714	1,559	1	0	2	0	0
Greenberg et al. (2010)	2	638	597	1,235	1	2	2	1	3
Griffith and West (2013)	2	441	–	441	0	0	0	0	0
Hammarberg and Silver (1994)	6	39	26	65	1	0	3	3	0
Hammermeister, Pickering, and Ohlson (2009)	2	27	–	27	0	0	2	1	0
Harms, Herian, Krasikova, Vanhove, and Lester (2013)	2	4,983	2,247	7,230	1	1	3	1	2
Harris et al. (2011)	6	26	29	55	1	3	2	1	0
Jakupcak et al. (2006)	6	10	–	10	0	0	3	1	0
Jakupcak, Wagner, Paulson, Varra, and McFall (2010)	6	7	–	7	0	0	3	2	1
Jensen (1994)	6	13	12	25	1	3	3	1	1
Jha et al. (2010)	3	29	17	46	1	0	3	1	0

Jha, Morrison, Parker, and Stanley (2017)	3	31	24	55	1	0	3	1	0
Johnson et al. (2014)	3	153	134	287	1	2	2	1	0
Johnston et al. (2015)	2	10	–	10	0	0	3	1	0
Jones, Perkins, Cook, and Ong (2008)	4	326	–	326	0	0	2	2	0
Kahn, Collinge, and Soltysik (2016) Mission reconnect	6	78	79	157	1	3	2	2	1
Kahn et al. (2016) MR + PREP	6	77	155	232	2	3	2	2	1
Kahn et al. (2016) PREP	6	77	79	156	1	3	2	2	1
Keane, Fairbank, Caddell, and Zimering (1989)	6	13	11	24	1	3	3	2	2
Kearney, McDermott, Malte, Martinez, and Simpson (2012)	6	66	–	66	0	0	2	2	2
Kees, Nerenberg, Bachrach, and Sommer (2015)	7	14	–	14	0	0	2	1	1
Larsson, Michel, and Lundin (2000) Peer support	4	29	56	85	1	0	2	1	2
Larsson et al. (2000) Peer support + defusing	4	60	56	116	2	0	2	1	2
Larsson et al. (2000) Peer support + defusing + debriefing	4	36	89	125	2	0	2	1	2
Lester, Harms, Herian, Krasikova, and Beal (2011)	2	6,739	3,215	9,954	1	1	2	1	2
Lester et al. (2012)/Saltzmann et al. (2011)	7	488	–	488	0	0	2	1	0
Litz, Engel, Bryant, and Papa (2007)	2	9	9	18	2	3	3	3	2
Lunasco et al. (2010)	4	320	–	320	0	0	0	0	1
McLay et al. (2011)	6	10	10	20	2	3	3	1	0
McLay et al. (2012)	6	17	–	17	0	0	2	2	1
Monk et al. (2016)	7	47	–	47	0	0	2	2	2
Monson et al. (2006)	6	23	26	49	1	3	2	3	1
Morland et al. (2010)	6	61	64	125	2	3	2	3	2
Mulligan et al. (2012)	4	724	872	1,596	1	2	2	1	1
Murphy et al. (2009)	6	44	31	75	2	3	3	1	3
Nakamura, Lipschitz, Landward, Kuhn, and West (2011)	6	33	25	58	2	3	2	2	0
Niederhauser, Maddock, LeDoux, and Arnold (2005)	2	50	41	91	1	0	2	2	2
Pinna, Hanson, Zhang, and Gewirtz (2017)	7	156	–	156	0	3	0	0	0
Pischke and Hallman (2008)	4	396	–	396	0	0	0	0	0
Polusny et al. (2015)	6	47	57	104	2	3	3	3	1
Potter, Baker, Sanders, and Peterson (2009)	4	38	–	38	0	0	2	1	0
Ragsdale, Cox, Finn, and Eisler (1996)	6	32	24	56	1	0	2	1	0
Ramsberger, Legree, and Mills (2002)	1	214	207	421	1	0	3	0	0
Rizzo, Difede et al. (2009/2010)	5	20	–	20	0	0	2	2	1
Rizzo, Newman et al. (2009)	5	13	7	20	2	0	2	2	0

Table 1. *(Continued)*

Study	Sub-Pop.	Treat *n*	Control *n*	Total *N*	Control Group Type	Part. Assign.	Outcome Quality	No. of Measurements	Follow-up
Rosenthal, Grosswald, Ross, and Rosenthal (2011)	6	5	–	5	0	0	3	2	1
Rothbaum, Hodges, Ready, Graap, and Alarcon (2001)	6	10	–	10	0	0	3	3	2
Roy, Highland, and Costanzo (2015)	6	13	13	26	2	3	2	2	1
Saltzman et al. (2016)	7	434	–	434	0	0	2	2	2
Shalev, Peri, and Rogel-Fuchs (1998)	4	39	–	39	0	0	2	1	0
Sharpley et al. (2008)	3	279	456	735	1	0	2	0	3
Sherman, Fischer, Sorocco, and McFarlane (2011)	7	70	–	70	0	0	0	1	0
Sherman, Fischer, Owen, Lu, and Han (2015)	6	83	–	83	0	0	3	2	3
Smith-Osborne, Maleku, and Morgan (2017)	3	131	–	131	0	0	2	1	0
Stanley, Schaldach, Kiyonaga, and Jha (2011)	3	30	17	47	1	0	2	1	0
Stecker, Fortney, and Sherbourne (2011)	2	27	–	27	0	0	0	3	1
Tan, Dao, Farmer, Sutherland, and Gevirtz (2011)	6	10	10	20	2	3	3	0	0
Taylor, Stanfill et al. (2011)	2	18	10	28	1	3	2	1	1
Tenhula et al. (2014)	6	416	–	416	0	0	2	1	0
Van Breda (1999)	7	24	–	24	0	0	2	1	0
Van Voorhees and Sweis (2010)	6	50	–	50	0	0	2	3	2
Vella, Milligan, and Bennett (2013)	6	74	–	74	0	0	2	2	1
Williams et al. (2004)	1	100	100	200	1	3	3	1	0
Williams et al. (2007)	1	583	616	1,199	1	2	3	3	0
Williams, Hagerty, Brasington, Clem, and Williams (2010)	2	142	–	142	0	0	0	0	0
Zamorski, Guest, Bailey, and Garber (2012)	5	3,024	19,089	22,113	2	0	0	1	0

Table 2. Frequencies of Study Scores on Each of the Four Evaluative Rigor Scales.

	k	%
Control group type		
No control group = 0	44	39.6
Non-intervention control group = 1	39	35.1
Active comparison control group = 2	28	25.2
Participant assignment		
Non-random assignment = 0	61	55
Matched assignment = 1	3	2.7
Clustered randomized assignment = 2	14	12.6
Random assignment = 3	33	29.7
Outcome quality		
Reactions = 0	10	9
Learning = 1	0	0
Self-report psychosocial/behavioral = 2	66	59.5
Other report psychosocial/behavioral or objective = 3	35	31.5
Number of measurement time points		
No pre-test = 0	42	37.8
Pre-test and one additional = 1	31	27.9
Pre-test and two additional = 2	26	23.4
Pre-test and three or more additional = 3	12	10.8
Follow-up distality		
Post-intervention = 0	42	37.8
≤3 months = 1	31	27.9
≤6 months = 2	26	23.4
>6 months = 3	12	10.8

Note: $k = 111$.

Table 3. Chi-square Tests of Independence between Evaluative Rigor Scale Values.

	1	2	3	4
1. Control group type				
2. Participant assignment	71.77*			
3. Outcome quality	14.90*	18.09*		
4. Number of measurement time points	7.99	18.34*	27.54*	
5. Follow-up distality	9.84	15.10†	11.02†	37.82*

Notes: Cell values represent Chi-square (χ^2) values.
χ^2 estimates are based on maximum likelihood due to sample sizes below $n = 5$ for some cells.
For each estimate, $df = 1$, $N = 111$.
*$p < 0.05$, †$p < 0.10$.

Finally, we estimated a series of multinomial logistic regression models to assess whether the rigor associated with any of the evaluative criterion scales has changed over time. Model results indicate that study publication year predicted coded rigor values for outcome quality, χ^2 (2, $N = 111$) = 12.23, $p < 0.05$, pseudo-$R^2_{\text{Cox \& Snell}} = 0.10$. Publication year did not predict coded rigor values on control group type, χ^2 (2, $N = 111$) = 5.17, ns, pseudo-$R^2_{\text{Cox \& Snell}} = 0.05$, participant assignment, χ^2 (3, $N = 111$) = 4.49, ns, pseudo-$R^2_{\text{Cox \& Snell}} = 0.04$, number of measurement time points, χ^2 (3, $N = 111$) = 3.91, ns, pseudo-$R^2_{\text{Cox \& Snell}} = 0.04$, or follow-up distality, χ^2 (3, $N = 111$) = 5.54, ns, pseudo-$R^2_{\text{Cox \& Snell}} = 0.05$. Parameter estimates are shown in Table 4, with odds ratio (OR) greater than 1 indicating more recent evaluative research having a higher likelihood of scoring lower on evaluative rigor. As depicted in Table 4, few binomial comparisons are statistically significant, suggesting that the evaluative rigor of psychosocial health intervention research has neither decreased nor increased over time. However, all effects that are statistically significant at $p < 0.05$ indicate that evaluative rigor has decreased over time.

These findings provide a number of insights into the current state of methodological rigor among studies evaluating psychosocial health interventions among military populations. First, findings suggest that the majority of studies have been designed with less-than-ideal evaluative rigor on one or more methodological design facets. Second, findings suggest that evaluative rigor values on the majority of criterion scales are interrelated. Thus, those with greater (weaker) evaluative rigor on a given criterion also tend to possess greater (weaker) evaluative rigor on other criteria. Third, findings suggest that the rigor of evaluative evidence has not improved over time. In fact, findings suggest that the change that has taken place over time has been in the direction of decreased evaluative rigor. The meta-analyses described above combine studies targeting different military sub-populations (e.g., soldiers preparing for deployment, combat veterans, and military families). We examine whether evaluative rigor differs across sub-populations and whether different sub-populations may be associated with different methodological hurdles.

Sub-population Evaluative Rigor Analysis

Mean scores by sub-population are shown in Table 5. Of the seven sub-populations examined, interventions conducted among three appeared to demonstrate stronger evaluative rigor relative to other sub-populations: soldiers completing basic training, soldiers returning from deployment, and combat veterans. Studies evaluating psychosocial health interventions conducted among these sub-populations produced the three highest mean scores on all five evaluative rigor criterion scales, with three exceptions. The mean score for studies conducted among soldiers returning from deployment ranked fourth highest on the outcome quality scale, and the mean score for studies conducted among soldiers completing basic training ranked second lowest on the number of measurement time points and lowest on the follow-up distality scale.

Psychosocial health interventions conducted among the remaining four sub-populations (active duty soldiers not deployed on combat duty, soldiers preparing for or on combat deployment, and military families) demonstrated relatively weaker evaluative rigor. However, intervention studies among some of these latter four sub-populations were not without their relative strengths. Studies of interventions conducted among active duty soldiers not deployed on combat duty

Table 4. Multinomial Logistic Regression Parameter Estimates Regressing Evaluation Rigor Categories on Year of Study Publication.

Predictor category	Reference category	*b*	*SE*	Wald	OR
Control group type					
No control group	Non-intervention control group	0.07	0.03	4.18*	1.07
No control group	Active comparison group	0.06	0.04	2.81†	1.06
Non-intervention control group	Active comparison group	–0.01	0.03	0.07	0.99
Participant assignment					
Non-random assignment	Matched assignment	–0.15	0.15	1.00	0.86
Non-random assignment	Clustered randomized assignment	–0.09	0.06	2.32	0.92
Non-random assignment	Random assignment	0.00	0.03	0.00	1.00
Matched assignment	Clustered randomized assignment	0.06	0.16	0.16	1.07
Matched assignment	Random assignment	0.15	0.15	0.98	1.16
Clustered randomized assignment	Random assignment	0.09	0.06	2.15	1.09
Outcome quality					
Reactions	Self-report psych./behavioral	0.11	0.08	1.66	1.11
Reactions	Other-report psych./behavior/objective	0.19	0.09	4.81*	1.21
Self-report psych./behavioral	Other-report psych./behavior/objective	0.08	0.03	7.38*	1.08
Number of measurement time points					
No Pre-test	Pre-test and one additional	–0.06	0.04	2.54	0.94
No Pre-test	Pre-test and two additional	–0.07	0.04	3.06†	0.93
No Pre-test	Pre-test and three or more additional	–0.02	0.04	0.28	0.98
Pre-test and one additional	Pre-test and two additional	–0.01	0.03	0.07	0.99
Pre-test and one additional	Pre-test and three or more additional	0.04	0.04	0.88	1.04
Pre-test and two additional	Pre-test and three or more additional	0.05	0.04	1.24	1.05
Follow-up distality					
No follow-up	Less than 3 months	0.01	0.04	0.15	1.01
No follow-up	3–6 months	0.06	0.04	2.68	1.06
No follow-up	More than 6 months	0.08	0.04	4.02*	1.09
Less than 3 months	3–6 months	0.04	0.04	1.42	1.04
Less than 3 months	More than 6 months	0.07	0.04	2.64	1.07
3–6 months	More than 6 months	0.03	0.04	0.42	1.03

Notes: $N = 110$ and Wald(df) = 1 for all estimates.
$^{*}p < 0.05$, $^{\dagger}p < 0.10$.

Table 5. Means and Standard Deviations for Each Evaluative Rigor Scale by Sub-Population.

Type of Sample	*k*	Control Group Type	Participant Assignment	Outcome Quality	Number of Measurement Time Points	Follow-up Distality
		M (SD)	*M* (SD)	*M* (SD)	*M* (SD)	*M* (SD)
Basic training	9	1.44 (0.53)	1.44 (1.24)	2.67 (0.50)	1.11 (1.27)	0.67 (0.50)
Active duty non-deployed	15	0.67 (0.62)	0.80 (1.15)	1.80 (1.01)	1.20 (0.94)	0.93 (1.03)
Preparing for deployment	8	0.63 (0.52)	0.25 (0.71)	2.25 (0.46)	1.13 (0.64)	0.88 (1.25)
On deployment	15	0.67 (0.82)	0.53 (0.92)	1.73 (0.70)	1.00 (0.76)	1.20 (1.21)
Returning from deployment	10	1.20 (0.92)	1.10 (1.20)	1.80 (1.03)	1.70 (0.67)	1.50 (1.08)
Combat veterans	40	0.95 (0.81)	1.73 (1.50)	2.50 (0.51)	1.88 (0.79)	1.15 (1.00)
Military families	14	0.50 (0.85)	1.07 (1.49)	1.71 (0.99)	1.43 (0.85)	0.93 (1.00)

showed consistently moderate evaluative rigor relative to other sub-populations. Studies of this sub-population ranked fourth in mean scores on the control group type, outcome quality, number of measurement time points, and follow-up distality scales. Moreover, the pre-deployment sub-population was associated with the third highest mean score on the outcome quality scale, the military families' sub-population was associated with the third highest mean score on the number of measurement time points scale, and the on-deployment sub-population was associated with the second highest mean score on the follow-up distality scale.

DISCUSSION

Efforts to enhance service member psychosocial health are high stakes endeavors, with critical implications for individuals, families, and health care systems. Thus, it is important that evidence regarding the effectiveness of relevant health interventions conducted among military populations be associated with strong evaluative rigor. The consequences of evidence that lacks validity, due to methodological shortcomings, can be as severe as (and possibly more so than) having no evidence at all. For example, low-quality evidence overstating an intervention's effectiveness at reducing stress among deployed soldiers can have far-reaching consequences if that evidence is used as the basis for implementing an intervention on a larger scale. Those consequences include the organization failing to see a meaningful return on the time and resource investments associated with greater implementation, as well as service members in need will not only not benefiting from the implemented intervention but potentially suffering further from organizational resources being diverted away from a potentially more beneficial intervention.

The purpose of this chapter was to assess the current state of the literature evaluating the methodological rigor of psychosocial health interventions conducted among military populations. Our findings highlight limitations associated with this literature. We propose two complimentary explanations for these findings that carefully consider factors associated with the rapid development of this evaluative literature. Further, we propose a multi-phase evaluation process aimed at improving the standardization of psychosocial health intervention research in this area moving forward.

Any discussion of the meaning and implications of these findings requires an understanding of the context within which much of the evidence summarized here was produced. Western allies' engagement in wars in Iraq and Afghanistan drew increased attention to the individual costs of combat duty (Hattenstone & Allison, 2014; Thompson & Gibbs, 2012) and the institutional costs of treating psychosocial health deficits (Armed Forces Health Surveillance Center, 2010). At the same time, there had begun a renaissance of scholarship on health and well-being throughout the social sciences (Seligman & Csikszentmihalyi, 2000). This renewed interest in prevention rather than treatment played an important role in psychosocial health programs becoming popular within organizations (Aldana, Merrill, Price, Hardy, & Hager, 2005). This has been particularly true with regard to military organizations as evidenced by the large proportion of studies in our sample (approximately 70%) that were published within the last decade.

Our findings of the apparently weak evaluative rigor associated with these interventions may be explained by the importance organizations place on managing stakeholder perceptions. Influencing the perceptions of stakeholders is often a primary reason for organizational behavior regardless of the explicit purpose of the behavior. As an extreme example, research has shown that even when organizations do not intend to implement business practices, they may communicate their intentions to do so to elicit a positive response from stakeholders (Zajac & Westphal, 2004). Similarly, organizations often proclaim their commitment to effective human resource management, while frequently failing to demonstrate that commitment in practice (Hammonds, 2005). More often, however, the disconnect between stated intentions and actual business practice is more subtle, as the literature has repeatedly observed trendy management practices being implemented more as a means to achieving organizational legitimacy than organizational efficiency (Staw & Epstein, 2000).

Given the widespread attention to soldier mental health and the growing popularity of preventive health interventions, perhaps military organizations satisfied stakeholders' perceptions of an adequate response to the mental health crisis simply by implementing such interventions. Moreover, in the case that one or more of these interventions were truly not effective, rigorous evaluation may be likely to accurately evidence this and potentially produce a negative impact on stakeholder perceptions. There is precedence for this explanation, as evidence from the broader organizational literature has demonstrated that while preventive health programs have not necessarily improved worker health, they have increased stakeholders' perceptions of the organizations that offer them (Nigam, Murphy, & Swanson, 2003).

The second way of explaining these findings may speak to the (lack of) effectiveness that existing interventions have shown. We disagree with Slomski's (2014) depiction of a lack of evidence evaluating the effects of psychosocial health interventions among military populations, and we believe that the sample sizes associated with our analyses support our position. However, our data cannot speak to another of Slomski's key conclusions – that the evidence that does exist regarding intervention effectiveness has been highly underwhelming. Existing reviews of interventions conducted in military settings are largely consistent with this conclusion, showing small and often inconsistent intervention effects (Mulligan et al., 2011; Vanhove et al., 2016). It is possible that evidence of both weak effects and relatively weak evaluative rigor are symptoms of the (lack of) maturity of the field. Given this explanation, the relatively weak evaluative rigor we observed, along with the rate at which empirical evidence is being produced on this topic, may actually be a sign for optimism.

One might be hard-pressed to identify another field of study that has produced the quantity of evidence summarized here in such a short period of time. For example, Slomski (2014) noted that, at the time, the Department of Defense was funding 39 separate studies of resilience-building interventions. It may not be practical to assume, however, that each of these studies would be using highly rigorous field evaluations. Studies of interventions farther along in the evaluation process may be expected to do so. However, one would assume that some studies would be at a more preliminary stage of the evaluation process, involving less rigorous conditions, prior to implementing interventions on larger scales or with more elaborate designs. Interestingly, we found no evidence that publication year was positively associated with increased levels of evaluative rigor, which contrasts what one might expect if interventions progressed toward more rigorous evaluations as a result of positive findings at prior stages. However, if existing interventions have failed to demonstrate meaningful effects, this finding may indicate that military organizations are continuing to pilot test novel interventions, rather than continuing with research on interventions that do not work.

Although failure up to this point to identify highly effective interventions is certainly a problem in terms of military organizations' ability to minimize the individual and organizational costs of service, it may indicate that military organizations are committed to finding a viable solution. From this interpretation, we might expect that, as the existing evidence and the literature continues to develop, so will theory around the tenets that are most consistently observed among interventions producing the strongest effects. Of course, this idea only reinforces the importance of highly rigorous evaluative designs moving forward to ensure the validity of evidence used for development of such an inductive theory.

Placing these two overarching explanations for our findings of relatively weak evaluative rigor back into the broader context, we might conclude that there is some truth in both explanations. Due to external pressures, military organizations have been forced to act on a problem for which there does not yet appear to be a clear set of solutions. This type of situation is not unique in military settings (Yerkes, 1921), nor is it unique for non-military organizations faced with decisions to implement psychosocial health interventions based on theory that is not developed fully (see Masten, 2007). Perhaps, there is some credence in the possibility that military organizations, while implementing imperfect and imperfectly evaluated interventions, continue to seek out more viable solutions.

Nonetheless, enhancing the health of service members and their families is a high stakes endeavor, and based on our findings we provide the following recommendations to enhance evaluative rigor and the quality of evidence moving forward.

Military organizations may benefit from establishing greater standardization in phasing intervention evaluation, such as a model similar to that used in clinical trial research. As Slomski (2014) points out, interventions have been implemented on a large scale within military organizations without sufficient pilot testing or even strong evidence supporting their effects in other populations. To avoid such opportunities moving forward, we propose a flexible evaluation process consisting of no fewer than four phases (see Table 6).

The first phase establishes clear and highly rigorous evidence of effectiveness in a non-military population, as well as a clear rationale for the generalizability of this evidence to target military populations. The second phase establishes preliminary evidence of intervention efficacy within a military setting. Although rigor in methodological design is important, the purpose of this initial pilot-testing phase is to determine not only whether the intervention has the potential to be effective among broad or specific military populations but also to identify needed revisions to content and delivery components. As such, tests during this phase may sacrifice some aspects of methodological rigor (e.g., randomized assignment, control condition, and follow-up measurement) in order to efficiently obtain preliminary evaluative evidence. Moreover, qualitative feedback may be useful at this point to determine whether changes to the intervention are needed prior to conducting more rigorous evaluations. Once preliminary evidence has been established and revisions have been made to improve the efficacy of implementation, the third phase establishes clear evidence of the intervention's impact on intended outcomes (e.g., building resilience or stress management skills; reducing depressive symptoms; and reducing diagnoses of post-traumatic stress disorder, PTSD).

Table 6. Possible Four-phase Process of Intervention Evaluation.

Phase	Focus	Design Features
Pre-evaluation	Establish clear evidence of effectiveness of effectiveness in non-military population and rationale for generalizability to target military populations	Literature review; randomized experiment or time series quasi-experiment to establish clear internal validity
Preliminary evaluation	Establish initial evidence of effectiveness and identify needed revisions to intervention content and delivery	Convenience sampling of low-risk military population; pre- and post-test designs; reaction and learning criteria; qualitative participant feedback
Intermediate evaluation	Establish clear evidence of internal validity of intervention with regard to intended intervention outcomes	Randomized assignment of low-risk military participants to intervention and control groups; control over extraneous variables; behavioral and organizational results criteria
Advanced evaluation	Establish generalizability of intervention with regard to intended intervention outcomes among target population	Quasi-experimental design of target high-risk military participants; behavioral and organizational results criteria; multiple pre- and post-test measurement time points that capture the long-term effects of intervention

The focus of this phase should be on establishing strong internal validity and, as such, possesses high evaluative rigor. Randomized field experiments or regression discontinuity designs may be ideal for this intermediate evaluation phase. The fourth phase focuses on external validity. While establishing internal validity is critical during the intermediate testing phase, certain elements of evaluative rigor may not be feasible among target populations (e.g., soldiers preparing for or on deployment). Having established clear evidence of internal validity, the focus should turn to whether those effects generalize to intended target populations. This phase should also include certain components of high evaluative rigor, such as the inclusion of intended outcomes of the intervention (e.g., reducing diagnoses of PTSD) and multiple and distal post-intervention measurement time points to assess the long-term effects of the intervention. Time-series quasi-experimental designs may be ideal for this advanced testing phase.

Specific issues facing investigators appear to differ based on the military sub-population being studied. Study findings provide insight into the feasibility of sampling different military sub-populations during the different proposed phases of intervention evaluation. Further, findings provide insight into the opportunity to capitalize on the methodological strengths afforded in different military settings.

Studies conducted among basic trainees scored high on the majority of the evaluative rigor criteria. Since the stakes are much lower relative to units on combat deployment, military organizations may be more willing to accommodate evaluative design components such as the random assignment of individual trainees to intervention with control conditions. In addition, the basic training context provides a viable objective outcome – successful completion of basic training. However, once basic training is complete, many trainees disperse to assignments in different localities. This can make tracking longer-term outcomes among participants more difficult, an aspect reflected in the low mean score on the follow-up distality criterion. Basic training may be an ideal setting for intermediate evaluation of interventions. Intensive basic training activities give trainees ample opportunity to demonstrate resilience and cope with novel stressors. Moreover, the relatively low-consequence setting provides the opportunity for highly rigorous testing to determine whether an intervention warrants advanced testing with high-risk military populations where some aspects of high evaluative rigor may be less feasible.

Studies conducted among combat veterans demonstrated the most consistently high rigor scores across evaluative criteria. One key factor likely influencing the rigor of these studies is the fact that they are typically carried out in health care organization settings. Consequently, interventions conducted among combat veterans likely entail fewer methodological barriers than those conducted in military organizations, where interventionists must work around military organizational operations and service members' occupational duties. However, interventions conducted among combat veterans also present a unique caveat – participants in these interventions are typically those voluntarily seeking help for clinical-level mental health diagnoses (e.g., post-traumatic stress). Thus, while the goal of interventions conducted with active duty sub-populations and military families primarily focus on preventing the development of clinical-level mental health conditions, interventions conducted among combat veterans tend to focus on treating these conditions. Given the unique nature of interventions conducted among combat veterans, a traditional clinical trial framework of treatment evaluation is likely most suitable.

The sub-population findings described above highlight an important observation – that is, the evaluative rigor in psychosocial health intervention studies is highest at the ends of the military service cycle. Unfortunately, most psychosocial risk factors appear in between the basic training and post-career phases. It should be a cause for concern that greater effort has not been made to evaluate rigorously the efficacy of interventions implemented in between these phases, particularly phases surrounding combat deployment. That said, combat missions represent extremely high-stake contexts, which likely contribute to our observation that evaluative rigor mean scores on most scales examined among psychosocial health intervention studies of the pre-deployment and on-deployment sub-populations were low.

Psychosocial health interventions conducted among both sub-populations are not without their strengths. Studies conducted among pre-deployment service members demonstrated high outcome quality. This may reflect the seriousness of the pre-deployment context. Since pre-deployment soldiers have an intensive preparation schedule, implementing largely untested interventions to gather preliminary evidence with weak outcome measures may not be appropriate and requiring service members to complete extensive batteries of self-report outcome measures after completing interventions may not be feasible. Studies conducted among on-deployment service members demonstrated high scores on the follow-up distality scale. One explanation is that deployed units remain intact for the duration of the deployment (6–12 months), allowing for increased opportunity to track participants and measure outcomes at distal time points (such as when the intact unit returns from deployment). Pre- and on-deployment military sub-populations are key populations targeted by psychosocial health interventions and represent ideal candidates for advanced intervention evaluation. It is perhaps encouraging that our findings suggest that intervention evaluations conducted among these sub-populations, although generally low in evaluative rigor, possess at least some key evaluative design features associated with advanced evaluation.

Relative to intervention studies conducted pre-deployment and on-deployment, studies conducted post-deployment showed high evaluative rigor. This likely underscores a shift in strategic priorities – because the high-stakes mission has come to an end – from operational readiness to the maintenance of psychosocial health and recovery. This is largely consistent with the previously discussed explanation for the high evaluative rigor among psychosocial health interventions conducted among combat veterans. Due to the relatively high evaluative rigor scores associated with studies conducted among the post-deployment sub-population coupled with post-deployment transitions being critical points at which resilience-building and stress-coping can minimize the development of clinical-level symptoms, this sub-population may represent a strong candidate for both intermediate and advanced evaluation.

It is more difficult to draw any clear conclusions from our findings regarding the potential barriers to designing highly rigorous evaluations of psychosocial interventions conducted among active duty service members not deployed on combat duty or those including service members' families. These sub-populations are themselves broad and diverse. For example, studies coded as non-combat active duty include September 11th Pentagon attack survivors (Litz et al., 2007), British Royal Naval personnel serving on warships, and a range of otherwise broadly described in-tact small units (Cacioppo et al., 2015) or a mix of individuals from different military branches (Gould et al., 2007) with little or no occupational duty information. Studies coded as representing intervention evidence from the military families sub-population included samples of military couples pre-deployment (Van Breda, 1999) and post-deployment (Baddeley & Pennebaker, 2011), military parents and their children (Saltzman, et al., 2016), and veteran and family member dyads (Monk, Ogolsky, & Bruner, 2016; Sherman et al., 2015).

Active duty service members not deployed on combat duty may be appropriate for any of the phases of evaluation, depending on the goals of the intervention, the psychosocial risk factors associated with the specific sampling pool, and the feasibility of including appropriate evaluative design features. Although our findings indicate interventions conducted among military families demonstrate relatively weak evaluative rigor, these interventions may be particularly well suited for the evaluation process proposed here. Similar to interventions among combat veterans, participation in these interventions is often voluntary and potentially presents less interference with military operations. As such, interventions conducted among military families present the opportunity for highly rigorous design. Perhaps the reason for relatively weak evaluative rigor scores is due to many of these interventions not having matured past the preliminary phase of evaluation, rather than there being considerable barriers to implementing methodological designs with the rigor necessary for intermediate or advanced evaluation.

Limitations and the Future Research Directions

As with any quantitative review, the summary conclusions we make regarding the evidence of psychosocial health intervention evaluative rigor represent a simplification of a dynamic body of literature. Nowhere is this clearer than with regard to the evidence relating to the sub-populations of active duty service members not deployed on combat duty and those involving military families. Studies of these two sub-populations were so diverse that conclusions about evaluative rigor practices in these contexts could not be drawn reliably. Research on interventions targeting military families, as opposed to only the service members themselves, is a growing area of interest and the context in which the study of psychosocial interventions is least mature. The future research may consider more closely examining the different evaluative design characteristics used among studies with more nuanced sub-samples (e.g., military couples preparing for deployment, post-deployment, or post-military career).

The five evaluative criteria on which we report are by no means exhaustive. Further, the categories representing different levels of evaluative rigor inherently represent a simplification of complex design features, and involve some level of subjectivity. Moreover, categories of relatively high and low rigor were in some cases partially determined by the distribution of rigor levels across studies. For example, it is recommended that longitudinal assessment involves as many measurement time points as feasible to capture accurately the nature of change. However, the highest rigor value on the number of measurement time points was defined as four or more due to the nature of the designs in our sample, as opposed to best practices that exist, and only approximately half of the studies met the minimum number (3) necessary to produce longitudinal effects (Ployhart & Vandenberg, 2010). In such cases, our interpretation of the relative rigor of the literature may have been lenient.

Finally, while research within the broader organizational context has demonstrated evaluative rigor to be negatively related to intervention effectiveness (Vanhove et al., 2016), the current study focused only on assessing the evaluative rigor of existing psychosocial health intervention studies conducted among military populations. It remains unclear whether less rigorous studies conducted among these populations produce stronger effects. Evidence indicating that evaluative rigor is inversely related to intervention effectiveness could have significant consequences for both science and practice within this literature.

CONCLUSION

Given the rapid growth of evidence-evaluating psychosocial health interventions conducted among military populations, this study sought to assess the methodological rigor used in evaluating psychosocial health interventions conducted among military populations. Results indicate that, in general, the evaluative rigor of such intervention studies is relatively weak, which should raise considerable concern over the validity of evidence regarding intervention effects. Moreover, the contexts in which evaluative rigor is greatest are those at the beginning and end phases of the military service cycle, while those during key periods of the military service cycle, when psychosocial health intervention may be expected to have important effects (i.e., pre-combat deployment and during combat deployment), have suffered from weak evaluative rigor. Consequently, we put forth recommendations aimed at increasing standardization of the evaluation process.

REFERENCES

(*Indicates the study was included in analyses.)

*Adler, A. B., Bliese, P. D., McGurk, D., Hoge, C. W., & Castro, C. A. (2009). Battlemind debriefing and battlemind training as early interventions with soldiers returning from Iraq: Randomization by platoon. *Journal of Consulting and Clinical Psychology*, *77*(5), 928–940.

*Adler, A. B., Litz, B. T., Castro, C. A., Suvak, M., Thomas, J. L., Burrell, L., … & Bliese, P. D. (2008). A group randomized trial of critical incident stress debriefing provided to US peacekeepers. *Journal of Traumatic Stress*, *21*(3), 253–263.

*Adler, A. B., Williams, J., McGurk, D., Moss, A., & Bliese, P. D. (2015). Resilience training with soldiers during basic combat training: randomisation by platoon. *Applied Psychology: Health and Well-Being*, *7*(1), 85–107.

Aldana, S. G., Merrill, R. M., Price, K., Hardy, A., & Hager, R. (2005). Financial impact of a comprehensive multisite workplace health promotion program. *Preventive Medicine*, *4*, 131–137.

Armed Forces Health Surveillance Center. (2010). Selected mental health disorders among active component members, U.S. Armed Forces, 2007–2010. *Medical Surveillance Monthly Report*, *17*(11), 2–5.

*Baddeley, J. L., & Pennebaker, J. W. (2011). A postdeployment expressive writing intervention for military couples: A randomized controlled trial. *Journal of Traumatic Stress*, *24*, 581–585.

Bagalman, E. (2013). *Mental disorders among OEF/OIF veterans using VA health care: Facts and figures*. Congressional Research Service Report for Congress, No. R41921. Retrieved from http://deploymentpsych.org/system/files/member_resource/Mental%20Disorders%20Among%20OEF-OIF%20Veterans%20Using%20VA%20Healthcare_0.pdf

*Beidel, D. C., Frueh, B. C., Uhde, T. W., Wong, N., & Mentrikoski, J. M. (2011). Multicomponent behavioral treatment for chronic combat-related posttraumatic stress disorder: A randomized controlled trial. *Journal of Anxiety Disorders*, *25*(2), 224–231.

*Bormann, J. E., Thorp, S., Wetherell, J. L., & Golshan, S. (2008). A spiritually based group intervention for combat veterans with posttraumatic stress disorder: Feasibility study. *Journal of Holistic Nursing*, *26*(2), 109–116.

*Bormann, J. E., Thorp, S. R., Wetherell, J. L., Golshan, S., & Lang, A. J. (2013). Meditation-based mantram intervention for veterans with posttraumatic stress disorder: A randomized trial. *Psychological Trauma: Theory, Research, Practice, and Policy*, *5*(3), 259.

*Boudewyns, P. A., & Hyer, L. (1990). Physiological response to combat memories and preliminary treatment outcome in Vietnam veteran PTSD patients treated with direct therapeutic exposure. *Behavior Therapy*, *21*(1), 63–87.

*Boudewyns, P. A., & Hyer, L. A. (1996). Eye movement desensitization and reprocessing (EMDR) as treatment for post-traumatic stress disorder (PTSD). *Clinical Psychology & Psychotherapy*, *3*(3), 185–195.

*Boudewyns, P. A. Hyer, L., Woods, M. G., Harrison, W. R., & McCranie, E. (1990). PTSD among Vietnam veterans: An early look at treatment outcome using direct therapeutic exposure. *Journal of Traumatic Stress*, *3*(3), 359–368.

Bowles, S. V., & Bates, M. J. (2010). Military organizations and programs contributing to resilience building. *Military Medicine*, *175*, 382–385.

*Brief, D. J., Rubin, A., Keane, T. M., Enggasser, J. L., Roy, M., Helmuth, E., … Rosenbloom, D. (2013). Web intervention for OEF/OIF veterans with problem drinking and PTSD symptoms: A randomized clinical trial. *Journal of Consulting and Clinical Psychology*, *81*(5), 890–900.

*Bryan, C. J., & Morrow, C. E. (2011). Circumventing mental health stigma by embracing the warrior culture: Lessons learned from the Defender's Edge program. *Professional Psychology: Research and Practice*, *42*(1), 16–23.

*Bush, N. E., Smolenski, D. J., Denneson, L. M., Williams, H. B., Thomas, E. K., & Dobscha, S. K. (2017). A virtual hope box: Randomized controlled trial of a smartphone app for emotional regulation and coping with distress. *Psychiatric Services*, *68*(4), 330–336.

*Cacioppo, J. T., Adler, A. B., Lester, P. B., McGurk, D., Thomas, J. L., Chen, H. Y., & Cacioppo, S. (2015). Building social resilience in soldiers: A double dissociative randomized controlled study. *Journal of Personality and Social Psychology*, *109*(1), 90–105.

*Carr, W., Bradley, D., Ogle, A. D., Eonta, S. E., Pyle, B. L., & Santiago, P. (2013). Resilience training in a population of deployed personnel. *Military Psychology*, *25*(2), 148–155.

*Castro, C. A., Adler, A. B., McGurk, D., & Bliese, P. D. (2012). Mental health training with soldiers four months after returning from Iraq: Randomization by platoon. *Journal of Traumatic Stress*, *25*(4), 376–383.

*Chard, K. M., Schumm, J. A., Owens, G. P., & Cottingham, S. M. (2010). A comparison of OEF and OIF veterans and Vietnam veterans receiving cognitive processing therapy. *Journal of Traumatic Stress*, *23*(1), 25–32.

*Chemtob, C. M., Tomas, S., Law, W., & Cremniter, D. (1997). Postdisaster psychosocial intervention: A field study of the impact of debriefing on psychological distress. *American Journal of Psychiatry*, *154*(3), 415–417.

*Chongruksa, D., Prinyapol, P., Sawatsri, S., & Pansomboon, C. (2015). Integrated group counselling to enhance mental health and resilience of Thai army rangers. *Asia Pacific Journal of Counselling and Psychotherapy*, *6*(1–2), 41–57.

*Cigrang, J. A., Rauch,.S. A., Avila, L. L., Bryan, C. J., Goodie, J. L., Hryshko-Mullen, A., & Peterson, A. L. (2011). Treatment of active-duty military with PTSD in primary care: Early findings. *Psychological Services*, *8*(2), 104–113.

*Cigrang, J. A., Todd, S. L., & Carbone, E. G. (2000). Stress management training for military trainees returned to duty after a mental health evaluation: Effect on graduation rates. *Journal of Occupational Health Psychology*, *5*(1), 48–55.

*Cohn, A., & Pakenham, K. (2008). Efficacy of a cognitive-behavioral program to improve psychological adjustment among soldiers in recruit training. *Military Medicine*, *173*(12), 1151–1157.

*Cooper, N. A., & Clum, G. A. (1989). Imaginal flooding as a supplementary treatment for PTSD in combat veterans: A controlled study. *Behavior Therapy*, *20*(3), 381–391.

*Deahl, M. P., Gillham, A. B., Thomas, J., Searle, M. M., & Srinivasan, M. (1994). Psychological sequelae following the Gulf War: Factors associated with subsequent morbidity and the effectiveness of psychological debriefing. *British Journal of Psychiatry*, *165*, 60–65.

*Deahl, M. P., Srinivasan, M., Jones, N., Neblett, C., & Jolly, A. (2000). Preventing psychological trauma in soldiers: The role of operational stress training and psychological debriefing. *British Journal of Medical Psychology*, *73*, 77–85.

*Doss, B. D., Mitchell, A., Georgia, E. J., Biesen, J. N., & Rowe, L. S. (2015). Improvements in closeness, communication, and psychological distress mediate effects of couple therapy for veterans. *Journal of Consulting and Clinical Psychology*, *83*(2), 405–415.

*Fischer, E. P., Sherman, M. D., Han, X., & Owen, R. R., Jr. (2013). Outcomes of participation in the REACH multifamily group program for veterans with PTSD and their families. *Professional Psychology: Research and Practice*, *44*(3), 127–134.

*Foran, H. M., Adler, A. B., McGurk, D., & Bliese, P. D. (2012). Soldiers' perceptions of resilience training and postdeployment adjustment: Validation of a measure of resilience training content and training process. *Psychological Services*, *9*(4), 390.

*Forbes, D., Lewis, V., Parslow, R., Hawthorne, G., & Creamer, M. (2008). Naturalistic comparison of models of programmatic interventions for combat-related post-traumatic stress disorder. *Australian & New Zealand Journal of Psychiatry*, *42*(12), 1051–1059.

*Fornette, M.-P., Bardel, M.-H., Lefrançois, C., Fradin, J., El Massioui, F., & Amalberti, R. (2012). Cognitive-adaptation training for improving performance and stress management of Air Force pilots. *International Journal of Aviation Psychology*, *22*, 203–223.

*Frappell-Cooke, W., Gulina, M., Green, K., Hacker Hughes, J., & Greenberg, N. (2010). Does trauma risk management reduce psychological distress in deployed troops? *Occupational Medicine*, *60*(8), 645–650.

*Frueh, B. C., Turner, S. M., Beidel, D. C., Mirabella, R. F., & Jones, W. J. (1996). Trauma management therapy: A preliminary evaluation of a multi-component behavioral treatment for chronic combat-related PTSD. *Behaviour Research and Therapy*, *34*(7), 533–543.

*Gewirtz, A. H., Pinna, K. L., Hanson, S. K., & Brockberg, D. (2014). Promoting parenting to support reintegrating military families: After deployment, adaptive parenting tools. *Psychological Services*, *11*(1), 31–40.

*Githens, W. H., & Zalinski, J. (1983). *Marine corps recruit training attrition: The effect of realistic job preview and stress-coping films* (NPRDC TR 83-18). San Diego, CA: Navy Personnel Research and Development Center.

*Glynn, S. M., Eth, S., Randolph, E. T., Foy, D. W., Urbaitis, M., Boxer, L., ... Katzman, J. W. (1999). A test of behavioral family therapy to augment exposure for combat-related posttraumatic stress disorder. *Journal of Consulting and Clinical Psychology*, *67*(2), 243–251.

*Gould, M., Greenberg, N., & Hetherton, J. (2007). Stigma and the military: Evaluation of a PTSD psychoeducational program. *Journal of Traumatic Stress*, *20*(4), 505–515.

*Gray, M. J., Schorr, Y., Nash, W., Lebowitz, L., Amidon, A., Lansing, A., ... Litz, B. T. (2012). Adaptive disclosure: An open trial of a novel exposure-based intervention for service members with combat-related psychological stress injuries. *Behavior Therapy*, *43*(2), 407–415.

*Greenberg, N., Langston, V., Everitt, B., Iversen, A., Fear, N. T., Jones, N., & Wessely, S. (2010). A cluster randomized controlled trial to determine the efficacy of Trauma Risk Management (TRiM) in a military population. *Journal of Traumatic Stress*, *23*(4), 430–436.

*Greenberg, N., Langston, V., Fear, N. T., Jones, M., & Wessely, S. (2009). An evaluation of stress education in the Royal Navy. *Occupational Medicine*, *59*(1), 20–24.

*Griffith, J., & West, C. (2013). Master resilience training and its relationship to individual well-being and stress buffering among Army National Guard soldiers. *The Journal of Behavioral Health Services & Research*, *40*(2), 140–155.

*Hammarberg, M., & Silver, S. M. (1994). Outcome of treatment for post-traumatic stress disorder in a primary care unit serving Vietnam veterans. *Journal of Traumatic Stress*, *7*(2), 195–216.

*Hammermeister, J., Pickering, M. A., & Ohlson, C. J. (2009). Teaching mental skills for self-esteem enhancement in a military health care setting. *Journal of Instructional Psychology*, *36*, 203–209.

Hammonds, K. H. (2005). Why we hate HR. *Fast Company*, *97*(8), 40–47.

*Harms, P. D., Herian, M. N., Krasikova, D. V., Vanhove, A. J., & Lester, P. B. (2013). *The comprehensive soldier and family fitness program evaluation. Report #4: Evaluation of resilience training and mental and behavioral health outcomes.* Retrieved from http://csf2.army.mil/supportdocs/TR4.pdf

Harms, P. D., Krasikova, D. V., Vanhove, A. J., Herian, M. N., & Lester, P. B. (2013). Stress and emotional well-being in military organizations. *Research in Occupational Stress and Well-Being*, *11*, 103–132.

*Harris, J. I., Erbes, C. R., Engdahl, B. E., Thuras, P., Murray-Swank, N., Grace, D., … Malec, C. (2011). The effectiveness of a trauma-focused spiritually integrated intervention for veterans exposed to trauma. *Journal of Clinical Psychology*, *67*(4), 425–438.

Hattenstone, S., & Allison, E. (2014, October 18). 'You don't ever get over it': Meet the British soldiers living with post-traumatic stress disorder. *The Guardian*. Retrieved from https://www.theguardian.com/society/2014/oct/18/collateral-damage-ex-soldiers-living-with-ptsd.

Hoge, C. W., & Castro, C. A. (2005). Impact of combat duty in Iraq and Afghanistan on the mental health of US soldiers: Findings from the Walter Reed Army Institute of Research Land Combat Study. In *Strategies to maintain combat readiness during extended deployments – A human approach* (pp. 11-1–11-16). *Meeting proceedings RTO-MP-HFM-124, paper 11.* Neuilly-sur-Seine, France: RTO. Retrieved from http://www.cvltf.org/files/96551903.pdf

*Jakupcak, M., Roberts, L. J., Martell, C., Mulick, P., Michael, S., Reed, R., … McFall, M. (2006). A pilot study of behavioral activation for veterans with posttraumatic stress disorder. *Journal of Traumatic Stress*, *19*(3), 387–391.

*Jakupcak, M., Wagner, A., Paulson, A., Varra, A., & McFall, M. (2010). Behavioral activation as a primary care-based treatment for PTSD and depression among returning veterans. *Journal of Traumatic Stress*, *23*(4), 491–495.

*Jensen, J. A. (1994). An investigation of eye movement desensitization and reprocessing (EMD/R) as a treatment for posttraumatic stress disorder (PTSD) symptoms of Vietnam combat veterans. *Behavior Therapy*, *25*, 311–325.

*Jha, A. P., Morrison, A. B., Parker, S. C., & Stanley, E. A. (2017). Practice is protective: Mindfulness training promotes cognitive resilience in high-stress cohorts. *Mindfulness*, *8*, 46–58.

*Jha, A. P., Stanley, E. A., Kiyonaga, A., Wong, L., & Gelfand, L. (2010). Examining the protective effects of mindfulness training on working memory capacity and affective experience. *Emotion*, *10*(1), 54–64.

*Johnson, D. C., Thom, N. J., Stanley, E. A., Haase, L., Simmons, A. N., Shih, P. A. B., … & Paulus, M. P. (2014). Modifying resilience mechanisms in at-risk individuals: A controlled study of mindfulness training in Marines preparing for deployment. *American Journal of Psychiatry*, *171*(8), 844–853.

*Johnston, J. M., Minami, T., Greenwald, D., Li, C., Reinhardt, K., & Khalsa, S. B. S. (2015). Yoga for military service personnel with PTSD: A single arm study. *Psychological Trauma: Theory, Research, Practice, and Policy*, *7*(6), 555–562.

*Jones, D. E., Perkins, K., Cook, J. H., & Ong, A. L. (2008). Intensive coping skills training to reduce anxiety and depression for forward-deployed troops. *Military Medicine*, *173*, 241–246.

*Kahn, J. R., Collinge, W., & Soltysik, R. (2016). Post 9/11 veterans and their partners improve mental health outcomes with a self-directed mobile and web-based wellness training program: A randomized controlled trial. *Journal of Medical Internet Research*, *18*(9), e255.

*Keane, T. M., Fairbank, J. A., Caddell, J. M., & Zimering, R. T. (1989). Implosive (flooding) therapy reduces symptoms of PTSD in Vietnam combat veterans. *Behavior Therapy*, *20*, 245–260.

*Kearney, D. J., McDermott, K., Malte, C., Martinez, M., & Simpson, T. L. (2012). Association of participation in a mindfulness program with measures of PTSD, depression and quality of life in a veteran sample. *Journal of Clinical Psychology*, *68*(1), 101–116.

*Kees, M., Nerenberg, L. S., Bachrach, J., & Sommer, L. A. (2015). Changing the personal narrative: A pilot study of a resiliency intervention for military spouses. *Contemporary Family Therapy*, *37*(3), 221–231.

Kirkpatrick, D. L. (1994). *Evaluating training programs: The four levels*. San Francisco, CA: Berrett-Koehler.

*Larsson, G., Michel, P. O., & Lundin, T. (2000). Systematic assessment of mental health following various types of posttrauma support. *Military Psychology*, *12*(2), 121–135.

*Lester, P. B., Harms, P. D., Herian, M. N., Krasikova, D. V., & Beal, S. J. (2011). *The comprehensive soldier fitness program evaluation. Report 3: Longitudinal analysis of the impact of master resilience training on self-reported resilience and psychological health data*. Retrieved from http://digitalcommons.unl.edu/publicpolicyfacpub/32

*Lester, P., Saltzman, W. R., Woodward, K., Glover, D., Leskin, G. A., Bursch, B., ... Beardslee, W. (2012). Evaluation of a family-centered prevention intervention for military children and families facing wartime deployments. *American Journal of Public Health*, *102*(S1), S48–S54.

*Litz, B. T., Engel, C. C., Bryant, R. A., & Papa, A. (2007). A randomized, controlled proof-of-concept trial of an Internet-based, therapist-assisted self-management treatment for posttraumatic stress disorder. *American Journal of Psychiatry*, *164*(11), 1676–1684.

*Lunasco, T. K., Goodwin, E. A., Ozanian, A. J., & Loflin, E. M. (2010). One shot-one kill: A culturally sensitive program for the warrior culture. *Military Medicine*, *175*(7), 509–513.

Martin, A., Sanderson, K., & Cocker, F. (2009). Meta-analysis of the effects of health promotion intervention in the workplace on depression and anxiety symptoms. *Scandinavian Journal of Work, Environment, and Health*, *35*, 7–18.

Masten, A. S. (2007). Resilience in developing systems: Progress and promise as the fourth wave rises. *Development and Psychopathology*, *19*, 921–930.

*McLay, R. N., Graap, K., Spira, J., Perlman, K., Johnston, S., Rothbaum, B. O., ... Rizzo, A. (2012). Development and testing of virtual reality exposure therapy for post-traumatic stress disorder in active duty service members who served in Iraq and Afghanistan. *Military Medicine*, *177*(6), 635–642.

*McLay, R. N., Wood, D. P., Webb-Murphy, J. A., Spira, J. L., Wiederhold, M. D., Pyne, J. M., & Wiederhold, B. K. (2011). A randomized, controlled trial of virtual reality-graded exposure therapy for post-traumatic stress disorder in active duty service members with combat-related post-traumatic stress disorder. *Cyberpsychology, Behavior, and Social Networking*, *14*(4), 223–229.

Meredith, L. S., Sherbourne, C. D., Gaillot, S., Hansell, L., Ritschard, H. V., Parker, A. M., & Wrenn, G. (2011). *Promoting psychological resilience in the U.S. military*. Santa Monica, CA: RAND.

Meyers, M. C., van Woerkom, M., & Bakker, A. B. (2013). The added value of the positive: A literature review of positive psychology interventions in organizations. *European Journal of Work and Organizational Psychology*, *22*, 618–632.

*Monk, J. K., Ogolsky, B. G., & Bruner, V. (2016). Veteran couples integrative intensive retreat model: An intervention for military veterans and their relational partners. *Journal of Couple and Relationship Therapy*, *15*, 158–176.

*Monson, C. M., Schnurr, P. P., Resick, P. A., Friedman, M. J., Young-Xu, Y., & Stevens, S. P. (2006). Cognitive processing therapy for veterans with military-related posttraumatic stress disorder. *Journal of Consulting and Clinical Psychology*, *74*(5), 898–907.

*Morland, L. A., Greene, C. J., Rosen, C. S., Foy, D., Reilly, P., ... Frueh, B. C. (2010). Telemedicine for anger management therapy in a rural population of combat veterans with posttraumatic stress disorder: A randomized non-inferiority trial. *Journal of Clinical Psychiatry*, *71*, 855–863.

*Mulligan, K., Fear, N. T., Jones, N., Alvarez, H., Hull, L., Naumann, U., ... Greenberg, N. (2012). Postdeployment battlemind training for the U.K. armed forces: A cluster randomized controlled trial. *Journal of Consulting and Clinical Psychology*, *80*(3), 331–341.

Mulligan, K., Fear, N. T., Jones, N., Wessely, S., & Greenberg, N. (2011). Psycho-educational interventions designed to prevent deployment-related psychological ill-health in armed forces personnel: A review. *Psychological Medicine*, *41*, 673–686.

*Murphy, R. T., Thompson, K. E., Murray, M., Rainey, Q., & Uddo, M. M. (2009). Effect of a motivation enhancement intervention on veterans' engagement in PTSD treatment. *Psychological Services*, *6*(4), 264–278.

*Nakamura, Y., Lipschitz, D. L., Landward, R., Kuhn, R., & West, G. (2011). Two sessions of sleep-focused mind-body bridging improve self-reported symptoms of sleep and PTSD in veterans: A pilot randomized controlled trial. *Journal of Psychosomatic Research*, *70*, 335–345.

National Institutes of Health. (2009, Winter). A growing epidemic. *NIH Medline Plus*, *4*(1), 11–15.

*Niederhauser, V. P., Maddock, J., LeDoux, F., & Arnold, M. (2005). Building strong and ready army families: A multi-risk reduction health promotion pilot study. *Military Medicine*, *170*, 227–233.

Nigam, J. A. S., Murphy, L. R., & Swanson, N. G. (2003). Are stress management programs indicators of good places to work? Results of a national survey. *International Journal of Stress Management*, *10*, 345–360.

*Pinna, K. L., Hanson, S., Zhang, N., & Gewirtz, A. H. (2017). Fostering resilience in National Guard and Reserve families: A contextual adaptation of an evidence-based parenting program. *American Journal of Orthopsychiatry*, *87*(2), 185–193.

*Pischke, P. J., & Hallman, C. J. (2008). Effectiveness of critical event debriefings during Operational Iraqi Freedom II. *United States Army Medical Department Journal* (July–September), 18–23.

Ployhart, R. E., & Vandenberg, R. J. (2010). Longitudinal research: The theory, design, and analysis of change. *Journal of Management*, *36*, 94–120.

*Polusny, M. A., Erbes, C. R., Thuras, P., Moran, A., Lamberty, G. J., Collins, R. C., … Lim, K. O. (2015). Mindfulness-based stress reduction for posttraumatic stress disorder among veterans: A randomized clinical trial. *JAMA*, *314*(5), 456–465.

*Potter, A. R., Baker, M. T., Sanders, C. S., & Peterson, A. L. (2009). Combat stress reactions during military deployments: Evaluation of the effectiveness of combat stress control treatment. *Journal of Mental Health Counseling*, *31*(2), 137–148.

*Ragsdale, K. G., Cox, R. D., Finn, P., & Eisler, R. M. (1996). Effectiveness of short-term specialized inpatient treatment for war-related posttraumatic stress disorder: A role for adventure-based counseling and psychodrama. *Journal of Traumatic Stress*, *9*(2), 269–283.

*Ramsberger, P. F., Legree, P., & Mills, L. (2002). *Evaluation of the buddy team assignment program* (No. HUMRRO-FR-02-20). Alexandria, VA: Human Resources Research Organization.

Richardson, K. M., & Rothstein, H. R. (2008). Effects of occupational stress management intervention programs: A meta-analysis. *Journal of Occupational Health Psychology*, *13*, 69–93.

*Rizzo, A. A., Difede, J., Rothbaum, B. O., Johnston, S., McLay, R. N., Reger, G., … Pair, J. (2009). VR PTSD exposure therapy results with active duty OIF/OEF combatants. *Medicine Meets Virtual Reality*, *17*, 277–282.

*Rizzo, A. A., Difede, J., Rothbaum, B. O., Reger, G., Spitalnick, J. Cukor, J., & McLay, R. (2010). Development and early evaluation of the Virtual Iraq/Afghanistan exposure therapy system for combat-related PTSD. *Annals of the New York Academy of Sciences*, *1208*(1), 114–125.

*Rizzo, A. A., Newman, B., Parsons, T., Difede, J., Reger, G., Holloway, K., … Rothbaum, B. (2009). Development and clinical results from the Virtual Iraq Exposure Therapy Application for PTSD. In *Virtual rehabilitation international conference* (pp. 8–15). Piscataway, NJ: IEEE.

*Rosenthal, J. Z., Grosswald, S., Ross, R., & Rosenthal, N. (2011). Effects of transcendental meditation in veterans of Operation Enduring Freedom and Operation Iraqi Freedom with posttraumatic stress disorder: A pilot study. *Military Medicine*, *176*, 626–630.

*Rothbaum, B. O., Hodges, L. F., Ready, D., Graap, K., & Alarcon, R. D. (2001). Virtual reality exposure therapy for Vietnam veterans with posttraumatic stress disorder. *The Journal of Clinical Psychiatry*, *62*(8), 617–622.

*Roy, M. J., Highland, K. B., & Costanzo, M. A. (2015). GETSmart: Guided education and training via smart phones to promote resilience. *Annual Review of Cybertherapy and Telemedicine*, *13*, 123–128.

*Saltzman, W. R., Lester, P., Beardslee, W. R., Layne, C. M., Woodward, K., & Nash, W. P. (2011). Mechanisms of risk and resilience in military families: Theoretical and empirical basis of a family-based resilience enhancement program. *Clinical Child and Family Psychology Review*, *14*(3), 213–230.

*Saltzman, W. R., Lester, P., Milburn, N., Woodward, K., & Stein, J. (2016). Pathways of risk and resilience: Impact of a family resilience program on active-duty military parents. *Family Process*, *55*, 633–646.

Sammons, M. T. (2005). Psychology in the public sector: Addressing the psychological effects of combat in the U.S. Navy. *American Psychologist*, *60*(8), 899–909.

Seligman, M. E. P., & Csikszentmihalyi, M. (2000). Positive psychology: An introduction. *American Psychologist*, *55*, 5–14.

*Shalev, A. Y., Peri, T., & Rogel-Fuchs, Y. (1998). Historical group debriefing after combat exposure. *Military Medicine*, *163*, 494–498.

*Sharpley, J. G., Fear, N. T., Greenberg, N., Jones, M., & Wessely, S. (2008). Pre-deployment stress briefing: Does it have an effect? *Occupational Medicine*, *58*, 30–34.

Sherman, J. J. (1998). Effects of psychotherapeutic treatments for PTSD: A meta-analysis of controlled clinical trials. *Journal of Traumatic Stress*, *11*, 413–435.

*Sherman, M. D., Fischer, E. P., Owen, R. R., Jr, Lu, L., & Han, X. (2015). Multifamily group treatment for veterans with mood disorders. *Couple and Family Psychology: Research and Practice*, *4*, 136–149.

*Sherman, M. D., Fischer, E. P., Sorocco, K., & McFarlane, W. R. (2011). Adapting the multifamily group model to the Veterans Affairs system: The REACH program. *Couple and Family Psychology: Research and Practice*, *1*(S), 74–84.

Skeffington, P. M., Rees, C. S., & Kane, R. (2013). The primary prevention of PTSD: A systematic review. *Journal of Trauma and Dissociation*, *14*, 404–422.

Slomski, A. (2014). IOM: Military psychological interventions lack evidence. *JAMA*, *311*, 1487–1488.

*Smith-Osborne, A., Maleku, A., & Morgan, S. (2017). Impact of applied suicide intervention skills training on resilience and suicide risk in army reserve units. *Traumatology*, *23*(1), 49–55.

*Stanley, E. A., Schaldach, J. M., Kiyonaga, A., & Jha, A. P. (2011). Mindfulness-based mind fitness training: A case study of a high-stress predeployment military cohort. *Cognitive and Behavioral Practice*, *18*, 566–576.

Staw, B. M., & Epstein, L. D. (2000). What bandwagons bring: Effects of popular management techniques on corporate performance, reputation, and CEO pay. *Administrative Science Quarterly*, *45*, 523–556.

*Stecker, T., Fortney, J. C., & Sherbourne, C. D. (2011). An intervention to increase mental health treatment engagement among OIF veterans: A pilot trial. *Military Medicine*, *176*, 613–619.

*Tan, G., Dao, T. K., Farmer, L., Sutherland, R. J., & Gevirtz, R. (2011). Heart rate variability (HRV) and posttraumatic stress disorder (PTSD): A pilot study. *Applied Psychophysiology and Biofeedback*, *36*, 27–35.

Taylor, A. H., & Schatz, S. (2011). Measuring the effectiveness of stress prevention programs in military personnel. In D. D. Schmorrow & C. M. Fidopiastis (Eds.), *Foundations of augmented cognition: Directing the future of adaptive systems* (pp. 636–646). Berlin, Germany: Springer-Verlag.

Taylor, A. H., Schatz, S., Marino-Carper, T. L., Carrizales, M. L., & Vogel-Walcutt, J. (2011). A review of military predeployment stress tolerance training. *Proceeding of the Human Factors and Ergonomics Society Annual Meeting*, *55*, 2153–2157.

*Taylor, M. K., Stanfill, K. E., Padilla, G. A., Markham, A. E., Ward, M. D., Koehler, M. M., … Adams, B. D. (2011). Effect of psychological skills training during military survival school: A randomized, controlled field study. *Military Medicine*, *176*, 1362–1368.

*Tenhula, W. N., Nezu, A. M., Nezu, C. M., Stewart, M. O., Miller, S. A., Steele, J., & Karlin, B. E. (2014). Moving forward: A problem-solving training program to foster veteran resilience. *Professional Psychology: Research and Practice*, *45*(6), 416–424.

Thompson, M, & Gibbs, N. (2012, July). The insidious enemy: Why the pentagon is losing the war against military suicide. *Time*, *180*(4), 22–31.

*Van Breda, A. D. (1999). Developing resilience to routine separations: An occupational social work intervention. *Families in Society: The Journal of Contemporary Human Services*, *80*, 597–605.

Vanhove, A. J., Herian, M. N., Perez, A. U. L., Harms, P. D., & Lester, P. B. (2016). Can resilience be developed at work? A meta-analytic review of resilience-building program effectiveness. *Journal of Occupational and Organizational Psychology*, *89*, 278–307.

*Van Voorhees, B., & Sweis, R. (2010). *Improving combat stress and depressive symptoms in veterans and post-deployment service members of OEF/OIF: Assessing the potential benefits of a web-based* *computerized cognitive behavioral therapy and peer-to-peer support intervention.* Brief Research Report, RISE Consulting and Prevail Health Solutions, LLC, Chicago, IL.

*Vella, E. J., Milligan, B., & Bennett, J. L. (2013). Participation in outdoor recreation program predicts improved psychosocial well-being among veterans with post-traumatic stress disorder: A pilot study. *Military Medicine, 178*(3), 254–260.

*Williams, R. A., Hagerty, B. M., Andrei, A. C., Yousha, S. M., Hirth, R. A., & Hoyle, K. S. (2007). STARS: Strategies to assist Navy recruits' success. *Military Medicine*, *172*, 942–949.

*Williams, R. A, Hagerty, B. M., Brasington, S. J., Clem, J. B., & Williams, D. A. (2010). Stress gym: Feasibility of deploying a web-enhanced behavioral self-management program for stress in a military setting. *Military Medicine*, *175*, 487–493.

*Williams, R. A., Hagerty, B. M., Yousha, S. M., Horrocks, J., Hoyle, K. S., & Liu, D. (2004). Psychosocial effects of the Boot Strap intervention in Navy recruits. *Military Medicine*, *169*, 814–820.

Yerkes, R. M. (1921). Psychological examining in the United States Army. In R. M. Yerkes (Ed.), *Memoirs of the National Academy of Sciences* (Vol. 15, pp. 1–180). Washington, DC: US Government Printing Office.

Zajac, E. J., & Westphal, J. D. (2004). The social construction of market value: Institutionalization and learning perspectives on stock market reactions. *American Sociological Review*, *69*(3), 433–457.

*Zamorski, M. A., Guest, K., Bailey, S., & Garber, B. G. (2012). Beyond battle mind: Evaluation of a new mental health training program for Canadian forces personnel participating in third-location decompression. *Military Medicine*, *177*(11), 1245–1253.

PAIN IN THE CIVILIAN AND MILITARY WORKPLACE

Ethan W. Gossett and P. D. Harms

ABSTRACT

Acute and chronic pain affects more Americans than heart disease, diabetes, and cancer combined. Conservative estimates suggest the total economic cost of pain in the United States is $600 billion, and more than half of this cost is due to lost productivity, such as absenteeism, presenteeism, and turnover. In addition, an escalating opioid epidemic in the United States and abroad spurred by a lack of safe and effective pain management has magnified challenges to address pain in the workforce, particularly the military. Thus, it is imperative to investigate the organizational antecedents and consequences of pain and prescription opioid misuse (POM). This chapter provides a brief introduction to pain processing and the biopsychosocial model of pain, emphasizing the relationship between stress, emotional well-being, and pain in the military workforce. We review personal and organizational risk and protective factors for pain, such as post-traumatic stress disorder, optimism, perceived organizational support, and job strain. Further, we discuss the potential adverse impact of pain on organizational outcomes, the rise of POM in military personnel, and risk factors for POM in civilian and military populations. Lastly, we propose potential organizational interventions to mitigate pain and provide the future directions for work, stress, and pain research.

Keywords: Pain; stress; military; protective factors; PTSD; opioid

Pain is the most expensive medical condition in the United States (Gaskin & Richard, 2012; Institute of Medicine Committee on Advancing Pain Research & Education, 2011). At an annual cost between $560 and $635 billion, pain costs

Occupational Stress and Well-being in Military Contexts
Research in Occupational Stress and Well-being, Volume 16, 157–186
Copyright © 2018 by Emerald Publishing Limited
All rights of reproduction in any form reserved
ISSN: 1479-3555/doi:10.1108/S1479-355520180000016012

more than the combined cost for heart disease ($309 billion) and cancer ($243 billion) (Gaskin & Richard, 2012). Furthermore, the cost of lost work productivity associated with pain ($299–335 billion), not medical treatment, has the greatest economic impact.

Most of the early investigations into the impact of pain on lost productivity focused on absenteeism (Blyth, March, Nicholas, & Cousins, 2003). However, mounting evidence suggests reduced productivity at work due to chronic pain, or presenteeism, has a much larger impact on overall work effectiveness than absenteeism (Blyth et al., 2003; Gaskin & Richard, 2012; Leeuwen, Blyth, March, Nicholas, & Cousins, 2006; Pohling, Buruck, Jungbauer, & Leiter, 2016). Chronic pain may impact productivity in direct and obvious ways, such as limiting physical activity or interfering with attention. Or, it may indirectly reduce work productivity by decreasing emotional well-being, given prior work suggests that poor emotional well-being is associated with detriments in job performance (Adler et al., 2006). Although investigation into the avenues through which chronic pain influences presenteeism, absenteeism, and other organizational outcomes is still in its infancy, a few recent studies have begun investigating these mechanisms (Byrne & Hochwarter, 2006; Christian, Eisenkraft, & Kapadia, 2015; Ferris, Rogers, Blass, & Hochwarter, 2009).

Pain is a dynamic process influenced by biological, psychological, and social factors (Edwards, Dworkin, Sullivan, Turk, & Wasan, 2016; Gatchel, Peng, Peters, Fuchs, & Turk, 2007). Biological factors (e.g., biomechanical stress) undoubtedly impact pain conditions, but biological factors alone have proven to be poor predictors of pain and disability, particularly in chronic conditions. Decades of clinical and experimental pain research strongly suggests that emotional well-being influences pain processing. In addition, prior work suggests organizational factors (e.g., occupational stress, leadership, and job demands) affect emotional well-being (Harms, Krasikova, Vanhove, Herian, & Lester, 2013; Tetrick & Winslow, 2015). Thus, organizational factors which impact emotional well-being may also indirectly impact pain.

The military provides an ideal population to study the biopsychosocial model of pain as it relates to the work environment for three primary reasons: (1) serving in the military is commonly associated with heavy physical demands and elevated risks for musculoskeletal injuries; (2) consistently rated as one of the most stressful occupations, military personnel are vulnerable to determinants in emotional well-being and psychological functioning, such as post-traumatic stress disorder (PTSD) and depression; and (3) prescription opioid misuse (POM) in current and former military service members has risen dramatically in recent years and may be associated with physical and psychosocial work hazards.

DYNAMICS OF PAIN

Pain is an unpleasant subjective sensory and affective experience influenced by biological, psychological, and social factors (Edwards et al., 2016; Staud, 2012;

Woolf, 2010). Although commonly seen as nuisance, perception of pain is an adaptive function essential for survival. This is evident in patients who frequently injure themselves unintentionally, develop infections, and even die due to medical conditions which cause deficits in pain perception. In contrast, chronic pain patients suffer from severe and intractable pain that can last for months, years, or even decades (Gatchel et al., 2007). This can lead to significant decrease in physical, psychological, and social functioning. Patients with chronic pain often become disabled and unable to work, which furthers the distress associated with chronic pain.

Pain was initially viewed by medical professionals as a symptom of actual or potential tissue injury proportional to the degree of injury or noxious stimulation (Edwards et al., 2016; Gatchel et al., 2007). Early experimental research discovered pain receptor fields and pathways which activated and elicited pain when stimulated with various noxious stimuli (Melzack, 1996). Although pain pathways have biological underpinnings (e.g., pain receptors and sensory neurons), cognitive and effective brain processes modulate and influence the culminated pain experience (Garcia-Larrea & Peyron, 2013). Beecher (1946) first noticed the discrepancy between injury and pain when treating World War II soldiers. Despite suffering severe physical trauma on the battlefield, many soldiers reported little or no pain and required relatively low levels of pain medication. This was in stark contrast to military patients he treated in domestic clinics who required greater pain medication for lesser injuries. Thus, he surmised that additional contextual mechanisms must also influence pain perception.

Melzack and Wall (1965) supported Beecher's speculation with their Gate-Control Theory of Pain. While this theory has since been amended and elaborated upon (see Staud, 2012), it posited that additional mechanisms modulate pain at the level of the spinal cord. Input from other neurons in the peripheral and central nervous system could either open or close the gate (i.e., activate or block spinal transmission neurons). An open gate would transmit nociceptive signals to the brain and a closed gate would prevent transmission. Thus, activation of nociceptive fibers in the peripheral nervous systems may or may not translate to conscious pain perception (Staud, 2012).

From an evolutionary perspective, pain modulation is an adaptive trait (Staud, 2012). When trying to fight or escape from a predator, it may be advantageous to inhibit pain, since immediate survival takes precedence over tending to tissue damage. In contrast, facilitating pain to heal and avoid further tissue damage may be more advantageous after the passing of threat. Thus, the context in which pain occurs influences the perception and evaluation of pain and, in turn, directs behavior. Psychological factors (e.g., attention and emotion) and social factors (e.g., social support and work stress) associated with pain modulation will be discussed in subsequent sections (Edwards et al., 2016).

Classification of Pain

Pain can be categorized in different ways, such as duration and body site, but the most concise way to conceptualize pain may be by a mechanism-based classification system (Loeser & Melzack, 1999; Woolf, 2010). In this respect, pain can be separated into three categories: nociceptive (transient), acute (inflammatory), and chronic (pathological). The antecedents and consequences of each type of pain vary, and biopsychosocial factors influence all types of pain. Pain that progresses into a chronic state appears to be strongly influenced by psychological and social factors (Gatchel et al., 2007).

Nociceptive Pain

Nociceptive pain is the immediate and overwhelming pain associated with intense noxious stimuli, such as heat, cold, pressure, or chemical (Woolf, 2010). Nociceptive pain is transmitted through a series of neurons that stretches from sensory receptors (nociceptors) in tissue to transmission neurons in the spinal cord and ultimately to a matrix of multiple brain centers, collectively known as the pain matrix (Garcia-Larrea & Peyron, 2013). Garcia-Larrea and Peyron (2013) conceptualize the pain matrix as a composite of three interdependent neural networks and their psychological correlates: the nociceptive, perceptive-attentional, and reappraisal-emotional networks.

The nociceptive network, or sensory-discriminative network, conveys the location and intensity of the stimulus and is associated primarily with increased activation in the somatosensory cortex of the brain. Stimulation of the nociceptive network alone does not elicit pain and is not associated with the unpleasantness or emotional response to pain. Conscious perception of pain is dependent on integration of noxious stimuli by the second-order perceptive-attentional network. Initial cognitive evaluation, appraisal, and modulation of pain are also associated with activation in the perceptive-attentional network. This network, which is also activated during other cognitive and effective processes independent of pain, conveys the unpleasant emotional experience of pain.

The third-order level of pain processing occurs in the reappraisal-emotional network of the pain matrix. This network involves higher-level cognitive processing which attaches meaning and consequence to pain, draws on previous pain experiences, and is heavily involved in descending modulation of nociceptive signals. Emotional and attentional modulations are important characteristics of the pain experience and underpin many of the risk and protective factors (e.g., depression and mindfulness) associated with chronic pain. The impact of cognitive and effective processes on pain perception will be discussed further in subsequent sections.

Acute Pain

Acute pain is pain which results from tissue damage and is normal part of the healing process (Gatchel et al., 2007; Woolf, 2010). After tissue damage, a cascade of inflammatory responses results in restructuring of the cellular membrane of nociceptive fibers around the injury site (Woolf, 2010). In addition, prolonged stimulation of nociceptors causes local molecular changes, such as release of substance P (Besson, 1999). Together these structural and molecular changes lower the activation threshold for noxious stimuli and increase the rate of firing. Increased input to transmission neurons in the spinal cords from nociceptive neurons induces similar changes in cellular structure and excitability of transmission neurons. Previously innocuous sensory stimuli, such as mild pressure or heat, become more likely to elicit pain. In non-pathological states, the structure and function of the pain pathway returns to its original state after the affected tissue heals, and medical treatment for pain is no longer needed.

Chronic Pain

Pain that persists after the normal healing process (typically no greater than three months) is considered chronic (Gatchel et al., 2007). Chronic pain disorders include a multitude of medical conditions with different etiology, mechanisms, symptoms, and treatment strategies. Osteoarthritis, rheumatoid arthritis, chronic musculoskeletal pain (e.g., low back pain, neck pain, and wrist pain), phantom limb pain, chronic headache, irritable bowel syndrome, and fibromyalgia are examples of chronic pain conditions (Lumley et al., 2011). Furthermore, it is common for patients to suffer from more than one chronic pain conditions at a time. In military populations, the most prevalent and germane forms of chronic pain tend to be musculoskeletal pain, osteoarthritis, and phantom limb pain.

The etiology of chronic pain is significantly more complex than nociceptive or inflammatory pain, and biomedical models have been less effective in treating chronic pain (Gatchel et al., 2007; Turk, Fillingim, Ohrbach, & Patel, 2016). Psychological and sociocultural factors have greater influence in chronic pain conditions. In some cases, no precipitating anatomical abnormality, such as a herniated intervertebral disc or damaged cartilage, can be identified (Beattie, Meyers, Stratford, Millard, & Hollenberg, 2000). Furthermore, anatomical abnormalities are not strongly correlated with patient ratings of pain severity or life dysfunction (Staud, 2012). For example, some patients with severely damaged intervertebral discs report no back pain, while others report severe back pain without disc damage or any other identifiable abnormality (Beattie et al., 2000). In other words, injury is often not directly associated with the extent of symptoms (Staud, 2012). Furthermore, surgery to correct an anatomical abnormality frequently fails to alleviate pain (Chan & Peng, 2011). In fact, conservative estimates suggest 20% of spinal surgeries fail to significantly reduce pain and improve function. Thus, the connection between stimulus, physiology, and pain is more complex in chronic pain than nociceptive or inflammatory pain.

BIOPSYCHOSOCIAL MODEL OF ACUTE AND CHRONIC PAIN

Determining the occupational risk factors of acute or chronic pain as well as developing prevention and treatment methods requires a multifactorial model. The biopsychosocial model of pain encompasses physiological correlates of pain (i.e., potential or actual damage to the body) with psychological and social constructs associated with pain (Edwards et al., 2016; Gatchel et al., 2007). Physiological factors associated with pain in the workplace include strains, sprains, stress fractures, degenerative disc disease, spinal stenosis (narrowing of the spinal canal), and joint degeneration (Bartynski, 2009; Bernard, 1997; Kumar, 2001; Neogi, 2013). While other occupational injuries incite pain (e.g., lacerations, burns, and abrasions), our review of biological risk factors will focus on musculoskeletal injury, since it is the most common type of non-fatal occupational injury in the civilian and military workforce (Bernard, 1997; Hauret, Jones, Bullock, Canham-Chervak, & Canada, 2010; Ruscio et al., 2010). Psychosocial factors include attention and memory, mood, emotion, job stress, and social support (Edwards et al., 2016; Garcia-Larrea & Peyron, 2013).

Biological Risk Factors

Injuries to the musculoskeletal system may be acute or have a chronic progression (Kumar, 2001). Acute musculoskeletal injuries are associated with a specific and discernable incident, such as overexertion, slip and fall, crushing, laceration, etc., in which excessive biomechanical stress leads to rapid structural failure of muscles, ligaments, bones, tendons, or other musculoskeletal components (Coenen, Kingma, Boot, Bongers, & van Dieën, 2014; Hauret et al., 2010; Kumar, 2001). In contrast, musculoskeletal disorder (MSD) may develop from damage to musculoskeletal tissue that occurs gradually through repeated and cumulative exposure to smaller biomechanical stressor, or micro-trauma (tendonitis, lumbar disc degeneration, carpal tunnel syndrome; Bernard, 1997; Coenen et al., 2014; Forde, Punnett, & Wegman, 2002). A systematic review of work-related MSD risk factors in the civilian workforce identified multiple biomechanical risk factors, such as heavy physical work, awkward posture, frequent lifting, and repetitive work, although the risk factors may vary according the type of MSD (da Costa & Vieira, 2010). In some occupations, biomechanical factors associated with work were related to approximately 50% of hospitalizations due to lumbar disc disease, a type of back injury (Wahlström, Burström, Nilsson, & Järvholm, 2012). Prior work suggests that firefighters, nurses, and bus drivers have elevated rates of MSD, which may be related to biomechanical risk factors encountered in these occupations (Bernard, 1997).

Injury in the Military

Few occupations are as physically demanding or as potentially dangerous as serving in the military. At a minimum, all military personnel must participate in physical training and maintain a moderate level of physical fitness. However, many occupations within the military require heavy physical work. Thus, personnel are exposed to multiple biomechanical risk factors. In addition, service members engaged in combat operations may be wounded in battle and suffer severe musculoskeletal trauma. Although the prevalence of blast injuries suffered in battle by military personnel are not observed in the civilian workforce, police officers and other first-responders may also encounter comparable violence and injury.

Non-Battle Injury. In 2006, there were over 743,000 injury-related musculoskeletal conditions among non-deployed, active duty military personnel, with a rate of 628 injuries per 1,000 person-years (Hauret et al., 2010). Inflammation and pain (overuse) accounted for 82% of injury-related musculoskeletal conditions, including both acute and chronic. Regarding body site, lower extremity overuse injuries were most common, such as stress fractures, Achilles tendonitis, and plantar fasciitis. Most musculoskeletal injuries in the military parallel civilian work populations – falls, trips and slips, repetitive movement, and over-exertion. These injuries occur during exercise, road marching, hiking, while entering or exiting a vehicle, and mounting or climbing an object (Anderson, Grier, Canham-Chervak, Bushman, & Jones, 2015; Ruscio et al., 2010). Owing to high standards of physical fitness, military personnel experience high rates of overuse injury resulting from physical training (i.e., exercise), which are commonly observed in sports medicine but less frequently in most civilian occupations (Bernard, 1997; Hauret et al., 2010; Lauder, Baker, Smith, & Lincoln, 2000). Unfortunately, injuries because of overuse and overexertion are unavoidable given the strenuous weight-bearing physical activities required of service members (Jones, Canham-Chervak, Canada, Mitchener, & Moore, 2010). Although motor vehicle accidents are a common reason for all-cause injury, these injuries most commonly occur off-duty in privately owned motor vehicles. Thus, the motor vehicle accidents that occurred at work were responsible for only a small portion of the total injury burden.

Battle Injury. Battle injuries are significantly less common than non-battle injuries (Cohen, Griffith, Larkin, Villena, & Larkin, 2005). However, injuries suffered during battle can cause severe physical trauma (Geiling, Rosen, & Edwards, 2012). The nature of enemy combat tactics as well as advances in medical technology and personal protective equipment has led to an increased rate of survival from injuries which would have been fatal in previous wars (Geiling et al., 2012). For instance, the ratio of wounded versus dead service members was 8.2 in Operation Eduring Freedom (OEF) and 7.2 in Operation Iraqi Freedom (OIF) compared to just 2.3 in World War II and 3.2 in Vietnam war. Although service members injured in OEF and OIF may survive such severe injuries, these wounded veterans face significant physical and psychological challenges on the path to recovery.

There has been a proliferation in the use of improvised explosive devices (IEDs; e.g., car, roadside, and suicide bombs) by enemy combatants during OIF and OEF. The rise in IED attacks has pertinent implications on health outcomes (Clark, Walker, Gironda, & Scholten, 2009; Cohen et al., 2005; Geiling et al., 2012; Lew et al., 2009). Explosive blast and projectiles from IEDs typically have a different profile than traditional battlefield wounds, such as gunshots. IED injuries are associated with a combination of trauma types (e.g., soft tissue injury, fracture, burn, and concussion) to multiple body sites, also known as polytraumatic injury (Clark et al., 2009; Lew et al., 2009). Individuals with blast injuries have significantly higher rates of amputation, penetrating head injury, and psychiatric diagnosis compared to non-blast or non-battle injury (Clark et al., 2009). In a sample of 29 spinal injury patients from OIF, over 90% of the injuries were caused by

IEDs (Cohen et al., 2005). In comparison, only one spinal injury was a result of a gunshot wound, the most common source of spinal cord injury in prior conflicts. The 7.4% incidence of spine injuries in a study of OIF soldiers was higher than any previous American military conflict in 60 years. Prior work reported service members injured by blasts received two to four times the prescription opioid (PO) pain medication dosage compared to other injuries upon admission to the hospital, and they continued to have significantly higher opioid dosage at discharge (Clark et al., 2009). These veterans may also face multiple surgeries, prolonged hospitalization, and long-term rehabilitation (Geiling et al., 2012).

Psychosocial Factors

Pain and Emotion

As we have emphasized thus far, pain is not simply a sensory experience. Pain is an aversive experience which motivates behaviors intended to protect against tissue damage and promote survival (Navratilova & Porreca, 2014; Rhudy, 2015). By eliciting an unpleasant emotional experience, pain motivates immediate withdrawal and avoidance of noxious stimuli. Furthermore, pain facilitates learning and reinforces future behavior that avoids identical or similar painful stimuli. In addition, relief from pain reduces negative effect and increases positive effect via the dopaminergic reward system, further reinforcing avoidance learning.

The relationship between pain and emotion is also bidirectional (Rhudy, 2015). Thus, emotions can influence pain perception as well by facilitating (i.e., enhancing) or inhibiting pain. In general, negative emotions facilitate pain and positive emotions inhibit pain (Rhudy, 2015; Rhudy et al., 2010). Rhudy et al. (2010) exposed participants to the International Affective Picture System (IAPS) and found that showing participants unpleasant pictures increased sensitivity to experimental pain (i.e., pain facilitation), while showing participants pleasant pictures decreased pain sensitivity (i.e., pain inhibition). Furthermore, the degree of pain inhibition or facilitation is commensurate with the arousal elicited by emotion. The most unpleasant pictures in the IAPS (mutilated bodies) elicited the greatest pain facilitation, and the most pleasant pictures (erotica) elicited the greatest pain inhibition. However, this dynamics may be altered in cases of extremely high unpleasant emotional arousal, such as a life-threatening situation or phobic response (Rhudy, 2015). Highly unpleasant emotional states may lead to dramatic inhibition of pain, which most likely evolved to enhance fighting or evasion behaviors during threatening situations. In contrast, no prior research suggests that any level of pleasant emotional arousal is associated with pain facilitation.

The association between emotion and pain is essential to motivating avoidance behavior and ensuring survival. However, the reciprocal ability of emotional states to modulate pain also makes the pain system vulnerable to dysfunctional emotional processing and may lead to exaggerated pain facilitation, as observed in chronic pain conditions (Bushnell, Ceko, & Low, 2013 Edwards et al., 2016). On the other hand, positive emotional styles may protect individuals against biological and social vulnerabilities to chronic pain by inhibiting pain (Edwards et al., 2016; Goodin et al., 2013).

Psychosocial Risk and Protective Factors

Psychosocial risk factors for chronic pain do not necessarily incite acute or chronic pain (Lumley et al., 2011). However, they may modify pain processes (e.g., central sensitization) and contribute to the transition from acute to persistent pain following initial physical insult (Lumley et al., 2011; Tracey, 2010). Many psychosocial risk factors have been identified (Edwards et al., 2016; Gatchel et al., 2007; Turk et al., 2016). Psychological risk factors include persistent mood disorders, such as depression and PTSD, as well as other maladaptive psychological schema associated with chronic pain, such as pain catastrophizing and injury sensitivity. Social risk factors include solicitous social responses (i.e., encouraging rest and disuse), workplace bullying, and role conflict at work (Christensen & Knardahl, 2014; Edwards et al., 2016; Kivimaki et al., 2004).

In contrast to identifying risk factors, researchers have also begun investigating so-called protective factors which may prevent chronic pain and disability, such as optimism, mindfulness, and positive effect (Edwards et al., 2016; Finan & Garland, 2015; Goodin et al., 2013; McCracken & Vowles, 2014). Risk and protective factors also influence the success rate of treatment and degree of functional disability. Given their bidirectional relationship with chronic pain, psychosocial factors will first be discussed as an antecedent to chronic pain. In a subsequent section, reduced psychosocial function will be interpreted as a consequence of chronic pain when discussing its impact on organizational outcomes.

Psychological Risk Factors.

Depression. Pain is strongly associated with emotion, and thus influenced by healthy or maladaptive emotional functioning (Gatchel et al., 2007). Mood disorders are the most common comorbidities of chronic pain (Banks & Kerns, 1996; Gatchel et al., 2007; Turk et al., 2016). The unpleasantness and persistent disruption due to chronic pain can wear on even the most resilient individuals. Patients can transition from a healthy and active lifestyle prior to chronic pain to severe disability and functional impairment after onset. Unsurprisingly, the incidence of depression is significantly higher in chronic pain patients (Bair, Robinson, Katon, & Kroenke, 2003; Goulet et al., 2016). Although depression and other mood disorders were originally thought to be a consequence of chronic pain, it appears that the relationship between chronic pain and psychological functioning is bidirectional (Edwards et al., 2016; Gatchel et al., 2007; Jarvik et al., 2005; Turk et al., 2016).

Jarvik et al. (2005) reported in a prospective study that depression predicted pain better than anatomical abnormality three years following the initial assessment. Depressed patients were more than twice as likely to report back pain. Other research suggests that depression symptoms may increase disengagement from daily activities and lead to greater perceived pain interference and chronic disability (Casey, Greenberg, Nicassio, Harpin, & Hubbard, 2008; Morasco et al., 2013). Thus, depression may be both an antecedent and consequence of chronic pain.

Fear and Anxiety. Fear and anxiety are emotions which promote avoidance behavior of immediate or potential threats to the self (Turk et al., 2016; Vlaeyen & Linton, 2000, 2012). Fear is caused by immediate threats which call for decisive action (i.e., fight or flight), while anxiety is elicited by potential impending threats and promotes future avoidance. Pain is intended to signal the imminent or actual threat of bodily damage and is thus capable of eliciting significant fear and anxiety. Furthermore, pain can signal a physical threat from an external stimulus (e.g., heat from a flame) or internal stimulus (e.g., putting pressure on a fractured leg). An important distinction between anxiety and fear is that anxiety is a future-oriented emotion associated with worry and rumination which does not require actual exposure to the threatening stimulus to cause distress and prompt avoidance (Vlaeyen, 2000).

After an injury, engaging in certain physical activities or movements (e.g., joint pressure or spine flexion) may be painful, appraised as physically threatening, and, in turn, evoke fear of (re)injury (Edwards et al., 2016; Gatchel et al., 2007; Vlaeyen & Linton, 2000, 2012). Over time, movements which elicit pain will be avoided in favor of positions or activities which reduce pain (Edwards et al., 2016; Turk et al., 2016; Vlaeyen & Linton, 2000, 2012).

During the phase of acute pain, this promotes rest and healing of damaged tissue. However, prolonged and/or exaggerated fear and anxiety toward physical activity may contribute to the development of chronic pain and disability. Furthermore, heightened vigilance to pain associated with pain-related fear may increase somatic awareness and focus attention toward noxious stimuli, thus increasing pain sensitivity (Crombez, Van Damme, & Eccleston, 2005; Vlaeyen & Linton, 2000). As a result, activities which elicit pain may be avoided or discontinued, resulting in reduced function and increased disability. Pain-related fear and anxiety are integral components of psychiatric anxiety disorders, such as PTSD.

Post-Traumatic Stress Disorder. Military organizations are unique in that their occupational hazards include, among other things, fire fights, mortar attacks, and IEDs. The danger associated with this occupation put service members at a heightened risk for traumatic injuries to themselves and fellow service members and even death. Furthermore, military personnel may have to directly injure or kill enemy combatants or witness others killing combatants.

Exposure to these life-threatening situations and traumatic injuries puts service members at an elevated risk of PTSD. Furthermore, there is a strong association between PTSD and pain (Brennstuhl, Tarquinio, & Montel, 2015). In a nationally representative sample, McWilliams, Cox, and Enns (2003) found that the rate of PTSD in patients with chronic pain was more than three times higher than patients without pain. Furthermore, prior work suggests that the relationship between chronic pain and PTSD is even stronger in veterans (Edwards et al., 2016). A recent review by Fishbain et al. (2017) determined prevalence of PTSD in subgroups of chronic pain patients (e.g., chronic low back pain, fibromyalgia, headache, and motor vehicle accident). Approximately 50% of the veteran group had a comorbid diagnosis of chronic pain and PTSD compared to 10% of the general population group.

PTSD, such as depression, is also associated with poorer treatment outcomes for chronic pain, and patients may benefit from concurrent treatment of the disorders (Bosco, Gallinati, & Clark, 2013). Patients with pain diagnosed with concurrent PTSD were three times more likely to be prescribed opioids, in higher doses, and for a longer period (Seal et al., 2012). This is especially alarming, given prior work suggesting that PTSD is a significant risk factor for POM (Rigg & DeCamp, 2014; Seal et al., 2011).

The mechanisms underlying PTSD and chronic pain are still being investigated; however, multiple models have been proposed to explain strong association between PTSD and chronic pain (Asmundson, Coons, Taylor, & Katz, 2002; Brennstuhl et al., 2015). Two prominent models are the mutual maintenance model and the shared vulnerability model, both of which draw from cognitive-behavioral models of chronic pain and PTSD (Asmundson et al., 2002; Brennstuhl et al., 2015; Sharp & Harvey, 2001; Vlaeyen & Linton, 2000).

The mutual maintenance model theorizes seven cognitive and emotional processes associated with each disorder and influences the expression of the other: attention biases, anxiety sensitivity, persistent reminders of trauma, avoidance-coping, depression, perception of anxiety and pain, and limited adaptive coping strategies (Asmundson et al., 2002; Brennstuhl et al., 2015; Sharp & Harvey, 2001). Attentional biases are activated when painful stimuli remind the patient of the original trauma (Sharp & Harvey, 2001). Consequentially, patients will become hypervigilant and hypersensitive to pain sensations, since experiencing pain becomes associated with the trauma. Anxiety sensitivity disposes individuals to misinterpret anxiety symptoms as an indication of harm. As a result, pain and bodily sensations associated with PTSD (e.g., arousal) elicit catastrophic thoughts. Chronic pain also becomes a persistent reminder of the trauma and may lead to reviviscence of the trauma (i.e., flashbacks) and arousal which, in turn, may sustain the connection between pain and the trauma. Both disorders encourage avoidance behaviors toward activities which elicit symptoms of the disease (i.e., avoidant coping styles). In chronic pain, a patient may avoid walking down stairs because it elicits pain, and a patient with PTSD may avoid crowded areas because it elicits anxiety and arousal. As a result, both disorders lead to reduced function and social interaction. Depression is also common in both disorders and promotes lack of engagement and exposure to aversive situations which may be necessary for treating PTSD and chronic pain. Anxiety often increases pain, possibly due to elevated arousal and muscle tension (Gatchel et al., 2007). Given that PTSD elicits anxiety and hyperarousal, it may increase pain sensitivity also (Vlaeyen & Linton, 2000, 2012). Lastly, the overwhelming and persistent nature of chronic pain and PTSD may exhaust cognitive resources, thereby reducing the ability to employ adaptive pain-management strategies (Sharp & Harvey, 2001). The impact of chronic pain symptoms on PTSD and the impact of PTSD on chronic pain symptoms may lead to a mutually reinforcing process which persist and worsen symptoms. Thus, interventions which consider both disorders may be the most impactful.

The shared vulnerability model posits that individuals with certain psychological tendencies (e.g., elevated fear response and lower threshold for physiological responsiveness to stressors) who are exposed to certain environmental conditions will develop PTSD and chronic pain concurrently (Asmundson et al., 2002; Brennstuhl et al., 2015). Individuals with psychological vulnerability who suffer a physical injury will develop chronic pain. In contrast, individuals with psychological vulnerability who experience a life-threatening traumatic event will develop PTSD. Thus, an individual with a psychological vulnerability will develop chronic pain and PTSD if the individual is exposed to an event that (1) causes physical injury that elicits pain and (2) is traumatic and life-threatening (Asmundson et al., 2002).

The directionality of PTSD and chronic pain is still being investigated, but there is a mounting evidence that PTSD, especially combat-related PTSD in veterans, is a risk factor for chronic pain (Brennstuhl et al., 2015; Edwards et al., 2016). Also, the mutual maintenance and shared vulnerability model of PTSD and chronic pain implicate certain psychological processes that may be intervention targets. Targeting these maladaptive processes may concurrently reduce symptoms and disability associated with both disorders, regardless of directionality. Indeed, Shipherd et al. (2007) demonstrated that pain was reduced by 50% after treatment for PTSD without ever being directly targeted by the intervention. Prior work suggests that treatment of PTSD may lead to more positive coping strategies, reduced avoidant behaviors, and better emotion regulation, all of which are also effective treatment strategies for chronic pain (Shipherd et al., 2007; Turk et al., 2016).

Social Risk Factors.

Solicitous Social Responses. Although pain is ultimately a private and subjective experience, pain perception may influence and may be influenced by the behavior of others (Gatchel et al., 2007; Hadjistavropoulos et al., 2011; Turk et al., 2016). Friends, family, co-workers, or acquaintances may react to an individual's outward expressions of pain, or pain behaviors (e.g., grimacing or verbalization) by offering social support (Hadjistavropoulos et al., 2011; Turk et al., 2016). Certain types of social support may be detrimental to chronic pain depending on the qualities of support offered (Turk et al., 2016).

Solicitous social responses to pain are actions that discourage patients from performing daily functions and task, such as taking over responsibilities and encouraging patients to rest (Edwards et al., 2016; Jensen, Moore, Bockow, Ehde, & Engel, 2011; Turk et al., 2016). Although caregivers may intend this as a kind and sympathetic gesture toward someone living with chronic pain, solicitous responses may promote avoidance of certain activities that elicit pain and, as a consequence, learning to adapt or cope. Indeed, patients with family members or spouse with solicitous pain responses reported higher pain intensity and lower levels of functioning (Jensen et al., 2011; McGeary et al., 2016; Mohammadi, Dehghani, Sanderman, & Hagedoorn, 2017).

Negative spousal reactions may also be associated with emotional disturbances and affect the adjustment of chronic pain patients (Burns et al., 2013; McGeary et al., 2016). Patient perception of spouse criticism and hostility has been associated with increased pain intensity at the time of the perceived criticism and even three hours later (Burns et al., 2013). In a sample of active duty military with chronic musculoskeletal pain, perceived negative responses from a significant other were associated with work-related fear avoidance, increased pain interference, increased affective distress, and worse physical health-related quality of life (McGeary et al., 2016).

Job Stressors. Early investigation into the impact of psychosocial work factors on pain lacked construct specificity, or focused primarily on one theoretical model, thereby making it more difficult to design and implement effective interventions (Christensen & Knardahl, 2012; Linton, 2001). More recent investigations have investigated relationships between pain and psychosocial work factors in greater detail and with a diverse set of psychosocial work constructs (Christensen & Knardahl, 2014; Eatough, Way, & Chang, 2012; Herr et al., 2015).

There is some evidence that job characteristics and experiences can be risk factors for increased pain. For example, studies of role conflict have found that it is a significant risk factor for neck pain (Christensen & Knardahl, 2010, 2014). In addition, workplace bullying has been implicated in the development of chronic pain disorders (Kivimaki et al., 2004). Other research has demonstrated that low job control and high role conflict are associated with higher levels of job strain and, in turn, higher levels of pain (Eatough et al., 2012). These results are suggestive of a link between psychosocial work stressors and musculoskeletal pain.

Psychological Protective Factors. Psychosocial risk factors for pain have historically received the maximum attention in pain research. However, there has been an increase in research investigating psychosocial factors that may protect against chronic pain (Edwards et al., 2016; Finan & Garland, 2015; Gatchel et al., 2007; Goodin et al., 2013). Such protective factors may promote adaptive psychological functioning and buffer against external psychosocial stressors and biological vulnerabilities.

Optimism. Prior work suggests that optimism may buffer against chronic pain and poor pain outcomes (Goodin & Bulls, 2013; Hood, Pulvers, Carrillo, Merchant, & Thomas, 2012; Tracey, 2010). Hood et al. (2012) reported participants with higher levels of optimism and hope had lower pain catastrophizing and reduced pain reports. In addition, Goodin et al. (2013) reported that individuals with high dispositional optimism reported less catastrophizing and less facilitation of experimental pain. A study of experimentally induced optimism and pain reported that optimism protected against pain-induced determinants in task-shifting performance (Boselie, Vancleef, & Peters, 2017). In military populations, optimism and related positive psychological characteristics have been shown also to decrease the likelihood of substance abuse post-deployment (Krasikova, Lester, & Harms, 2015).

Positive Effect. Although negative effect has received considerable attention in pain research, there has been an increased interest in positive effect (Finan & Garland, 2015). Positive effect is associated with reduced pain sensitivity in experimental and clinical settings (Rhudy, 2015; Sibille et al., 2012). In an experimental pain study, participants with a healthy effective style (low negative effect and high positive effect) demonstrated less passive coping strategies (e.g., reduced physical activity and seeking help from others), endorsed lower somatic symptoms, and reduced ischemic pain (i.e., pain elicited by insufficient blood flow) sensitivity (Sibille et al., 2012). Prior work also suggests that individuals with higher positive effect may be more psychologically resilient to emotional disturbances elicited by increased pain, thereby leading to lower dysfunction and better pain outcomes (Zautra & Sturgeon, 2016).

Mindfulness. Cognitive appraisal of pain signals strongly influences pain processing. Exaggerated pain-related fear is associated with enhanced pain facilitation (Goodin et al., 2013). Thus, psychological states which attenuate negative appraisal and pain-related fear may also reduce pain intensity and protect against pain disorders.

Mindfulness can be roughly defined as a state of nonjudgmental awareness whereby individuals are aware and accept internal and external experiences without appraisal or mental elaboration (e.g., magnification and rumination; Grant, 2014; McCracken & Vowles, 2014). Thus, if an individual observes a painful sensation without exaggerated negative appraisal and pain-related fear, then the desire to avoid the pain is reduced, which may in turn reduce pain facilitation. Indeed, experienced meditators showed decreased activation in executive, evaluative, and affective brain networks, such as the prefrontal cortex and amygdala, while control participants did not (Grant, Courtemanche, & Rainville, 2011). In addition, a neuroimaging investigation of experimentally induced pain indicated a short mindfulness training intervention associated with altered neural activity and a significant reduction in pain ratings (Zeidan, Gordon, Merchant, & Goolkasian, 2010). Prior research also suggests that increased mindfulness may decrease pain-related anxiety and in turn improve functional outcomes (McCracken, Gauntlett-Gilbert, & Vowles, 2007).

Social Protective Factors.

Organizational Factors. Christensen and Knardahl (2010) reported that higher levels of the following organizational factors were associated with lower neck pain at baseline: decision control, support from immediate superior, empowering leadership, fair leadership, predictability during the next month, commitment to organization, and social climate. Furthermore, empowering leadership was one of the strongest predictors of neck pain. Participants reporting greater empowering leadership at baseline had lower odds of having neck pain at baseline and at follow-up. A prospective study of back pain reported that greater decision control, empowering leadership, and fair leadership were associated with less back pain (Christensen & Knardahl, 2012). Lastly, prior work reported that greater social support reduced the likelihood of persistent low back pain, and a better social climate at work predicted less neck pain (Christensen & Knardahl, 2014; Melloh et al., 2013).

IMPACT OF CHRONIC PAIN ON EMOTIONAL WELL-BEING

Chronic pain can be a devastating illness which spills over into multiple life domains. The persistent, unpleasant, and disruptive nature of chronic pain can be overwhelming and distressing (Banks & Kerns, 1996; Eccleston & Crombez, 1999). It may lead to disengagement from enjoyable activities and loss of meaningful social roles (Banks & Kerns, 1996; Gatchel et al., 2007; Harris, Morley, & Barton, 2003). The burden of chronic pain may be particularly devastating to young and previously active veterans with greater family responsibilities than older individuals (Matthias, Miech, Myers, Sargent, & Bair, 2014). Consequentially, reduced engagement and increased dysfunction due to pain may increase psychological distress (Banks & Kerns, 1996; Ojala et al., 2015). As a result, patients with chronic pain often suffer significant detriments in emotional well-being (Dersh, 2002; Gatchel et al., 2007).

Prior work suggests that over 40% of chronic pain patients have depression (Bair et al., 2003; Banks & Kerns, 1996; Dersh, 2002; Gatchel et al., 2007; Turk et al., 2016). In addition, chronic pain may elicit anger, anxiety, and hopelessness (Dersh, 2002; Gatchel et al., 2007; Matthias et al., 2014; Trost, Vangronsveld, Linton, Quartana, & Sullivan, 2012). Chronic pain may also influence behavioral health outcomes, such as increased risk of suicide, sleep impairment, and opioid misuse (Hooten, 2016; Ilgen et al., 2013; Seal et al., 2012; Turk et al., 2016). Thus, chronic pain has a significant impact on well-being and may indirectly impact work outcomes, such as presenteeism and absenteeism.

ORGANIZATIONAL OUTCOMES

Absenteeism

The relationship between pain and absenteeism is clear. Prior work has reported that osteoarthritis (OA) patients were absent three times as often versus controls and were significantly more likely to work part-time (Ricci et al., 2005). In a sample of Spanish workers, those reporting chronic pain had a significantly greater chance and period of absenteeism compared to individuals without pain (Mesas et al., 2014). Furthermore, younger workers had significantly higher incidence and duration of absenteeism due to chronic lower back or neck pain. A systematic review has reported that chronic pain had a consistent association with increased rates of pain and greater pain intensity was associated with greater sickness absenteeism (Patel et al., 2012).

There also appears to be a strong relationship between pain, psychological functioning, and absenteeism. Prior research has reported that chronic pain patients with depression were 2.9 times more likely to be absent than non-depressed individuals (Munce, Stansfeld, Blackmore, & Stewart, 2007). There may also be a synergistic relationship between psychological dysfunction and pain (Saastamoinen, Leino-Arjas, Rahkonen, & Lahelma, 2016). A recent study has found that emotional exhaustion and pain were independently associated with increased absenteeism (Saastamoinen et al., 2016). However, co-occurring pain and emotional exhaustion were associated with absenteeism in excess of the additive risk of each condition. Both pain and emotional exhaustion are associated with reduced coping resources, so the two conditions may compound and perpetuate each other. In addition, chronic pain patients with depression may use absenteeism as a coping strategy (Munce et al., 2007).

Disability Discharge

For the military, chronic pain not only limits function and increases absenteeism but it can also lead to medical disability and discharge, thereby creating greater turnover (Feuerstein, Berkowitz, & Peck, 1997; Gubata, Piccirillo, Packnett, & Cowan, 2013; Lincoln, Smith, Amoroso, & Bell, 2002). Indeed, musculoskeletal conditions are by far the most common reasons for disability discharge, and this trend is increasing at an alarming rate (Bell, Schwartz, Harford, Hollander, & Amoroso, 2008; Feuerstein et al., 1997; Gubata et al., 2013; Lincoln et al., 2002). Prior research suggests that MSDs are responsible for over 50% of disability discharge, and soldiers hospitalized for a MSD had a five-year cumulative risk of 13.2% disability discharge (Lincoln et al., 2002). In addition, the prevalence of musculoskeletal-related disability increased from 70 per 100,000 in 1985 to 950 per 100,000 in 2005 (Bell et al., 2008). Unlike psychiatric conditions, which are more common in previously deployed service members, prior research suggests that musculoskeletal conditions occur at similar rates in both deployed and non-deployed populations, thereby adding to the organizational burden even during peacetime or limited military engagement (Gubata et al., 2013). In addition, these disorders are not limited to older service members at the end of their career. Lincoln et al. (2002) reported that disability discharge rates due to musculoskeletal conditions in the Army were highest among 21–34-year olds, those with a year or less of service, and lower pay grades. In addition, disability discharge was higher among soldiers reporting high job stress and lower job satisfaction.

Presenteeism

Although absenteeism represents a significant source of lost productivity associated with pain, this may only represent a small proportion of the actual cost. Many workers may still attend work despite experiencing pain (Agaliotis et al., 2013; Goetzel et al., 2004). However, this may result in detriments to job performance, such as reduced output, errors, and failure to meet production standards. This is known as presenteeism (Schultz, Chen, & Edington, 2009).

Prior work found presenteeism costs dwarfed other costs related to chronic illnesses (Goetzel et al., 2004). In addition, the impact of presenteeism on total health costs is likely a function of disease characteristics as some conditions are associated with more consistent work task interference, such as musculoskeletal pain (Goetzel et al., 2004; Schultz et al., 2009). Goetzel et al. (2004) found chronic pain conditions, compared to other health conditions, also had the greatest ratio of cost due to presenteeism versus all overall costs (i.e., presenteeism plus absenteeism, prescription, outpatient care, and hospitalization). By comparison, heart disease is likely more associated with medical costs and absenteeism, such as surgery and hospitalization, rather than presenteeism. Studies investigating pain interference specifically support these assertions. Patients with arthritis lost twice as much productive time compared to individuals without arthritis (Ricci et al., 2005). Agaliotis et al. (2013) found 80% of patients with chronic knee pain reported some reduction in work productivity, particularly in occupations with greater physical demands. Pohling et al. (2016) devised a study to investigate the relationship between psychosocial work stressors, musculoskeletal complaints, and productivity losses. They reported that higher rates of musculoskeletal complaints were associated with higher productivity losses. Furthermore, they found evidence for the mediating role of musculoskeletal complaints on the relationship between work-related factors and presenteeism. A low-risk work condition in the area of work life (e.g., manageable workload, control, reward, and values) was associated with fewer musculoskeletal complaints, which in turn was associated with lower productivity loss due to health-related conditions.

Two population-based studies estimated the impact of chronic pain in Australia (Blyth et al., 2003; Leeuwen et al., 2006). Blyth et al. (2003) found 28.6% of chronic pain patients reported that their work was restricted by pain, 68% of participants reported working with pain, and 60% of males and 54% of females reported some pain interference with work effectiveness. When the effect of working with pain was included, lost productivity (absenteeism plus reduced on-the-job productivity) was more than three times greater. Interestingly, they found patients with a legal claim (e.g., worker's compensation or accident compensation) not only had greater pain complaints and dysfunction but also took narcotic pain medication at a rate three times higher than individuals without legal claims (12.5% vs 34.7%).

A few recent studies have attempted to understand the impact of pain on specific organizational outcomes apart from general measures of presenteeism (Byrne & Hochwarter, 2006; Christian et al., 2015; Ferris et al., 2009). Christian et al. (2015) investigated the relationship between pain and discretionary behaviors at work. Their findings suggest that greater pain is associated with greater avoidance behaviors and lower promotive extra-role behaviors. They also found association between pain and resource depletion and job engagement. Days spent working with pain (83.8 days in six months) was much greater days than lost work days (4.5 days). Byrne and Hochwarter (2006) investigated the relationship between pain, perceived organizational support (POS), and job performance outcomes (i.e., effectiveness, work intensity, citizenship behaviors, and task performance). When POS was low, high levels of chronic pain were associated with low performance, low perceived citizenship, and low perceived effectiveness. However, when POS was average or high, this effect was attenuated. Ferris et al. (2009) investigated the impact of pain interference at work, or job-limiting pain (JLP) on organizational outcomes. JLP significantly predicted job satisfaction and citizenship behavior. Furthermore, they found that as pain increased, job satisfaction decreased in individuals with low political skill. Also, individuals with high JLP and low political skill had lower citizenship behavior.

PAIN, OPIOIDS, AND OVERDOSE

Few issues in mental health have attracted more public attention than opioid abuse, and rightly so (Katz, 2017). To say it's an epidemic seems too cautious. Drug overdose in the United States was responsible for 52,404 deaths in 2015, the most ever recorded (Rudd, Seth, David, & Scholl, 2016). The dramatic increase in overall drug overdose deaths is associated with a concomitant rise in the number of patients prescribed opioid medication for pain, deaths attributed to POs, and the transition of PO users to heroin (Banerjee et al., 2016; Hedegaard, Warner, & Miniño, 2017; Rudd et al., 2016). Opioids were involved in 33,091 of the overdose deaths (63.1%) in 2015. From 2000 to 2015, the rate of opioid overdose tripled, rising at an average of 5% annually (Hedegaard et al., 2017; Rudd et al., 2016). Furthermore, approximately 165,000 persons died from an overdose related to POs between 1999 and 2014 (Dowell, Haegerich, & Chou, 2016). Although the rate of PO overdose has shown some improvement in recent years, the rate of heroin overdose increased three-fold from 2010 to 2015 (Banerjee et al., 2016; Hedegaard et al., 2017; Rudd et al., 2016).

The military and veterans have not been spared from this epidemic. If anything, this crisis has been more harmful to this population (Bray, Olmsted, & Williams, 2012; Bohnert, Ilgen, Galea, McCarthy, & Blow, 2011). Prior work suggests that overdose deaths related to POs in the military may be twice the deaths in civilian population (Bohnert et al., 2011). Illicit drug use in the military steadily declined from 27.6% in 1980 to 3.4% in 2002, largely due to implementation of drug testing (Bray et al., 2010, 2012). However, illicit drug use increased to 5% in 2002 and 12% in 2008 (Bray et al., 2012). The reason for this dramatic increase appears to be due to increase in prescription drug misuse, particularly POM. In fact, when prescription drugs were excluded, rates of any illicit drug use stayed at approximately 2% from 2002 to 2008. In contrast, POM increased from 2% to 11% during the same period. Further, during this period there were very low rates of drug use across most categories except for pain relievers, which showed a marked increase from 1% in 2002 to 10% in 2008. Notably, heavy alcohol use increased from 1988 (15%) to 2008 (20%), which is in contrast with the relatively stable rate in the previous 10 years (Bray et al., 2010). This may signify the use of intoxicating substances to cope with stressors and other mental health problems. Recent trends in POM suggest that service members and veterans may be using opioids in a similar fashion.

A recent survey from one Army infantry brigade obtained three months after return from Afghanistan corroborates some of the prior findings (Toblin, Quartana, Riviere, Walper, & Hoge, 2014). Of the entire cohort, 15.1% reported past-month opioid use. Among soldiers prescribed opioids, 5.6% reported no past-month pain, 38.5 % reported mild pain, 37.7% reported moderate pain, and 18.2% reported severe pain. In addition, 44.0% of soldiers reported chronic pain and 51.2% reported moderate to severe pain. These two findings are surprising, given the relatively young age of the sample.

Prior research suggests that there is a strong relationship between POM, psychological distress, and drug availability. Bray et al. (2012) found that the strongest predictors of prescription pain medication misuse were positive PTSD screening, engaging in heavy drinking, and having a prescription for pain medication. Prior work also found individuals who reported having been prescribed a prescription pain reliever within the last month were twice more likely to misuse a pain reliever than individuals having been prescribed a pain reliever during the past year (Jeffery, Babeu, Nelson, Kloc, & Klette, 2013). In addition, patients who received at least a 211-day supply of POs had a greater risk for opioid abuse or dependence than those with a 91–120-day supply (Edlund, Steffick, Hudson, Harris, & Sullivan, 2007). This may suggest a "dose–response" relationship between number of days for which opioids are prescribed and risk of POM. Furthermore, prior research noted that symptoms of distress had a widespread association with prescription medication misuse, which suggests service members may be self-medicating to reduce distress and control mental health symptoms instead of utilizing legitimate health services and/or nonpharmacological treatments, such as counseling and relaxation techniques (Jeffery et al., 2013).Thus, the increased availability of POs obtained through legitimate prescriptions for pain medications from a doctor may increase the risk of POM, especially in patients on long-term opioid therapy who experience high psychological distress (Bray et al., 2012; Jeffery et al., 2013).

POs are the primary therapy for acute and chronic pain. Although POs are moderately effective in treating acute pain, the efficacy of long-term opioid therapy has not been demonstrated (Kissin, 2013; Manchikanti, Fellows, Ailinani, & Pampati, 2010). Surprisingly, Kissin (2013) was unable to find a single randomized controlled trial (RCT) study of POs lasting longer than six months published in a top-ranked medical journal. Considering the standard of evidence-based medicine and the ubiquity of long-term opioid therapy, the lack of a single long-term RCT is astounding and troubling.

The harm associated with exposure to opioid therapy, on the other hand, is well established (Sullivan & Howe, 2013). Interviews with inner-city veterans in New York revealed that most veterans did not use POs prior to military service, and PO use was often initiated during deployment (Golub & Bennett, 2013). Most veterans who reported POM during deployment also misused opioids after separating from the military. Furthermore, some veterans who used opioids during deployment as prescribed started misusing opioids after separation.

The relationship between psychological dysfunction and POM may be bidirectional (Scherrer et al., 2016). Scherrer et al. (2016) used a three-wave prospective cohort study to investigate whether opioid use was associated with depression in a sample of chronic low back pain patients. Baseline depression was significantly associated with Morphine Equivalent Dose (MED). During follow-up, the probability of having depression was significantly greater when subjects were taking more than a 50-mg MED compared to taking no opioids, and developing depression was associated with a more than two-fold increased chance of increasing rather than decreasing MED.

THE ROLE OF ORGANIZATIONS IN COMBATING PAIN

Pain is a complex biopsychosocial process, and managing it requires an equally interdisciplinary approach (Gatchel, McGeary, McGeary, & Lippe, 2014). It is now clear that biomedical treatments for chronic pain, such as POs and/or surgery, are insufficient and potentially dangerous (Chan & Peng, 2011; Gatchel et al., 2014; Kissin, 2013; Loeser, 2012; Turk et al., 2016). When referencing decades of treating patients at pain clinics, Loeser (2012, p. 2) bluntly stated, "It did not enter our minds that there could be significant numbers of chronic pain patients who were successfully managed on opioids, because if there were any, we almost never saw them." Considered within the context of the 20-year opioid epidemic, this observation is gut-wrenching: Despite little if any treatment efficacy and in the presence of overwhelming risks, millions of patients were nonetheless prescribed opioids, and as a result hundreds of thousands lost their lives. It seems that the call to prevent and manage pain using psychosocial approaches has never been louder.

Many individuals and organizations see pain as a biomedical problem which can only be treated in health care settings (Kristman et al., 2016). However, given the influence of workplace factors on employee's health, the workplace also plays a significant role in prevention and treatment of pain (Blyth, Macfarlane, & Nicholas, 2007; Kristman et al., 2016; Shaw, Campbell, Nelson, Main, & Linton, 2013). This may be especially true of organizations with significant occupational risk factors for pain (e.g., high stress and high injury rate), such as the military. In addition, prior work suggests that unaddressed occupational risk factors may hinder clinical pain treatment (Shaw et al., 2013). Thus, employers may need to communicate and collaborate with patients and clinicians to create a plan conducive to the worker's recovery (Kristman et al., 2016; Shaw et al., 2013). This may entail modifications to the work environment or schedule. However, intervening before the condition of worker deteriorates to this point is preferred. Once pain becomes chronic, it is difficult to treat, and complete amelioration is improbable (Gatchel, 2004; Gatchel et al., 2014; Jensen & Turk, 2014; Turk, Wilson, & Cahana, 2011). The goal of most chronic pain treatments is to manage and cope with chronic pain, not cure it.

Most organizations are limited in their capacity to aid treatment efforts. However, they may be positioned to facilitate pain-prevention efforts. As we have emphasized thus far, emotional processes are intrinsic to pain perception (Edwards et al., 2016; Gatchel et al., 2007). Furthermore, emotional distress is associated with greater pain and poorer outcomes (Chou & Shekelle, 2010; Edwards et al., 2016; Gatchel et al., 2007). As such, interventions which reduce emotional distress and enhance well-being may play a significant role in preventing pain disorders (Eatough et al., 2012; Pohling et al., 2016). One method to combat emotional distress is by reducing job stressors and/or increasing psychosocial resources (Tetrick & Winslow, 2015).

Prior research identified organizational factors which may increase the risk of pain conditions. These include low control, high quantitative demand, low social support, high role conflict, and low supervisor support (Christensen & Knardahl, 2012, 2014; Herr et al., 2015; Melloh et al., 2013). Interventions which target these risk factors may reduce the incidence or progression of pain disorders. Organizations may also mitigate some job performance deficits related to pain by increasing job resources. Prior findings suggest that increasing POS, political skill, job engagement, and job satisfaction may protect against decrease in performance associated with pain disorders (Byrne & Hochwarter, 2006; Christian et al., 2015; Ferris et al., 2009).

In addition to enhancing job resources, organizations may also protect against pain disorders by enhancing personal resources (e.g., psychological resiliency). Although workplace risk factors may increase vulnerability to pain, the workplace may also be a vehicle for interventions which increase resiliency to pain and other physical and mental health conditions (Glomb, Duffy, Bono, & Yang, 2011; Harms et al., 2013; Tetrick & Winslow, 2015). Many workplace interventions have been developed to promote resiliency to stressors, particularly in the military (Glomb et al., 2011; Harms et al., 2013; Johnson et al., 2014; Tetrick & Winslow, 2015; Vanhove, Herian, Perez, Harms, & Lester, 2016). In recent years, there has been a surge in research and implementation of mindfulness-based workplace interventions to cope with occupational stress (Glomb et al., 2011; Roeser et al., 2013; Tetrick & Winslow, 2015).

Mindfulness training teaches practitioners to reduce aversive thoughts, emotions, and behaviors by developing an attitude of open and nonjudgmental awareness toward everyday experiences (Garland, Hanley, Baker, & Howard, 2017; Glomb et al., 2011; Grant, 2014; Kabat-Zinn & Hanh, 2009). Mindfulness may protect against maladaptive chronic stress by reducing stress reactivity and enhancing top-down self-regulation (Garland et al., 2017). Similarly, Glomb et al. (2011) suggest that mindfulness exerts its positive influence on well-being by decoupling the self from thoughts, emotions, events, and experiences (i.e., decentering); reducing automatic and reactive mental process that constrain thinking; and increasing awareness and regulation of physiological systems. Prior work suggests that these core processes may increase active coping, counteract learned helplessness, increase perceived control, reduce rumination, and increase reward responsiveness (Garland et al., 2017; Glomb et al., 2011).

A prior study investigated the impact of a 20-hour mindfulness intervention, Mindfulness-Based Mind Fitness Training (MMFT), with a non-clinical sample of U.S. Marines prior to pre-deployment training (Johnson et al., 2014). Following a stressful combat training task, Marines who underwent the mindfulness training intervention demonstrated better heart rate and breathing recovery compared to controls. In addition, the MMFT group showed changes in brain activation associated with cognitive control, emotion-regulation, reward-monitoring, and interoception. Pre-deployment stress is also associated with decrease in work memory capacity and positive effect and increase in negative effect (Jha, Stanley, Kiyonaga, Wong, & Gelfand, 2010). However, prior findings suggest a mindfulness-based intervention may protect against these deficits. Also, a recent investigation reported that acceptance-coping strategies were more consistent and effective in dealing with stressors in basic military training than active coping strategies (Britt, Crane, Hodson, & Adler, 2016). Furthermore, the authors suggested mindfulness training, given its emphasis on accepting rather than attempting to control experiences, may be especially effective in environments where job control is limited, such as military settings. Lastly, an experimental investigation utilizing repeated psychosocial stress reported that a mindfulness-based intervention attenuated anticipatory sensitization of the cortisol response in individuals with high initial reactivity (Turan et al., 2015). Collectively, these results suggest that mindfulness training may increase resiliency and stress-coping in healthy service members prior to stressful events, thereby preventing maladaptive psychological and physiological reactions.

Roeser et al. (2013) investigated the effects of mindfulness training on occupational stress and burnout in teachers at two separate test sites (United States and Canada) using a randomized, waitlist-control field trial. The intervention showed a significant positive impact on occupational well-being. Teachers who underwent mindfulness training had significant increase in mindfulness and self-compassion. Furthermore, the training group showed significant decreases in occupational stress and burnout, anxiety symptoms, and depression symptoms and a significant increase in attention/working memory capacity. In addition, mediation analyses suggesting decrease in stress, burnout, anxiety, and depression following the intervention were accounted for by increase in mindfulness and self-compassion. The intervention was not associated with improvements in physiological measures (blood pressure, cortisol, or heart rate), which may be due to methodological limitations.

Mindfulness-based interventions may also protect against POM in patients with comorbid chronic pain and POM (Garland et al., 2014). A prior investigation found that participants in a mindfulness training intervention for chronic pain and POM had greater reduction in pain severity and pain-related dysfunction compared to a traditional support group, and the mindfulness group had significant reductions in desire for opioid medication and opioid use disorder. Furthermore, increase in non-reactivity and reinterpretation of pain sensations mediated the relationship between the mindfulness intervention and pain reduction.

FUTURE DIRECTIONS AND CONCLUSION

Elucidating the complex and dynamic relationship between work, stress, and pain requires integration of literature from public health, occupational health psychology, industrial–organizational psychology, clinical psychology, organizational behavior, and organizational design (Tetrick & Winslow, 2015). Furthermore, designing interventions to mitigate the impact of pain on organizations would strongly benefit from a comprehensive model which incorporates these various domains. In addition, some methodological weaknesses could be improved upon in the future investigations of pain and disability (Kristman et al., 2016). These include a lack of random sample of workplaces for study (i.e., selection bias), over-reliance on large workplaces, over-reliance on worker self-report, lack of organizational perspective, and lack of investigation into etiologic mechanisms. More research is needed to understand in better way boundary conditions and the processes underlying the relationship between organizational factors and pain. Collecting a wide array of biological markers, including medical imaging, and using more rigorous pain measures may also increase the quality of findings. While most current research focuses on individual-level perspectives, the future research should strive to include whole workforce perspective, supervisor attitudes, and organizational practices and procedures.

Advances in pain treatment and prevention have been made, but the progress is slow, and the burden of an aging society continues to grow. Few of any organizations are more vulnerable to the consequences of pain and disability than the military. Pain clearly undermines force readiness by diminishing performance, escalating health care costs, and increasing attrition. Ineffective treatments for chronic pain contribute to an overreliance on PO therapy and the relentless and devastating opioid epidemic in the United States and elsewhere, while the high comorbidity of pain and PTSD leave military service members and veterans increasingly vulnerable. Furthermore, coping with pain and psychiatric illness creates additional challenges for veterans transitioning into the civilian workforce. Thus, we believe there is a palpable urgency for organizational researchers to familiarize themselves with the dynamics of pain and its implications for the workforce. Although clinical pain research is well developed, there needs to be a concerted effort to integrate pain with organizational outcomes, so the consequences of a pain epidemic can no longer be ignored.

REFERENCES

Adler, D. A., McLaughlin, T. J., Rogers, W. H., Chang, H., Lapitsky, L., & Lerner, D. (2006). Job performance deficits due to depression. *American Journal of Psychiatry*, *163*(9), 1569–1576.

Agaliotis, M., Fransen, M., Bridgett, L., Nairn, L., Votrubec, M., Jan, S., ... Mackey, M. (2013). Risk factors associated with reduced work productivity among people with chronic knee pain. *Osteoarthritis and Cartilage*, *21*(9), 1160–1169.

Anderson, M. K., Grier, T., Canham-Chervak, M., Bushman, T. T., & Jones, B. H. (2015). Occupation and other risk factors for injury among enlisted U.S. Army Soldiers. *Public Health*, *129*(5), 531–538. doi:10.1016/j.puhe.2015.02.003

Asmundson, G. J., Coons, M. J., Taylor, S., & Katz, J. (2002). PTSD and the experience of pain: Research and clinical implications of shared vulnerability and mutual maintenance models. *The Canadian Journal of Psychiatry*, *47*(10), 930–937.

Bair, M. J., Robinson, R. L., Katon, W., & Kroenke, K. (2003). Depression and pain comorbidity: A literature review. *Archives of Internal Medicine*, *163*(20), 2433–2445.

Banerjee, G., Edelman, E. J., Barry, D. T., Becker, W. C., Cerdá, M., Crystal, S., ... Kerns, R. D. (2016). Non-medical use of prescription opioids is associated with heroin initiation among US veterans: A prospective cohort study. *Addiction*, *111*(11), 2021–2031.

Banks, S. M., & Kerns, R. D. (1996). Explaining high rates of depression in chronic pain: A diathesis-stress framework. *Psychological Bulletin*, *119*(1), 95.

Bartynski, W. S. (2009). Clinical, anatomic, and imaging correlation in spine-related pain: The essential elements. *Techniques in Vascular and Interventional Radiology*, *12*(1), 2–10.

Beattie, P. F., Meyers, S. P., Stratford, P., Millard, R. W., & Hollenberg, G. M. (2000). Associations between patient report of symptoms and anatomic impairment visible on lumbar magnetic resonance imaging. *Spine*, *25*(7), 819–828.

Beecher, H. K. (1946). Pain in men wounded in battle. *Annals of Surgery*, *123*(1), 96.

Bell, N. S., Schwartz, C. E., Harford, T., Hollander, I. E., & Amoroso, P. J. (2008). The changing profile of disability in the US Army: 1981–2005. *Disability and Health Journal*, *1*(1), 14–24.

Bernard, B. P. (1997). *Musculoskeletal disorders an workplace factors: A critical review of epidemiologic evidence for work-related musculoskeletal disorders of the neck, upper extremity, and low back.* Washington, DC: U.S. Department of Health and Human Services, Public Health Service, Centers for Disease Control, and National Institute of Occupational Safety and Health.

Besson, J. (1999). The neurobiology of pain. *The Lancet*, *353*(9164), 1610–1615.

Blyth, F. M., Macfarlane, G. J., & Nicholas, M. K. (2007). The contribution of psychosocial factors to the development of chronic pain: The key to better outcomes for patients? *PAIN*, *129*(1–2), 8–11. doi:10.1016/j.pain.2007.03.009

Blyth, F. M., March, L. M., Nicholas, M. K., & Cousins, M. J. (2003). Chronic pain, work performance and litigation. *PAIN*, *103*(1–2), 41–47. doi:10.1016/S0304-3959(02)00380-9

Bohnert, A. S., Ilgen, M. A., Galea, S., McCarthy, J. F., & Blow, F. C. (2011). Accidental poisoning mortality among patients in the Department of Veterans Affairs Health System. *Med Care*, *49*(4), 393–396. doi:10.1097/MLR.0b013e318202aa27

Bosco, M. A., Gallinati, J. L., & Clark, M. E. (2013). Conceptualizing and treating comorbid chronic pain and PTSD. *Pain Research and Treatment*, *2013*, 174728. doi:10.1155/2013/174728

Boselie, J. J., Vancleef, L. M., & Peters, M. L. (2017). Increasing optimism protects against pain-induced impairment in task-shifting performance. *The Journal of Pain*, *18*(4), 446–455.

Bray, R. M., Olmsted, K. R., & Williams, J. (2012). Misuse of prescription pain medications in US active duty service members. *Pain Syndromes: From Recruitment to Returning Troops*, *91*, 3–16. doi:10.3233/978-1-60750-986-8-3

Bray, R. M., Pemberton, M. R., Lane, M. E., Hourani, L. L., Mattiko, M. J., & Babeu, L. A. (2010). Substance use and mental health trends among U.S. military active duty personnel: Key findings from the 2008 DoD health behavior survey. *Military Medicine*, *175*(6), 390–399. doi:10.7205/milmed-d-09-00132

Brennstuhl, M. J., Tarquinio, C., & Montel, S. (2015). Chronic pain and PTSD: Evolving views on their comorbidity. *Perspectives in Psychiatric Care*, *51*(4), 295–304.

Britt, T. W., Crane, M., Hodson, S. E., & Adler, A. B. (2016). Effective and ineffective coping strategies in a low-autonomy work environment. *Journal of Occupational Health Psychology*, *21*(2), 154–168. doi:10.1037/a0039898

Burns, J. W., Peterson, K. M., Smith, D. A., Keefe, F. J., Porter, L. S., Schuster, E., & Kinner, E. (2013). Temporal associations between spouse criticism/hostility and pain among patients with chronic pain: A within-couple daily diary study. *PAIN*, *154*(12), 2715–2721.

Bushnell, M.C., Ceko, M., & Low, L.A. (2013). Cognitive and emotional control of pain and its disruption in chronic pain. *Nature Reviews Neuroscience*, *14*, 502–511.

Byrne, Z. S., & Hochwarter, W. A. (2006). I get by with a little help from my friends: The interaction of chronic pain and organizational support on performance. *Journal of Occupational Health Psychology*, *11*(3), 215.

Casey, C. Y., Greenberg, M. A., Nicassio, P. M., Harpin, R. E., & Hubbard, D. (2008). Transition from acute to chronic pain and disability: A model including cognitive, affective, and trauma factors. *PAIN*, *134*(1), 69–79.

Chan, C.-W., & Peng, P. (2011). Failed back surgery syndrome. *Pain Medicine*, *12*(4), 577–606.

Chou, R., & Shekelle, P. (2010). Will this patient develop persistent disabling low back pain? *JAMA*, *303*(13), 1295–1302.

Christensen, J. O., & Knardahl, S. (2010). Work and neck pain: A prospective study of psychological, social, and mechanical risk factors. *PAIN*, *151*(1), 162–173. doi:10.1016/j.pain.2010.07.001

Christensen, J. O., & Knardahl, S. (2012). Work and back pain: A prospective study of psychological, social and mechanical predictors of back pain severity. *European Journal of Pain*, *16*(6), 921–933. doi:10.1002/j.1532-2149.2011.00091.x

Christensen, J. O., & Knardahl, S. (2014). Time-course of occupational psychological and social factors as predictors of new-onset and persistent neck pain: A three-wave prospective study over 4years. *PAIN*, *155*(7), 1262–1271.

Christian, M. S., Eisenkraft, N., & Kapadia, C. (2015). Dynamic associations among somatic complaints, human energy, and discretionary behaviors: Experiences with pain fluctuations at work. *Administrative Science Quarterly*, *60*(1), 66–102.

Clark, M. E., Walker, R. L., Gironda, R. J., & Scholten, J. D. (2009). Comparison of pain and emotional symptoms in soldiers with polytrauma: Unique aspects of blast exposure. *Pain Medicine*, *10*(3), 447–455.

Coenen, P., Kingma, I., Boot, C., Bongers, P., & van Dieën, J. (2014). Cumulative mechanical low-back load at work is a determinant of low-back pain. *Occupational and Environmental Medicine*, *71*(5), 332–337.

Cohen, S. P., Griffith, S., Larkin, T. M., Villena, F., & Larkin, R. (2005). Presentation, diagnoses, mechanisms of injury, and treatment of soldiers injured in operation Iraqi Freedom: An epidemiological study conducted at two military pain management centers. *Anesthesia & Analgesia*, *101*(4), 1098. doi:10.1213/01.ane.0000169332.45209.cf

Crombez, G., Van Damme, S., & Eccleston, C. (2005). Hypervigilance to pain: An experimental and clinical analysis. *PAIN*, *116*(1–2), 4–7.

Crombez, G., Vlaeyen, J. W., Heuts, P. H., & Lysens, R. (1999). Pain-related fear is more disabling than pain itself: Evidence on the role of pain-related fear in chronic back pain disability. *PAIN*, *80*(1), 329–339.

da Costa, B. R., & Vieira, E. R. (2010). Risk factors for work-related musculoskeletal disorders: A systematic review of recent longitudinal studies. *American Journal of Industrial Medicine*, *53*(3), 285–323.

Dersh, J. (2002). Chronic pain and psychopathology: Research findings and theoretical considerations. *Psychosomatic Medicine*, *64*(5), 773–786. doi:10.1097/01.psy.0000024232.11538.54

Dowell, D., Haegerich, T. M., & Chou, R. (2016). CDC guideline for prescribing opioids for chronic pain – United States, 2016. *JAMA*, *315*(15), 1624–1645. doi:10.1001/jama.2016.1464

Eatough, E. M., Way, J. D., & Chang, C.-H. (2012). Understanding the link between psychosocial work stressors and work-related musculoskeletal complaints. *Applied Ergonomics*, *43*(3), 554–563.

Eccleston, C., & Crombez, G. (1999). Pain demands attention: A cognitive–affective model of the interruptive function of pain. *Psychological Bulletin*, *125*(3), 356.

Edlund, M. J., Steffick, D., Hudson, T., Harris, K. M., & Sullivan, M. D. (2007). Risk factors for clinically recognized opioid abuse and dependence among veterans using opioids for chronic non-cancer pain. *PAIN*, *129*(3), 355–362. doi:10.1016/j.pain.2007.02.014

Edwards, R. R., Dworkin, R. H., Sullivan, M. D., Turk, D. C., & Wasan, A. D. (2016). The role of psychosocial processes in the development and maintenance of chronic pain. *Journal of Pain*, *17*(9 Suppl), T70–T92. doi:10.1016/j.jpain.2016.01.001

Ferris, G. R., Rogers, L. M., Blass, F. R., & Hochwarter, W. A. (2009). Interaction of job-limiting pain and political skill on job satisfaction and organizational citizenship behavior. *Journal of Managerial Psychology*, *24*(7), 584–608.

Feuerstein, M., Berkowitz, S. M., & Peck, C. A. (1997). Musculoskeletal-related disability in US Army personnel. *Journal of Occupational & Environmental Medicine*, *39*(1), 68–78. doi:10.1097/00043764-199701000-00013

Finan, P. H., & Garland, E. L. (2015). The role of positive affect in pain and its treatment. *The Clinical Journal of Pain*, *31*(2), 177.

Fishbain, D. A., Pulikal, A., Lewis, J. E., & Gao, J. (2017). Chronic pain types differ in their reported prevalence of post-traumatic stress disorder (PTSD) and there is consistent evidence that chronic pain is associated with PTSD: An evidence-based structured systematic review. *Pain Medicine*, *18*, 711–735.

Forde, M. S., Punnett, L., & Wegman, D. H. (2002). Pathomechanisms of work-related musculoskeletal disorders: Conceptual issues. *Ergonomics*, *45*(9), 619–630. doi:10.1080/00140130210153487

Garcia-Larrea, L., & Peyron, R. (2013). Pain matrices and neuropathic pain matrices: A review. *PAIN*, *154*, S29–S43.

Garland, E. L., Hanley, A. W., Baker, A. K., & Howard, M. O. (2017). Biobehavioral mechanisms of mindfulness as a treatment for chronic stress: An RDoC perspective. *Chronic Stress*, *1*, 2470547017711912.

Garland, E. L., Manusov, E. G., Froeliger, B., Kelly, A., Williams, J. M., & Howard, M. O. (2014). Mindfulness-oriented recovery enhancement for chronic pain and prescription opioid misuse: Results from an early-stage randomized controlled trial. *Journal of Consulting* and *Clinical Psychology*, *82*(3), 448–459. doi:10.1037/a0035798

Gaskin, D. J., & Richard, P. (2012). The economic costs of pain in the United States. *The Journal of Pain*, *13*(8), 715–724. doi:10.1016/j.jpain.2012.03.009

Gatchel, R. J. (2004). Musculoskeletal disorders: Primary and secondary interventions. *Journal of Electromyography & Kinesiology*, *14*(1), 161–170. doi:10.1016/j.jelekin.2003.09.007

Gatchel, R. J., McGeary, D. D., McGeary, C. A., & Lippe, B. (2014). Interdisciplinary chronic pain management: Past, present, and future. *American Psychologist*, *69*(2), 119–130. doi:10.1037/a0035514

Gatchel, R. J., Peng, Y. B., Peters, M. L., Fuchs, P. N., & Turk, D. C. (2007). The biopsychosocial approach to chronic pain: Scientific advances and future directions. *Psychological Bulletin*, *133*(4), 581–624. doi:10.1037/0033-2909.133.4.581

Geiling, J., Rosen, J. M., & Edwards, R. D. (2012). Medical costs of war in 2035: Long-term care challenges for veterans of Iraq and Afghanistan. *Military Medicine*, *177*(11), 1235–1244. doi:10.7205/milmed-d-12-00031

Glomb, T. M., Duffy, M. K., Bono, J. E., & Yang, T. (2011). Mindfulness at work. In Aparna, J., Hui, L., & Martocchio, J. J. *Research in personnel and human resources management* (pp. 115–157): Wagon Lane, Bingley: Emerald Group Publishing.

Goetzel, R. Z., Long, S. R., Ozminkowski, R. J., Hawkins, K., Wang, S., & Lynch, W. (2004). Health, absence, disability, and presenteeism cost estimates of certain physical and mental health conditions affecting US employers. *Journal of Occupational and Environmental Medicine*, *46*(4), 398–412.

Golub, A., & Bennett, A. S. (2013). Prescription opioid initiation, correlates, and consequences among a sample of OEF/OIF military personnel. *Substance Use & Misuse*, *48*(10), 811–820.

Goodin, B. R., & Bulls, H. W. (2013). Optimism and the experience of pain: Benefits of seeing the glass as half full. *Current Pain and Headache Reports*, *17*(5), 329.

Goodin, B. R., Glover, T. L., Sotolongo, A., King, C. D., Sibille, K. T., Herbert, M. S., ... Fillingim, R. B. (2013). The association of greater dispositional optimism with less endogenous pain facilitation is indirectly transmitted through lower levels of pain catastrophizing. *The Journal of Pain*, *14*(2), 126–135. doi:http://dx.doi.org/10.1016/j.jpain.2012.10.007

Goulet, J. L., Kerns, R. D., Bair, M., Becker, W. C., Brennan, P., Burgess, D. J., ... Fenton, B. T. (2016). The musculoskeletal diagnosis cohort: Examining pain and pain care among veterans. *PAIN*, *157*(8), 1696–1703.

Grant, J. A. (2014). Meditative analgesia: The current state of the field. *Annals of the New York Academy of Sciences*, *1307*(1), 55–63.

Grant, J. A., Courtemanche, J., & Rainville, P. (2011). A non-elaborative mental stance and decoupling of executive and pain-related cortices predicts low pain sensitivity in Zen meditators. *PAIN*, *152*(1), 150–156.

Gubata, M. E., Piccirillo, A. L., Packnett, E. R., & Cowan, D. N. (2013). Military occupation and deployment: Descriptive epidemiology of active duty US Army men evaluated for a disability discharge. *Military Medicine*, *178*(7), 708–714.

Hadjistavropoulos, T., Craig, K. D., Duck, S., Cano, A., Goubert, L., Jackson, P. L., ... Fitzgerald, T. D. (2011). A biopsychosocial formulation of pain communication. *Psychological Bulletin*, *137*(6), 910–939. doi:10.1037/a0023876

Harms, P. D., Krasikova, D. V., Vanhove, A. J., Herian, M. N., & Lester, P. B. (2013). Stress and emotional well-being in military organizations. In Perrewé, P. L., Rosen, C. C., & Halbesleben, J. R. B. *Research in Occupational Stress and Well-Being* (Vol. 11, pp. 103–132). Bingley, UK: Emerald.

Harris, S., Morley, S., & Barton, S. B. (2003). Role loss and emotional adjustment in chronic pain. *PAIN*, *105*(1), 363–370.

Hauret, K.G., Jones, B.H., Bullock, S.H., Canham-Chervak, M., & Canada, S. (2010). Musculoskeletal injuries description of an under-recognized injury problem among military personnel. *American Journal of Preventative Medicine, 38*, 61–70.

Hedegaard, H., Warner, M., & Miniño, A. M. (2017). Drug overdose deaths in the United States, 1999–2015. *NCHS Data Brief* (273), 1–8.

Herr, R. M., Bosch, J. A., Loerbroks, A., van Vianen, A. E., Jarczok, M. N., Fischer, J. E., & Schmidt, B. (2015). Three job stress models and their relationship with musculoskeletal pain in blue-and white-collar workers. *Journal of Psychosomatic Research*, *79*(5), 340–347.

Higgins, D. M., Kerns, R. D., Brandt, C. A., Haskell, S. G., Bathulapalli, H., Gilliam, W., & Goulet, J. L. (2014). Persistent pain and comorbidity among operation enduring freedom/operation Iraqi freedom/operation new dawn veterans. *Pain Medicine*, *15*(5), 782–790. doi:10.1111/pme.12388

Hollander, I. E., & Bell, N. S. (2010). Physically demanding jobs and occupational injury and disability in the U.S. Army. *Military Medicine*, *175*(10), 705–712. doi:10.7205/MILMED-D-09-00214

Hood, A., Pulvers, K., Carrillo, J., Merchant, G., & Thomas, M. D. (2012). Positive traits linked to less pain through lower pain catastrophizing. *Personality and Individual Differences*, *52*(3), 401–405.

Hooten, W. M. (2016). Chronic pain and mental health disorders: Shared neural mechanisms, epidemiology, and treatment. Paper presented at the Mayo Clinic Proceedings. Rochester, MN.

Ilgen, M. A., Kleinberg, F., Ignacio, R. V., Bohnert, A. S., Valenstein, M., McCarthy, J. F., ... Katz, I. R. (2013). Noncancer pain conditions and risk of suicide. *JAMA Psychiatry*, *70*(7), 692–697.

Institute of Medicine Committee on Advancing Pain Research, C., & Education. (2011). The National Academies Collection: Reports funded by National Institutes of Health. In *Relieving pain in America: A blueprint for transforming prevention, care, education, and research*. Washington, DC: National Academies Press (US), National Academy of Sciences.

Jarvik, J. G., Hollingworth, W., Heagerty, P. J., Haynor, D. R., Boyko, E. J., & Deyo, R. A. (2005). Three-year incidence of low back pain in an initially asymptomatic cohort: Clinical and imaging risk factors. *Spine*, *30*(13), 1541–1548.

Jeffery, D. D., Babeu, L. A., Nelson, L. E., Kloc, M., & Klette, K. (2013). Prescription drug misuse among U.S. active duty military personnel: A secondary analysis of the 2008 DoD survey of health-related behaviors. *Military Medicine*, *178*(2), 180–195. doi:10.7205/MILMED-D-12-00192

Jensen, M. P., Moore, M. R., Bockow, T. B., Ehde, D. M., & Engel, J. M. (2011). Psychosocial factors and adjustment to chronic pain in persons with physical disabilities: A systematic review. *Archives of Physical Medicine and Rehabilitation*, *92*(1), 146–160.

Jensen, M. P., & Turk, D. C. (2014). Contributions of psychology to the understanding and treatment of people with chronic pain: Why it matters to ALL psychologists. *American Psychologist*, *69*(2), 105.

Jha, A. P., Stanley, E. A., Kiyonaga, A., Wong, L., & Gelfand, L. (2010). Examining the protective effects of mindfulness training on working memory capacity and affective experience. *Emotion*, *10*(1), 54.

Johnson, D. C., Thom, N. J., Stanley, E. A., Haase, L., Simmons, A. N., Shih, P.-A. B., ... Paulus, M. P. (2014). Modifying resilience mechanisms in at-risk individuals: A controlled study of mindfulness training in Marines preparing for deployment. *American Journal of Psychiatry*, *171*(8), 844–853.

Jones, B. H., Canham-Chervak, M., Canada, S., Mitchener, T. A., & Moore, S. (2010). Medical surveillance of injuries in the U.S. Military: Descriptive epidemiology and recommendations for improvement. *American Journal of Preventive Medicine*, *38*(1, Supplement), S42–S60. doi:10.1016/j.amepre.2009.10.014

Kabat-Zinn, J., & Hanh, T. N. (2009). *Full catastrophe living: Using the wisdom of your body and mind to face stress, pain, and illness*. Crystal Lake, IL: Delta. New York.

Katz, J. (2017, June 5). Drug deaths in America are rising faster than ever. *New York Times*. Retrieved from https://www.nytimes.com/interactive/2017/06/05/upshot/opioid-epidemic-drug-overdose-deaths-are-rising-faster-than-ever.html?_r=0

Kissin, I. (2013). Long-term opioid treatment of chronic nonmalignant pain: Unproven efficacy and neglected safety? *Journal of Pain Research*, *6*, 513.

Kivimaki, M., Leino-Arjas, P., Virtanen, M., Elovainio, M., Keltikangas-Jarvinen, L., Puttonen, S., ... Vahtera, J. (2004). Work stress and incidence of newly diagnosed fibromyalgia: Prospective cohort study. *Journal of Psychosomatic Research*, *57*(5), 417–422.

Knapik, J. J., Reynolds, K. L., & Harman, E. (2004). Soldier load carriage: Historical, physiological, biomechanical, and medical aspects. *Military Medicine*, *169*(1), 45.

Krasikova, D., Lester, P. B., & Harms, P. D. (2015). Effects of psychological capital on mental health and substance abuse. *Journal of Leadership and Organizational Studies*, *22*, 280–291.

Kristman, V. L., Shaw, W. S., Boot, C. R., Delclos, G. L., Sullivan, M. J., & Ehrhart, M. G. (2016). Researching complex and multi-level workplace factors affecting disability and prolonged sickness absence. *Journal of Occupational Rehabilitation*, *26*(4), 399–416.

Kumar, S. (2001). Theories of musculoskeletal injury causation. *Ergonomics*, *44*(1), 17–47.

Lauder, T. D., Baker, S. P., Smith, G. S., & Lincoln, A. E. (2000). Sports and physical training injury hospitalizations in the Army. *American Journal of Preventive Medicine*, *18*(3), 118–128. doi:10.1016/S0749-3797(99)00174-9

Leeuwen, M. T., Blyth, F. M., March, L. M., Nicholas, M. K., & Cousins, M. J. (2006). Chronic pain and reduced work effectiveness: The hidden cost to Australian employers. *European Journal of Pain*, *10*(2), 161–161. doi:10.1016/j.ejpain.2005.02.007

Lew, H. L., Otis, J. D., Tun, C., Kerns, R. D., Clark, M. E., & Cifu, D. X. (2009). Prevalence of chronic pain, posttraumatic stress disorder, and persistent postconcussive symptoms in OIF/OEF veterans: Polytrauma clinical triad. *The Journal of Rehabilitation Research and Development*, *46*(6), 697. doi:10.1682/JRRD.2009.01.0006

Lincoln, A. E., Smith, G. S., Amoroso, P. J., & Bell, N. S. (2002). The natural history and risk factors of musculoskeletal conditions resulting in disability among US Army personnel. *Work*, *18*(2), 99–113.

Linton, S. J. (2001). Occupational psychological factors increase the risk for back pain: A systematic review. *Journal of Occupational Rehabilitation*, *11*(1), 53–66.

Loeser, J. (2012, January). Five crises in pain management. *Pain Clinical Updates*, *20*(1), 1–4. Retrieved from https://www.iasp- pain.org/PublicationsNews/NewsletterIssue.aspx?ItemNumber=2074

Loeser, J. D., & Melzack, R. (1999). Pain: An overview. *The Lancet*, *353*(9164), 1607–1609.

Lumley, M. A., Cohen, J. L., Borszcz, G. S., Cano, A., Radcliffe, A. M., Porter, L. S., … Keefe, F. J. (2011). Pain and emotion: A biopsychosocial review of recent research. *Journal of Clinical Psychology*, *67*(9), 942–968.

Manchikanti, L., Fellows, B., Ailinani, H., & Pampati, V. (2010). Therapeutic use, abuse, and non-medical use of opioids: A ten-year perspective. *Pain Physician*, *13*(5), 401–435.

Matthias, M. S., Miech, E. J., Myers, L. J., Sargent, C., & Bair, M. J. (2014). A qualitative study of chronic pain in operation enduring freedom/operation Iraqi freedom veterans: "A burden on my soul." *Military Medicine*, *179*(1), 26–30. doi:10.7205/milmed-d-13-00196

McCracken, L. M., Gauntlett-Gilbert, J., & Vowles, K. E. (2007). The role of mindfulness in a contextual cognitive-behavioral analysis of chronic pain-related suffering and disability. *PAIN*, *131*(1), 63–69.

McCracken, L. M., & Vowles, K. E. (2014). Acceptance and commitment therapy and mindfulness for chronic pain: Model, process, and progress. *American Psychologist*, *69*(2), 178.

McGeary, C. A., Blount, T. H., Peterson, A. L., Gatchel, R. J., Hale, W. J., & McGeary, D. D. (2016). Interpersonal responses and pain management within the US military. *Journal of Occupational Rehabilitation*, *26*(2), 216–228. doi:10.1007/s10926-015-9605-2

McWilliams, L. A., Cox, B. J., & Enns, M. W. (2003). Mood and anxiety disorders associated with chronic pain: An examination in a nationally representative sample. *PAIN*, *106*(1), 127–133.

Melloh, M., Elfering, A., Stanton, T. R., Käser, A., Salathé, C. R., Barz, T., … Theis, J.-C. (2013). Who is likely to develop persistent low back pain? A longitudinal analysis of prognostic occupational factors. *Work*, *46*(3), 297–311.

Melzack, R. (1996). Gate control theory. *Pain Forum*, *5*(2), 128–138. doi:10.1016/S1082-3174(96)80050-X

Melzack, R., & Wall, P. (1965). Pain mechanisms: A new theory. *Science (New York, NY)*, *150*(3699), 971–979.

Mesas, A. E., González, A. D., Mesas, C. E., de Andrade, S. M., Magro, I. S., & del Llano, J. (2014). The association of chronic neck pain, low back pain, and migraine with absenteeism due to health problems in Spanish workers. *Spine*, *39*(15), 1243–1253.

Mohammadi, S., Dehghani, M., Sanderman, R., & Hagedoorn, M. (2017). The role of pain behaviour and family caregiver responses in the link between pain catastrophising and pain intensity: A moderated mediation model. *Psychology & Health*, *32*(4), 422–438.

Morasco, B. J., Lovejoy, T. I., Lu, M., Turk, D. C., Lewis, L., & Dobscha, S. K. (2013). The relationship between PTSD and chronic pain: Mediating role of coping strategies and depression. *PAIN*, *154*(4), 609–616.

Munce, S. E., Stansfeld, S. A., Blackmore, E. R., & Stewart, D. E. (2007). The role of depression and chronic pain conditions in absenteeism: Results from a national epidemiologic survey. *Journal of Occupational and Environmental Medicine*, *49*(11), 1206–1211.

Navratilova, E., & Porreca, F. (2014). Reward and motivation in pain and pain relief. *Nature Neuroscience*, *17*(10), 1304–1312.

Neogi, T. (2013). The epidemiology and impact of pain in osteoarthritis. *Osteoarthritis and Cartilage*, *21*(9), 1145–1153.

Ojala, T., Häkkinen, A., Karppinen, J., Sipilä, K., Suutama, T., & Piirainen, A. (2015). Chronic pain affects the whole person – A phenomenological study. *Disability and Rehabilitation*, *37*(4), 363–371.

Ossipov, M. H., Dussor, G. O., & Porreca, F. (2010). Central modulation of pain. *The Journal of Clinical Investigation*, *120*(11), 3779.

Patel, A. S., Farquharson, R., Carroll, D., Moore, A., Phillips, C. J., Taylor, R. S., & Barden, J. (2012). The impact and burden of chronic pain in the workplace: A qualitative systematic review. *Pain Practice*, *12*(7), 578–589.

Pohling, R., Buruck, G., Jungbauer, K.-L., & Leiter, M. P. (2016). Work-related factors of presenteeism: The mediating role of mental and physical health. *Journal of Occupational Health Psychology*, *21*(2), 220.

Rhudy, J. L. (2015). Emotional modulation of pain. In al'Absi, M. & Flaten, M. A. *Neuroscience of pain, stress, and emotion: Psychological and clinical implications* (pp. 51–75). Academic Press: New York.

Rhudy, J. L., Bartley, E. J., Williams, A. E., McCabe, K. M., Chandler, M. C., Russell, J. L., & Kerr, K. L. (2010). Are there sex differences in affective modulation of spinal nociception and pain? *The Journal of Pain*, *11*(12), 1429–1441.

Ricci, J. A., Stewart, W. F., Chee, E., Leotta, C., Foley, K., & Hochberg, M. C. (2005). Pain exacerbation as a major source of lost productive time in US workers with arthritis. *Arthritis Care & Research*, *53*(5), 673–681.

Rigg, K. K., & DeCamp, W. (2014). Explaining prescription opioid misuse among veterans: A theory-based analysis using structural equation modeling. *Military Behavioral Health*, *2*(2), 210–216. doi:10.1080/21635781.2014.917011

Roeser, R. W., Schonert-Reichl, K. A., Jha, A., Cullen, M., Wallace, L., Wilensky, R., … Harrison, J. (2013). Mindfulness training and reductions in teacher stress and burnout: Results from two randomized, waitlist-control field trials. *Journal of Educational Psychology*, *105*(3), 787.

Rudd, R. A., Seth, P., David, F., & Scholl, L. (2016). Increases in drug and opioid-involved overdose deaths — United States, 2010–2015. *MMWR. Morbidity and Mortality Weekly Report*, *65*(50–51), 1445–1452. doi:10.15585/mmwr.mm655051e1

Ruscio, B. A., Jones, B. H., Bullock, S. H., Burnham, B. R., Canham-Chervak, M., Rennix, C. P., … Smith, J. W. (2010). A process to identify military injury prevention priorities based on injury type and limited duty days. *American Journal of Preventive Medicine*, *38*(1, Supplement), S19–S33. doi:10.1016/j.amepre.2009.10.004

Saastamoinen, P., Leino-Arjas, P., Rahkonen, O., & Lahelma, E. (2016). Separate and combined associations of pain and emotional exhaustion with sickness absence. *PAIN*, *157*(1), 186–193.

Scherrer, J. F., Salas, J., Copeland, L. A., Stock, E. M., Ahmedani, B. K., Sullivan, M. D., … Lustman, P. J. (2016). Prescription opioid duration, dose, and increased risk of depression in 3 large patient populations. *The Annals of Family Medicine*, *14*(1), 54–62. doi:10.1370/afm.1885

Schultz, A. B., Chen, C.-Y., & Edington, D. W. (2009). The cost and impact of health conditions on presenteeism to employers. *Pharmacoeconomics*, *27*(5), 365–378.

Seal, K. H., Cohen, G., Waldrop, A., Cohen, B. E., Maguen, S., & Ren, L. (2011). Substance use disorders in Iraq and Afghanistan veterans in VA healthcare, 2001–2010: Implications for screening, diagnosis and treatment. *Drug and Alcohol Dependence*, *116*(1–3), 93–101. doi:10.1016/j.drugalcdep.2010.11.027

Seal, K. H., Shi, Y., Cohen, G., Cohen, B. E., Maguen, S., Krebs, E. E., & Neylan, T. C. (2012). Association of mental health disorders with prescription opioids and high-risk opioid use in US veterans of Iraq and Afghanistan. *JAMA*, *307*(9), 940–947. doi:10.1001/jama.2012.234

Sharp, T. J., & Harvey, A. G. (2001). Chronic pain and post-traumatic stress disorder: Mutual maintenance? *Clinical Psychology Review*, *21*(6), 857–877.

Shaw, W. S., Campbell, P., Nelson, C. C., Main, C. J., & Linton, S. J. (2013). Effects of workplace, family and cultural influences on low back pain: What opportunities exist to address social factors in general consultations? *Best Practice & Research Clinical Rheumatology*, *27*(5), 637–648.

Shipherd, J. C., Keyes, M., Jovanovic, T., Ready, D. J., Baltzell, D., Worley, V., … Duncan, E. (2007). Veterans seeking treatment for posttraumatic stress disorder: What about comorbid chronic pain? *The Journal of Rehabilitation Research and Development*, *44*(2), 153. doi:10.1682/jrrd.2006.06.0065

Sibille, K. T., Kindler, L. L., Glover, T. L., Staud, R., Riley III, J. L., & Fillingim, R. B. (2012). Affect balance style, experimental pain sensitivity, and pain-related responses. *The Clinical Journal of Pain*, *28*(5), 410.

Staud, R. (2012). Abnormal endogenous pain modulation is a shared characteristic of many chronic pain conditions. *Expert Review of Neurotherapeutics*, *12*(5), 577–585. doi:10.1586/ern.12.41

Sullivan, M. D., & Ballantyne, J. C. (2016). Must we reduce pain intensity to treat chronic pain? *PAIN*, *157*(1), 65. doi:10.1097/j.pain.0000000000000336

Sullivan, M. D., & Howe, C. Q. (2013). Opioid therapy for chronic pain in the United States: Promises and perils. *PAIN*, *154*(Suppl 1), S94–S100. doi:10.1016/j.pain.2013.09.009

Tetrick, L. E., & Winslow, C. J. (2015). Workplace stress management interventions and health promotion. *Annual Review of Organzational Psychology and Organizational Behavior*, *2*(1), 583–603.

Toblin, R. L., Quartana, P. J., Riviere, L. A., Walper, K., & Hoge, C. W. (2014). Chronic pain and opioid use in US soldiers after combat deployment. *JAMA Internal Medicine*, *174*(8), 1400–1401. doi:10.1001/jamainternmed.2014.2726

Tracey, I. (2010). Getting the pain you expect: Mechanisms of placebo, nocebo and reappraisal effects in humans. *Nature Medicine*, *16*(11), 1277–1283.

Trost, Z., Vangronsveld, K., Linton, S. J., Quartana, P. J., & Sullivan, M. J. (2012). Cognitive dimensions of anger in chronic pain. *PAIN*, *153*(3), 515–517. doi:10.1016/j.pain.2011.10.023

Turan, B., Foltz, C., Cavanagh, J., Wallace, B., Cullen, M., Rosenberg, E., … Kemeny, M. (2015). Anticipatory sensitization to repeated stressors: The role of initial cortisol reactivity and meditation/emotion skills training. *Psychoneuroendocrinology*, *52*, 229.

Turk, D. C., Fillingim, R. B., Ohrbach, R., & Patel, K. V. (2016). Assessment of psychosocial and functional impact of chronic pain. *The Journal of Pain*, *17*(9), T21–T49.

Turk, D. C., Wilson, H. D., & Cahana, A. (2011). Treatment of chronic non-cancer pain. *The Lancet*, *377*(9784), 2226–2235.

Vanhove, A., Herian, M., Perez, A., Harms, P. D., & Lester, P. (2016). Can resilience be developed at work? A meta-analytic review of resilience-building program effectiveness. *Journal of Occupational and Organizational Psychology*, *89*, 278–307.

Vlaeyen, J. W., & Linton, S. J. (2000). Fear-avoidance and its consequences in chronic musculoskeletal pain: A state of the art. *PAIN*, *85*(3), 317–332.

Vlaeyen, J. W., & Linton, S. J. (2012). Fear-avoidance model of chronic musculoskeletal pain: 12 years on. *PAIN*, *153*(6), 1144–1147.

Wahlström, J., Burström, L., Nilsson, T., & Järvholm, B. (2012). Risk factors for hospitalization due to lumbar disc disease. *Spine*, *37*(15), 1334–1339.

Woolf, C. J. (2010). What is this thing called pain? *The Journal of Clinical Investigation*, *120*(11), 3742.

Zautra, A. J., & Sturgeon, J. A. (2016). Examining the complexities of affective experience will enhance our understanding of pain and inform new interventions designed to bolster resilience. *PAIN*, *157*(8), 1586–1587.

Zeidan, F., Gordon, N. S., Merchant, J., & Goolkasian, P. (2010). The effects of brief mindfulness meditation training on experimentally induced pain. *The Journal of Pain*, *11*(3), 199–209.

INDEX

9/11, 78

Absenteeism, 54, 171
Acute pain, 160–161
  biopsychosocial model of
    biological risk factors, 162–164
    psychosocial factors, 164–170
African-Americans and Hispanics, 6
After Deployment: Adaptive Parenting Tools (ADAPT), 104
Aggressive behaviors, 33–34, 100
Air Force's Extended Duty Care, 106
Alcohol, 95
Alcohol misuse, 80
Altruism, 14,
American Psychological Association, 10, 51
Antisocial personality disorder, 39
Anxiety, 3–5, 7, 10, 26–27, 33, 38, 61, 95, 99, 103, 166–167, 171
Armed force
  affiliation, 105, 108
  bases, 101, 105
  branches, 72, 78, 98, 123, 148
  careers, 74, 92, 95–96
  child care, 106
  children, 100, 104–105
  children change, 104
  community, 24–25, 52, 64, 70, 104
  couples, 75, 77–83, 85, 148
    married, 72–73
    outcomes of, 73, 82
    research on, 71, 73, 81
    understanding of, 71
  couples experience, 80
  culture, 77, 118, 120
Armitage, 96
Army
  community, 99–100, 106,
  families,100, 105,
  job performance, 61–62
  soldiers, 56–57, 63–64, 76
Armed Forces Surveillance Study, 96
Army Family Team Building (AFTB), 105
Army job performance
  data constraints, 63–64
  experience in, 61–62
  and health behaviors, 59–60
  and mental health, 60
  person-event data environment, 63
  and physical health, 58–59
  and stress, 56–58
Army vs.Civilian Metrics, 55
Assistance-based programs, 103
Attraction-selection-attrition (ASA) model, 29, 31, 36
Avoidance-based strategies, 13

Bipolar disorder, 95
Breastfeeding, 97–98
B-Scan, 28

Childbirth, 93–95
Child development centers, 106
Child-focused resources, 104–105
Children's Strain, 100–101

Chronic pain, 161
biopsychosocial model of
biological risk factors, 162–164
psychosocial factors, 164–170
impact on emotional well-being, 170–171
psychosocial risk factors for, 165
Civilian
employment, 118, 121
jobs, 71, 82–83, 118–119, 124–125
life, 50, 70, 74, 104, 118, 122–123
war survivors, 4, 11, 13, 16
women, 15, 94, 97–98
Civilian war survivors
coping with PTSD, 13
demographic predictors of PTSD, 11–12
individual factors predicting PTSD, 12–13
Cognitive-behavioral therapy, 10
Cognitive stressor, 31
Cognitive therapy, 10
Combat and Operational Stress Reactions (COSR), 24
Combat duty, 130–131, 134, 140, 143, 148
Combat-related PTSD, 30, 168
Combat stress reactions, 4
Combat veterans, 131, 134, 140, 146–148
Comorbidity, 3–5
Composite life cycle model, 74–75, 83–85
Comprehensive Soldier and Family Fitness (CSF2), 103
Conscientiousness, 24
Contextual behavior, 55
Contextual performance, 55
Convoy model, 84
Convoy Model of Social Relations, 84
Coping with PTSD
civilian war survivors, 13
military war survivors, 8–11
Critical military functions, 24
Dark Triad, 24
Defense Equal Opportunity Management Institute's Organizational Climate Survey (DEOCS), 54
Defense of Marriage Act (DOMA), 108
Demographic predictors of PTSD
civilian war survivors, 11–12
military war survivors, 5–7
Department of Defense (DoD), 39, 63, 72, 101, 102
Deployment
as a cycle, 79–81
female service members, 79
male service members, 79
marital satisfaction, 80
Military Family Life Project, 79
PTSD symptoms, 78
Depression, 2–5, 9–10, 51, 58–61, 99–100, 165, 167, 171, 175, 178
Deployment Cycle Study, 82
The Deployment Life Study, 80
Depression, 95, 165
Diagnostic and Statistical Manual of Mental Disorders-IV (DSM-IV), 27
Disability discharge, 172
Distress, 50
DoD Yellow Ribbon Reintegration Program, 104
Drill, 70
Drug abuse, 95
DSM-5, 2
Dual-military couples, 72

Emotional cycle of deployment model, 79
Emotional intelligence, 24
Emotional regulation, 14
Emotional stressor, 31
Employee job satisfaction, 28
Enhanced Extended Child Care program, 106
Eustress, 50
Evaluative rigor scale, 134
Experiential avoidance, 13

Exposure therapy, 10
Extreme temperatures, 23

Family and Medical Leave Act (FMLA), 102
Family Child Care, 106
Family Readiness Groups (FRG s), 105
Fear, 166
Federal policy and leave availability, 101–102
Fight-or-flight response, 51
Formal job performance measures, 52–53

Gating criteria, 64
Give an Hour, 103
Global Assessment Tool (GAT), 63

Hardiness, 24
Health, 57, 59, 61, 71, 73–74, 80–84, 119, 122, 143, 145
  behaviors, 52, 56, 58–59, 61
  conditions
    chronic, 59
    mental, 60–61, 177
  interventions, 130, 142
    evaluating psychosocial, 140
  of military couples, 71, 73, 75, 77, 79, 81, 83, 85
  relationships between PTSD and mental, 3, 5
Hierarchical mapping technique, 84
Hogan Development Survey (HDS), 27

IAPS. *see* International Affective Picture System (IAPS)
Improvised explosive devices (IED), 163
Individual factors predicting PTSD
  civilian war survivors, 12–13
  military war survivors, 7–8
Injuries
  non-battle, 163
  physical, 32, 168
  traumatic, 166
Integrative Method, 85
International Affective Picture System (IAPS), 164

Job-limiting pain (JLP), 173
Job performance metrics, 52, 54–55, 60, 62
Job stress, 56–58, 82, 162
Job stressors, 169
Joint Family Support Assistance Program, 104

Kirkpatrick taxonomy, 132

Lesbian, gay, bisexual, transgender, queer (LGBTQ), 107
Life stage theory, 74
Longitudinal panel studies, 82

Machiavellianism, 26
Marital satisfaction, 80
Mental health, 60
Metrics, army job performance
  within the Army
    formal job performance measures, 52–53
    semi-formal job performance measures, 53–54
    stress and health, 50–51
  in the civilian sector, 54–55
  vs civilian metrics, 55
Military Caregiver Leave (MCL), 102
Military Child Care in Your Neighborhood, 106
Military couples
  composite life cycle model, 83–85
  definition, 72–73
  expand research on, 81–83
  future directions
    expand research on, 81–83
    expand the composite life cycle model, 83–85
  military service and the life course, 73–75
  relocation effects on, 76–78

research on married, 73
systematic comparison of, 83
transitions in the military life course, 75–81
Military–family balance, 101
Military Family Life Project, 79, 82
Military life, 74
children's strain, 100–101
health interventions, 132, 140
pregnancy and childbirth, 93–95
trailing spouses, 76
transitions
deployment, 78–81
deployment as a cycle, 79–81
relocation, 75–78
work-family strain, 98–99
Military life and parenting
breastfeeding, 97–98
child-focused resources, 104–105
federal policy and leave availability, 101–102
gendered occupation, 93
localized military support programs, 105–108
parent–child relationships, 92
postpartum, 95–96
pregnancy and childbirth, 93–95
service member as parent, 98–101
support resources
whole-family functioning/parenting supports, 102–104
Military organizations
psychosocial health prevention programs, 130–131
support programs, 105–108
Military transition
approach
military and cultural factors, 119–120
nature of the transition, 122–123
personal characteristics, 121–122
civilian transition factors, 119
managing the
community/civilian transition support, 125
individual adjustment factors, 123
military transition management, 123–125
military transition theory, 118–119
Military war survivors
coping with PTSD, 8–11
demographic predictors of PTSD, 5–7
individual factors predicting PTSD, 7–8
Military workplace
battle injury, 163–164
IAPS, 164
injury in the, 162
non-battle injury, 163
pain and emotion, 164
Millenium Cohort Study, 81
Millennium Cohort Family Study, 82
Mindfulness-Based Mind Fitness Training (MMFT), 177
Motherhood penalty, 95
Multi-Source Assessment and Feedback (MSAF), 53
Musculoskeletal disorder (MSD), 162
Mutual maintenance model, 167

Narcissism, 26, 39
National Guard and Reserves (NG/R), 70, 78, 82, 83
National Military Family Association, 103
Navy's Child Development Group Homes, 106
NG/R. *See* National Guard and Reserves (NG/R)
Nociceptive pain, 160
Non-commissioned officer (NCO), 53
Non-Commissioned Officer Evaluation Reports (NCOER), 53
Not-for-profit organizations programs, 103

Occupational stress, 71, 158, 177–178
Officer Evaluation Reports (OER), 53
Operation enduring freedom (OEF), 11
Operation Homefront, 103
Operation Military Child Care, 106
Operation Purple Camp project, 103
Opioid, 164
Optimism, 144, 165, 169
Organization-based self-esteem (OBSE), 58
Osteoarthritis (OA), 171

Pain
  classification of
    acute pain, 160–161
    chronic pain, 161
    nociceptive pain, 160
  definition, 158
  dynamics of, 158–159
  and emotion, 164
  opioids and overdose, 173–175
  psychological protective factors, 169–170
    job stressors, 169
    mindfulness, 170
    optimism, 169
    positive effect, 169
  psychosocial risk factors for, 165
  role of organizations in, 175–178
  social protective factors, 170
  social risk factors, 168–169
Pain and prescription opioid misuse (POM), 158
Parent–child relationships, 92
Parent Management Training-Oregon (PMTO), 104
Part-time soldiers, 71
Perceived organizational support (POS), 173
Performance
  factors influencing stress, 58
  and health behaviors, 59–60
  and mental health, 60
  and physical health, 58–59
  and stress, 56–58
Person-event Data Environment (PDE), 63
Physical health, 58–59
Physical stress, 32
Postpartum, 95–96
Post-traumatic stress disorder (PTSD), 2, 24, 70, 95, 158, 166
  antecedents of, 15–16
  coping with PTSD, 8–11, 13
  demographic predictors of PTSD, 5–7, 11–12
  emotional regulation, 14
  individual factors predicting PTSD, 7–8, 12–13
  limitations and future directions, 16
  and mental health, 3–5
  protective factors in, 14
  psychopathy, in military, 37–38
  and psychopathy relationship, 38
  risk factors associated with, 5–13
Pre-birth conflict, 98
Pre-deployment stress, 177
Pregnancy, 93–95
Pregnant woman, 94
  and US Air Force, 96
  US Navy regulation, 95
Presenteeism, 54, 172–173
Preterm birth, 94
Protective factors in post-trauma response, 14
Psychological resiliency, 177
Psychological strain, 24
Psychological stress, 30–32
Psychopathic Personality Inventory – Revised (PPI-R), 27
Psychopathology, 13
Psychopathy, 24
  consequences at Work, 28–29
  definition, 25–27
  measurement, 27–28
  nonclinical personality, 26
  and PTSD relationship, 38
Psychopathy Checklist – Revised (PCL-R), 27
Psychopathy, in military
  gender, 32–34

leadership, 34–35
post-traumatic stress disorder, 37–38
stress
physical stress, 32
psychological stress, 30–32
suicide, 38–39
teams and teamwork, 35–36
turnover, 36–37
Psychopathy Measure–Management Research Version, 28
Psychosocial health interventions, 140
PTSD, 78, 122. *See* Post-traumatic stress disorder (PTSD)

Qualifying Exigency Leave (QEL), 102

Relocation
frequent, 77, 94, 98–99
periodic, 71, 75, 78
Resilience, 14, 75
Resilience-building family-based programs, 103
Resource-focused programs, 103
Rest and recuperation (R&R) leave, 102
Risk
for maternal and infant complications, 94
for pregnant military women, 96
of PTSD, 166
psychosocial, 147–148, 165

Schizophrenia, 95
School-Age Care, 106
Self-efficacy, 24
Self-rated performance surveys, 54
Self-Report Psychopathy Scale III, 28
Semi-formal job performance measures, 53–54
Shared vulnerability model, 167
Sleep deprivation, 23
Soldier life cycle, 74
Stress, 56–58
definition, 50
factors influencing performance, 58
negative connotation of, 57
and performance, 56–58
physical stress, 32
psychological stress, 30–32
Stress-buffer, 34
Stressors, 23
military-related, 95
physical, 32
pre-deployment, 8
traumatic, 37, 50–51
unique, 50, 95
work-related, 57
situations, external, 7
Stressor–strain relationships, 24
Stress-performance, 24
Study for Employment Retention of Veterans (SERVe), 75, 82
Suicide, 38–39

Teamwork-focused environment, 24
Trailing spouses, 76
Transitions
military-to-civilian life, 124
stressful, 77
Transition assistance program (TAP), 123–124
Trauma, 2–8, 11–12, 14–15, 38, 51, 130, 167
childhood, 7, 12–15
events, 2, 9–10, 14, 37, 95
exposure, 12, 14
multiple, 7, 15
prior, 8
victims, 14
wartime, 11–12, 15
Traumatic stressor, 37

United Service Organizations, and Families OverComing Under Stress (FOCUS), 103
Unit life cycle, 74
US Air Force, 95
U.S. Department of Veterans Affairs (2016), 38
U-shaped hypothesis, 56, 57
US military policy, 25
US Navy regulation, 95

9/11 veterans, 118, 124
Veterans' affairs (VA), 119
Veterans affairs National Center, 6
Vietnam veterans, 6, 11
Vietnam War, 14, 24
Violent behavior, 27, 30

War survivors, 5, 9, 11, 16
Wartime, 2, 11–13
Weekend warrior, 70
Widows, 12, 26–28, 31, 35–36, 38
Wives, 77, 79
Woman, 95, 107
  active duty, 94, 96–97,
Women service members, 93–94, 107
Women veterans, 95
Work–family conflict, 92, 93, 98
Work–family management programs, 105
Work-family strain, 98–99
Workforce, civilian, 70–71, 82, 125, 162
Work stress, 30, 159
Work–life conflict, 102
World War II (WWII), 24

Yerkes–Dodson effect, 56

Printed and bound by CPI Group (UK) Ltd, Croydon, CR0 4YY

15/09/2026

14962483-0001